P. Elsner H.F. Merk H.I. Maibach (Eds.)

Cosmetics –
Controlled Efficacy Studies and Regulation

Springer-Verlag Berlin Heidelberg GmbH

P. Elsner H.F. Merk H.I. Maibach (Eds.)

Cosmetics

Controlled Efficacy Studies and Regulation

With a Preface by Fritz H. Kemper

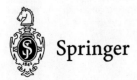 Springer

Prof. Dr. med. P. Elsner
Klinikum der
Friedrich Schiller-Universität Jena
Klinik für Hautkrankheiten
Erfurter Straße 35
D-07740 Jena, Germany

Prof. Dr. med. Hans F. Merk
Rheinisch-Westfälische Technische
Hochschule Aachen
Hautklinik
Pauwelsstraße 30
D-52074 Aachen, Germany

Howard I. Maibach, M.D.
Professor
University of California San Francisco
School of Medicine
Department of Dermatology
Box 0989, Surge 110
San Francisco, CA 94143-0989, U.S.A.

Library of Congress Cataloging–in–Publication Data

Cosmetics : controlled efficacy studies and regulation / P. Elsner ... (ed.) –
Berlin ; Heidelberg ; New York ; Barcelona ; Hong Kong ; London ; Milano ; Paris ; Singapore : Springer, 1999
   ISBN 978-3-642-64160-2   ISBN 978-3-642-59869-2 (eBook)
   DOI 10.1007/978-3-642-59869-2

© Springer-Verlag Berlin Heidelberg 1999
Originally published by Springer-Verlag Berlin Heidelberg New York in 1999
Softcover reprint of the hardcover 1st edition 1999

Cover design: design & production, Heidelberg
Typesetting: Goldener Schnitt, Sinzheim

SPIN: 10652697   22/3134   5 4 3 2 1 0   –   Printed on acid-free paper

Contents

List of Contributors

Prof. André O. Barel
Laboratory of General and Biological
Chemistry
Faculty of Physical Education and
Physiotherapy
Free University of Brussel (VUB)
B-1050 Brussel, Belgium

Saqib J. Bashir, MD
University of California
School of Medicine
Box 0989, Surge 110
San Francisco, CA 94143, U.S.A.

Enzo Berardesca, MD
Department of Dermatology
IRCCS Policlinico S. Matteo
1-27100 Pavia, Italy

Dr. B. Blömeke
Hautklinik der Medizinischen Fakultät
der RWTH Aachen
Pauwelsstraße 30
D-52074 Aachen

James P. Bowman
Hill Top Research, Inc.
P.O.Box 429501
Miamiville
Cincinnati, OH 45242, U.S.A.

Dr. Peter Clarys
Laboratory of General and Biological
Chemistry
Faculty of Physical Education and
Physiotherapy
Free University of Brussel (VUB)
B-1050 Brussel, Belgium

Dr. Robert D. Combes
FRAME
96-98 North Sherwood Street
NG 1 4EE
Nottingham, U.K.

Tamotsu Ebihara, M.D.
Saiseikai Central Hospital
Shinyo CK Building 6 F
3-3-5, Kam-hsaki, Shinagawer-ku
Tokyo 141-0021, Japan

Patricia G. Engasser, MD
Department of Dermatology
Kaiser Permanente Medical Center
1150 Veterans Blvd.
Redwood City, CA 94063-2037, U.S.A.

Dr. Bernard Gabard
Department of Biopharmacy
Spirig Ltd., Pharmaceuticals
CH-4622 Egerkingen, Switzerland

Prof. Dr. Uwe-Frithjof Haustein
Department of Dermatology
University of Leipzig
Liebigstraße 21
D-04103 Leipzig, Germany

Prof. Dr. M. Heinzel
Henkel KGa
Henkelstr. 67
D-40191 Düsseldorf, Germany

B. Homey
Department of Dermatology
Heinrich-Heine-University Düsseldorf
Moorenstr. 5
D-40225 Düsseldorf, Germany

Edward M. Jackson, Ph.D.
Jackson Research Associates, Inc.
20203 121st Street Court E
Sumner, WA 98390, U.S.A.

Tsuneo Jinnai
Sansho Seiyaku Co., LTD
2-26-7, Oh-ike, Ohnojo-shi
Fukuoka Prefecture, 816-8550, Japan

Prof. Dr.med. P. Lehmann
Heinrich-Heine-University of Düsseldorf
Department of Dermatology
Moorenstraße 5
D-40225 Düsseldorf, Germany

Stanley B. Levy, M.D.
Clinical Professor
Department of Dermatology
University of North Carolina at Chapel
Hill
891 Willow Drive
Chapel Hill, NC 27514, U.S.A.

Philippe Masson, Ph.D.
Expert Toxicoloque Pharmacologue
Président Directeur Général
Laborataire De recherche et
D'Experimentation
1, rue Massue
Vincennes F-94300, France

Gerald N. McEwen, Jr., Ph.D., J.D.
The Cosmetic, Toiletry, and Fragrance
Association
1101 17th St., N.W.
Suite 3000
Washington DC 20036–4702, USA

Prof. Dr. med. Hans F. Merk
Hautklinik der Medizinischen
Fakultät der RWTH Aachen
Pauwelsstraße 30
D-52074 Aachen , Germany

Emalee G. Murphy
Securing the Industry's Future Since 1894
1101 17th St., N.W.
Suite 3000
Washington DC 20036–4702, USA

Dr. Pietro Nenoff
Department of Dermatology
University of Leipzig
D-04103 Leipzig, Germany

Dr. N.J. Neumann
Department of Dermatology, Andrology
Heinrich-Heine-University Düsseldorf
Moorenstraße 5
D-40225 Düsseldorf, Germany

Linda P. Oddo
Hill Top Research, Inc.
Scottsdale, Arizona, U.S.A.

Prof. C. Piérard-Franchimont
Centre Hospitalier Universitaire de Liège
Service Dermatopathologie
Domaine Universitaire du Saint Tilmann
B. 35
B-4000 Liège 1, Belgien

Prof. G.E. Piérard
Centre Hospitalier Universitaire de Liège
Service Dermatopathologie
Domaine Universitaire du Saint Tilmann
B. 35
B-4000 Liège 1, Belgien

Ronald L. Rizer, Ph.D.
Thomas J. Stephens & Associates, Inc.
3310 Keller Springs Road
Suite 130
Carrollton TX 75006, U.S.A.

Luis Rodrigues, Ph.D.
Professor of Human Physiology
Laboratory of Experimental Physiology
Faculdade de Farmaçia da Universidade
de Lisboa
Av. Das Forças Armadas
1600 Lisboa, Portugal

Claudia Rona
Department of Dermatology
IRCCS Policlinico S. Matteo
1-27100 Pavia, Italy

Noriko Satoh, M.D.
Yanagihara Hospital
Shinyo CK Building 6 F
3-3-5, Kam-hsaki, Shinagawa-ku
Tokyo 141-0021, Japan

Dr. Karlheinz Schrader
Institutes Dr. Schrader
Max-Planck-Straße 6
D-37603 Holzminden, Germany

Dr. S. Sieben
Hautklinik der Medizinischen Fakultät
der RWTH Aachen
Pauwelsstraße 30
D-52074 Aachen, Germany

Hachiro Tagami, M.D.
Department of Dermatology
Tohoku University School of Medicine
Sendai 980-8574, Japan

H.W. Vohr
Bayer Vital GmbH & Co KG
D-51368 Leverkusen, Germany

Prof. Dr. med. V. Wienert
Universitätshautklinik
der RWTH Aachen
Pauwelsstraße 30
D-52074 Aachen, Germany

John E. Wild
Hill Top Research, Inc.
P.O.Box 429501
Miamiville
Cincinnati, OH 45242, U.S.A.

Leszek J. Wolfram, M.D.
666 Westover Rd.
Stamford, CT 06902, U.S.A.

Hongbo Zhai, M.D.
Assistant Research Dermatologist
Department of Dermatology
University of California
School of Medicine
San Francisco, CA 94143, U.S.A.

Dr. Valérie Zuang
European Centre for the Validation of
Alternative Methods (ECVAM)
Environment Institute
Joint Research Centre of the European
Commission
1-21020 Ispra (Va), Italy

Foreword of the editors

With the 6th Amendment of the European Cosmetics Directive, the producer or importer of a cosmetic product is required to make evidence of the claimed effect of a given product available to the competent authorities.

This is a new quality in legislation on cosmetics. While there is still no registration process for cosmetic finished products as it exists for drugs, for the first time cosmetic effects are taken seriously by the authorities instead of being just viewed under the perspective of truthful advertising.

Obviously, the legal situations in the United States and in Japan are different, but, as contributions in this book show, aspects of cosmetic efficacy are increasingly of interest to regulators and companies in these countries as well. Cosmetologists, pharmacists, toxicologists, and dermatologists all over the world are more and more confronted with the problem how to document and measure cosmetic efficacy.

Considering that a text was dearly needed gathering information on how to perform controlled efficacy studies in the perspective of cosmetic regulations, the editors gathered a panel of leading experts in the field to write this book.

We are glad that so many colleagues followed our invitation, and we would like to thank them for sharing their valuable experience. As the reader will notice, we did not superimpose strict standard chapter outlines, but we left the organization of the individual chapters widely to the authors. Thus, certain study methods that are of special interest to the authors may be treated with more detail than others, but we did not consider this to be a drawback, but to add to the livelihood of the book.

We hope that the reader will draw support for his daily work with cosmetics from this text. With the topic so new, it is natural that not all relevant aspects could be be covered in detail, and we would encourage our readership to send us suggestions and criticisms what to consider in future editions.

Finally, we would like to thank Ms. B. Merker for secretarial support and the staff of Springer Publishers, especially Ms. Fingerhuth, for their kind help with the project.

Jena, Aachen, San Francisco, June 1999   Peter Elsner
                                                     Hans F. Merk
                                                  Howard I. Maibach

Preface

Together with the 6th Amendment – Council Directive 93/35 EEC – to the Cosmetic Directive 76/768 EEC it was the first time that, according to Article 7b, special claims of efficacy could be legally attributed to cosmetic products but under the obligation to make evidence of the claimed effects; also an entirely new "controller" was introduced – the independent "safety assessor". This indeed means not only progress in reliable and honest marketing arguments but above all transparency as to the respective proof and thus protection of consumer's health. Such claims demand high standards in scientifically based methodology and their results in order to prove such demands evidently.

There are also within the 6th Amendment to the Cosmetic Directive in Article 4a strict restrictions as to the further use of conventional animal testing for cosmetic products and their ingredients and especially for finished products. Without doubt there is a competition between the necessity and expectations on consumer health on the one hand and the requirements of acknowledged protection of animals as done in Council Directive 86/609 EEC on the other. But at least, based on the present state of knowledge, tests in human beings cannot replace animal testing in all instances. Not only ethical reasons alone prohibit or impede testing in humans but also very often the lack of knowledge on functional and/or biological processes underlaying observed effects with the consequence that suitable experimental methodologies are missing.

In national and international laws and regulations it is widely accepted that cosmetic products and their ingredients must not be liable to cause damage to human health when they are applied under normal conditions of use. On the European level (EC-DG XXIV) the Scientific Committee on Cosmetic Products, and Non-Food Products intended for Consumers (SCCNFP) is responsible for the scientifically based valuation of cosmetic ingredients which is laid down in "opinions" those being the background for administrative and legislative regulations.

The valuation procedure is carried out following the *"Notes of Guidance for Testing of Cosmetic Ingredients for Their Safety Evaluation"*, which were already prepared in June 1982, followed by a revised adition in 1990, taking into account the experience developed within the SCC, in a safety assessment and the growing scientific knowledge in toxicology. A second revision has been adopted in 1997 by the SCC, now SCCNFP, and includes besides recent progress in scientific knowledge the concept of the 6th Amendment which implies the new mentioned aspects in the protection of consumer's health but also regarding methodology, e.g. animal experiments. Since then the SCCNFP is amending these *"Notes of Guidance"* regularly; the results are published in Internet (http://www.europa.eu.int/comm/dg24/health/sc/sccp/index_en.html).

In general, besides following GMP and GLP rules, especially a safety valuation is based on results of test procedures covering detailed statements on acute and subchronic toxicity, skin and eye irritation/corrosivity, skin sensitization and photosensitization, phototoxicity/photoirritation, mutagenicity/genotoxicity and photomutagenicity and preferably on percutaneous absorption and toxicokinetic studies followed by tolerance studies inclucing tests on compatibility and acceptability carried out mostly in human beings. In addition the microbiological quality of the finished product is of superior importance and has to follow acknowledged standards.

Special rules for a safety valuation of perfumes and their ingredients as well as for an assessment of ingredients of botanical origin or those derived from mineral or animal origin or from biotechnology procedures are also necessary and will lead after an intense scientific discussion to respective opinions and entries into the central catalogue of cosmetic ingredients, the INCI, as well as where necessary into the Cosmetic Directive.

The use of human volunteers in compatibility testing calls for high responsibilities especially regarding ethical considerations. Thus the SCCNFP has addressed recently in an appropriate opinion this sensible problem as a recommendation to the European Commission.

In this situation it is highly appreciated that three worldwide reputated scientists in the field of academic dermatology, acting as editors, had the idea to ask other well-known authors in basic and applied sciences to contribute to a compilation of the state-of-the-art of methods to be used in cosmetology in order to put tools at disposal to fulfill the basic demands of consumer health protection in the described sence.

It seems to be a good idea to have divided the contents of the book into three parts and to introduce this collection of scientifically based experimental methodologies of basic and applied cosmetology with a chapter on the legal and regulatory background of an application of the results of investigations which could lead to appropriate claims.

With pleasure it can be stated that within the "efficacy chapter" the single parts of the collection, contributions which begin with the evaluation of a hydratization of the skin, ranging over cleansing effects, the efficacy of barrier creams and others, are not limited to an enumeration of different methods but also lead into a sometimes even critical discussion on the usefulness of procedures in order to find out if a recommended method is applicable for a special purpose or not.

In the final "safety chapter" the editors succeeded to induce a debate on biological reactions not only emanating from cosmetic products and their ingredients but also from other influences of daily life. In modern risk assessment irritation phenomena play an important part as well as questions of a mutagenicity.

Even a compilation of methodologies used in cosmetology as collected with emphasis on supporting claims of efficacy in a book of this size, with more than 300 pages, cannot describe all possibilities but is aiming to elucidate in a kind of view through a kaleidoscope the different aspects of possible claims and affiliated methodologies suitable to prove such statements preferably in humans. With very few exeptions the basic toxicological evaluation of ingredients or their combinations in cosmetic products is not addressed in the book and should be found elsewhere. Moreover methodologies suitable for the latter purposes do not differ from general investigations in toxicology.

All good wishes accompany the intentions of this book and its distribution to all to whom it may concern.

Münster, June 1999   Fritz H. Kemper

General Background

CHAPTER 1

Cosmetic Claim Substantiation in the United States: Legal Considerations

G. N. McEwen Jr, E. G. Murphy

Introduction

Control of consumer product claims in the United States, including representations about cosmetic products, is governed by federal and state law, by private judicial actions against false and misleading advertising, and by programs administered by voluntary industry organizations. While with some exceptions, cosmetic labeling and advertising need not be approved prior to its use, a cosmetic marketer devising advertising and labeling statements for the United States must have a reasonable basis for, and be able to substantiate, claims. The potential penalties for making unsubstantiated claims include federal, state, and private sanctions. This chapter will identify the bases for claim substantiation requirements for cosmetic products in the United States.

Chief Federal Laws Governing Cosmetic Claims

The chief federal laws governing cosmetic claims in product labeling are the Federal Food, Drug, and Cosmetic Act (FDC Act) [1] and the Fair Packaging and Labeling Act (FPLA) [2] administered by the Food and Drug Administration (FDA). The Federal Trade Commission Act (FTC Act) [3][1] administered by the Federal Trade Commission (FTC), governs cosmetic claims in advertising. In addition, the Lanham Act [4] permits companies to bring private suits to stop false and misleading advertising and to seek monetary and other remedies for any resulting injuries.

State Laws Governing Cosmetic Claims

Although the Mail Fraud Act [5] is another federal law, which governs claims for products promoted through the US mail, it is actually enforced by the Attorney General's office in each individual state. The AG and district attorney offices may also bring actions based upon state consumer protection laws, including "little" FDA and FTC laws, related to false advertising and labeling of cosmetics.

---

[1] Section 5 of the Federal Trade Commission Act prohibits unfair methods of competition in or affecting commerce, and unfair or deceptive acts or practices in or affecting commerce. Section 12 of the FTC Act prohibits "false advertising for foods, drugs, devices and cosmetics", and defines false advertisement as one that is misleading to a material extent.

Non-judicial Private Actions

Non-judicial private actions are also available through unofficial industry groups such as the National Advertising Division (NAD) of the Council of Better Business Bureaus or broadcast and print advertising review boards. Most print and broadcast companies exercise prior control over the advertising claims made through the media. This is not the case with the other laws and programs addressing this issue.

Penalties for False Labeling and Advertising

An advertiser, promoter or labeler in the US market must keep all the standards for claim substantiation in mind when devising product representations, or risk substantial civil monetary and equitable penalties, removal of the product from the market, and possible criminal prosecution.

Distinguishing Between the FDA and the FTC

The FDA and FTC, as the chief enforcers of claim substantiation standards, have overlapping and concurrent jurisdiction over the advertising and labeling of foods, nonprescription drugs, medical devices and cosmetics.

The Food and Drug Administration

The Food and Drug Administration enforces the misbranding provisions of the FDC Act, prohibiting statements made in product labeling that are false or misleading in any particular [6]. The term "labeling," as defined in the FDC Act, includes not only the product label, containers, and package inserts, but also material that accompanies the product, such as booklets, catalogues, and even unaccompanying promotional pieces [7]. Although its jurisdiction extends to economic deceptions, the FDA is primarily concerned that the public health and safety are not endangered through consumer reliance on unsubstantiated claims for safety and effectiveness. In determining whether labeling is misleading, FDA takes into account not only the explicit and implied claims, but also the extent to which the labeling fails to reveal material facts about the product and its use [8].

The Federal Trade Commission

The FTC regulates advertising that is deceptive or unfair, including promotional claims that appear in broadcast, print, Internet, and other media. The Commission's chief concern is that the consumer have reliable, substantiated information upon which to base purchasing decisions [9], and it focuses primarily on consumer deception and economic injury. As a practical matter, however, the responsibilities of the two agencies overlap, and nothing in the law would prevent simultaneous FDA and FTC prosecution against deceptive, unfair and misleading labeling and promotional claims.

Coordination Between the FDA and the FTC

To avoid unwanted duplicate proceedings, the FDA and the FTC have entered into a liaison agreement [10], in which the FTC agrees to take primary responsibility for regulating "advertising" and the FDA agrees to take primary responsibility for regulating "labeling". As part of the Agreement, the FTC and FDA exchange information about enforcement proceedings, as needed.

Food and Drug Administration

The approach to claims substantiation by the Food and Drug Administration (FDA) is largely circumscribed by its statutory requirements. The Food and Drug Administration is involved with claim substantiation through its authority over cosmetic labeling. In this section, we will review the statutory authority of the FDA, in particular, between cosmetics and drugs, judicial interpretation, and FDA regulatory and enforcement actions.

Important Statutory Definitions

To understand the FDA's approach to cosmetic product claims, two statutory definitions are of primary importance, the definition of a cosmetic and the definition of a drug.

Definition of a Cosmetic

The FDC Act defines "cosmetic" as "(1) articles <u>intended</u> to be rubbed, poured, sprinkled, or sprayed on, introduced into, or otherwise applied to the human body or any part thereof for cleansing, beautifying, promoting attractiveness, or altering the appearance, and (2) articles <u>intended</u> for use as a component of any such articles, except that such terms shall not include 'soap'" [11].

Definition of a Drug

In contrast, the FDC Act defines "drug", in pertinent part, as "(B) articles <u>intended for use</u> in the diagnosis, cure, mitigation, treatment, or prevention of disease...; and (C) articles...intended to affect the structure or any function of the body...." [12].

Thus, it is the marketer's intent in selling the product to the public that is key to determining whether it is classified as a cosmetic or a drug. As a result, products represented in labeling for diagnostic or therapeutic purposes or as intended to affect an aspect of the body's structure or function, are no longer regulated by FDA as cosmetics and are held to the different, and more stringent, requirements for drug products.

Interpretation of "Intended Use"

FDA interprets the "intended use" of a product as the objective intent of the seller, as determined by statements made by the seller about the product and the circumstances surrounding the article's distribution[13].[2] A product represented as a drug, but which is not generally recognized by qualified experts as safe and effective for its intended purposes, is deemed to be both misbranded and an unapproved new drug. Accordingly, it may only be marketed for those purposes if its safety and effectiveness have been substantiated either through adherence to an applicable regulation for over-the-counter (non-prescription) drugs [14], or through approval of a New Drug Application (NDA).

Product Representations of Concern to FDA

FDA has for many years considered certain representations made for cosmetics as either false and misleading or as representations that fall within the FDC Act drug definition. As most companies faced with misbranding or new drug charges choose to modify product labeling rather than to develop the data required to support drug approval, therefore, only a few judicial decisions address cosmetic claims in any detail.

Historical Considerations

The three chief cases stem from the 1960s, at which time, FDA initiated civil seizures of skin care products widely promoted to smooth, reduce or prevent wrinkles.

Line Away
Line Away Temporary Wrinkle Smoother was advertised to "visibly smooth out fatigue lines, laugh lines, worry lines, frown lines, tiny age lines and crows feet, while discouraging new lines from forming". Advertising for Line Away contained statements that "Line Away is an amazing protein liquid. Contains no hormones or harmful drugs. It's the only wrinkle smoother packaged under biologically aseptic conditions in the pharmaceutical laboratories of (the manufacturer)" [15].

Sudden Change
Sudden Change was labeled and advertised as the "new and improved, dramatically different wrinkle-smoothing cosmetic. By simple, dynamic contraction, it lifts, firms, tones slack skin... smooths out wrinkles, lifts the puffs under the eyes, leaving your contours looking beautifully defined. It acts noticeably, visibly... not a hormone or chemical astringent, Sudden Change is a concentrated purified natural protein....". Sudden Change was also advertised as a "face lift without surgery!...[it] is the one cosmetic that can make you look years younger for hours...although it cannot eliminate wrinkles permanently... Just smooth it on and watch it smooth away crows' feet, laugh and frown lines – even under-eye puffiness... Sudden Change... does not change the structure or function of your skin in any way" [16].

---

[2] FDA has occasionally determined that articles are drugs even when the seller has made no statements as to the intended use of a product. This may occur if it is foreseeable that the article will be used predominantly for drug or device purposes. In such cases, courts have held that consumers must use the product predominantly and in fact nearly exclusively – with the appropriate intent before the requisite statutory intent can be inferred. *National Nutritional Food Association [NNFA] v. Mathews*, 557 F. 2d 325, 333–334 (2d Cir. 1977)

Magic Secret
Magic Secret, the third product, was advertised to "smooth away wrinkles in minutes... keep them away for hours", to "firm the skin", to "tighten and moisturize tired skin", to "smooth away crows' feet, puffy under eye circles, laugh, frown, and throat lines in just minutes". Users would "feel an astringent sensation...gently firming and toning the skin" [17].

Comparisons of These Early Cases
Although the representations for these products are quite similar, only the intended uses for Magic Secret were held to be within the FDC Act's cosmetic definition. The courts in Line Away and Sudden Change found these products to be represented as drugs based upon their promoted ability to affect the structure and function of the body by "lifting" the skin, by discouraging new wrinkle lines, and in the case of Line Away, by the therapeutic implications created by statements that the product was produced in a "pharmaceutical laboratory" and packed under "biologically aseptic conditions".

Once these products were removed from classification as cosmetics, FDA was relieved of any need to assess the level of substantiation for the claims as cosmetic effects, as the applicable standard became the demonstration of safety and efficacy appropriate to a new drug approval. FDA does not appear to have challenged the substantiation supporting the cosmetic claims for Magic Secret. FDA may have agreed with the statement by the court in Magic Secret, that "even the ignorant, unthinking and credulous consumer would not be led by these references to believe that Magic Secret would do other than alter their appearance". As the court in Line Away observed: "Some 'puffery' may not amount to representation of a cosmetic as a drug"...."but when 'puffery' contains the strong therapeutic implications we find in the Line Away promotional material, we think the dividing line has been crossed" [18].

Recent Claims for Skin Treatment Products

In 1987, FDA considered that the skin care industry had overstepped the dividing line between acceptable cosmetic "puffery" and drug claims. Between 1987 and 1989, FDA sent Regulatory Letters (similar letters today are called "Warning Letters") to over 30 companies informing them that: "We consider a claim that a product will affect the body in some physiological way to be a drug claim, even if the claim is that the effect is only temporary... therefore, we consider most of the anti-aging and skin physiological claims... to be drug claims" [19]. For example, claims that a product "counteracts", "retards", or "controls" aging or the aging process, as well as claims that a product "rejuvenates", "repairs", or "renews" the skin, are drug claims because they can be fairly understood as claims that a function of the body, or that the structure of the body, will be affected by the product. For this reason, all the examples, [that] allege an effect within the epidermis as the basis for a temporary beneficial effect on wrinkles, lines, or fine lines are unacceptable. A claim such as "molecules absorb... and expand, exerting upward pressure to 'lift wrinkles upward' is a claim for an inner, structural change".

FDA further stated that "...we would not object to claims that products will temporarily improve the appearance of ...outward signs of aging.[3] The label of such pro-

---

[3] Id.

ducts should state that the product is intended to cover up the signs of aging, to improve the appearance by adding color or luster to skin, or otherwise to affect the appearance through physical means.... We would consider a product that claims to improve or to maintain temporarily the appearance or the feel of the skin to be a cosmetic. For example, a product that claims to moisturize or soften the skin is a cosmetic".

"Puffery" vs. Drug Representations

Since 1987, the line between cosmetic "puffery" and drug representations has shifted as consumers have become more sophisticated. Today, even the most "credulous, ignorant and unthinking" consumers have become accustomed to product claims considerably stronger than those made about Sudden Change and Line Away. However, without any change in the statute, cosmetic regulations, or case law, the apparent permissible claims for cosmetics have been significantly limited, but, the limitations have assisted the industry by clearly identifying claims outside of the cosmetic category. These include all claims made for products subject to the OTC Drug Review Program, many of which were considered cosmetics prior to their OTC drug classification (such as skin protectants, skin lighteners, sunscreen, antiperspirants, hair growers). Also off-limits are claims approved by FDA for particular new drugs represented to improve the appearance. Any claims outside these boundaries, unless blatantly intended as otherwise therapeutic, appear to elicit little or no FDA response.

Representations Specifically Challenged by FDA

If FDA tends to shift the burden of enforcement from the cosmetic to the drug arena at one end of the spectrum, and to expand (at least for practical purposes) the scope of claims considered to be mere "puffery" at the other extreme, are there cosmetic claims that FDA considers to be false and misleading and which cause a cosmetic to be misbranded without reference to drug effectiveness?

Highlighting an Ingredient

Highlighting one ingredient in a multi-ingredient product may cause the product to be misbranded if it gives a false or misleading impression of the product [20]. The Agency's only formal attempt to quantify the level of a cosmetic ingredient necessary to avoid a false and misleading claim to product content dictates the amount of egg in an "egg shampoo" (one egg per shampoo). A shampoo containing less than that amount could not be identified as "egg shampoo", although "shampoo with egg" was considered acceptable. A shampoo with less than 2% egg content was deemed misbranded if egg was mentioned outside of the ingredient declaration. This regulation obviously has a limited application and in fact, was recently revoked [21]. Nevertheless, it is clear that the absence of an ingredient listed in the ingredient declaration or highlighted in the labeling would render the product misbranded.

Reference to "Hypoallergenicity"

In 1974 FDA proposed to define the term "hypoallergenic" used to describe cosmetics [22]. Although the proposal was subsequently withdrawn as the result of a judicial challenge by industry members [23], some of the concepts related to substantiating a claim to hypoallergenicity have subsequently been accepted by industry members. Thus, companies that claim product hypoallergenicity are generally prepared to show that each step in the formulation and production of the product was informed by special selection of ingredients and other procedures designed to minimize the creation or addition of allergens.

Reference to Inclusion of "Hormones"

One practice FDA has clearly identified as false and misleading for cosmetics is the use of drug and "near-drug" phrases and terms to describe cosmetics. For example, FDA has stated that the use of the word "hormone" in the text of labeling or in the cosmetic ingredient declaration is an implied claim to drug effectiveness [24]. Furthermore, any reference to hormones in cosmetics is false and misleading since any hormone ingredients used in cosmetics must be prepared from materials lacking biological activity.

Reference to Nutrient or Health Benefit

FDA has stated that a cosmetic represented as offering nutrient or health benefits based on its vitamin content may also be misbranded [25]. If FDA should at some future date revise its view of vitamins in light of increasing evidence that certain vitamins in topical preparations do have a beneficial cosmetic effect, the result may be to classify products with vitamin-related claims as drugs, rather than as effective cosmetics.

Reference to Government Approval

FDA considers reference in cosmetic labeling to "government" or "FDA approval" as false and misleading.

Federal Trade Commission

The Federal Trade Commission (FTC) is involved with cosmetic claims substantiation through its authority over advertising. In this section, we will review the statutory authority of the FTC, policy factors for determining when the FTC brings an action against a company, and the standards of support for advertising expected by the FTC.

Statutory Authority

The Commission's authority over advertising is found in three Sections of the Federal Trade Commission Act (FTC Act). Section 5 prohibits unfair methods of competition and unfair or deceptive acts or practices, Section 12 prohibits false advertising for cosmetics, and Section 15 defines false advertising as misleading to a material extent.

Section 5 Prohibits Unfair Methods of Competition and Unfair or Deceptive Acts or Practices

Section 5 of the FTC Act prohibits unfair methods of competition in or affecting commerce, and unfair or deceptive acts or practices in or affecting commerce [26]. In general, it is the prerogative of the FTC to determine what it will consider to be unfair or deceptive acts or practices, and to bring individual cases to illuminate these determinations. The Commission can also institute rulemaking proceedings to address general problems of an industry if it feels that this approach will achieve the purpose of restricting the activity more effectively.

Section 12 Prohibits False Advertising for Cosmetics

Section 12 of the FTC Act prohibits false advertising for foods, drugs, devices, and cosmetics specifically [27]. This section must be considered, however, in light of the overlapping responsibilities of the FDA and the FTC. Potential jurisdictional problems have been addressed by distinguishing between advertising and labeling, and by effective liaison between the two agencies.

Section 15 Defines False Advertising

Section 15 of the FTC Act defines false advertising as advertising that is misleading in a material respect [28]. Labeling is exempted (acknowledging the distinction between FDA and FTC jurisdiction). An advertisement will be considered false if it does not reveal facts that are material in light of the representations in the advertisement, or regarding possible consequences of use under conditions that are customary or are prescribed in the advertisement.

Policy Factors for Bringing Actions

As the amount of advertising in the United States is prodigious, the FTC staff developed criteria for determining when to bring an action against particular advertising. These criteria have been followed, more or less, since 1975, and were highlighted in a speech to the American Advertising Federation by FTC Chairman Miller in 1981 [29]. The criteria include: (1) consumer interpretation of the claim, (2) scale of the deception or lack of substantiation, (3) materiality, (4) adequacy of corrective market forces, (5) effect on flow of truthful information, (6) deterrence, (7) law enforcement efficiency, and (8) additional, social considerations.

Consumer Interpretation of the Claim

The consumer interpretation of the claim may be the single most important issue in the FTC's decision to bring a case. Often, the only contested issue is whether the advertising contains a particular implied claim that the FTC considers deceptive or unsubstantiated.

US courts have typically upheld the expertise of the FTC to make the judgment as to whether a particular advertisement contains an implied claim. Consumer research studies or consumer testimony were not required in the past [30]. However, there has been increasing criticism of this practice as the FTC staff are usually lawyers and economists and rarely have special expertise or training in interpreting advertisements. Consumer surveys as to the meaning of the advertising are an effective and increasingly common way to address questions of this nature.

Scale of the Deception or Lack of Substantiation

If the advertising reaches a large number of consumers, and if it is likely to affect their purchasing decisions in a significant manner, then the FTC is more likely to take action. Hence, national advertising is more likely to gain attention than a more localized campaign. Additionally, objective market claims will receive more scrutiny as to substantiation, since it is easier for the FTC to determine if there is adequate claim support.

Materiality

Although the FTC need not show an actual consumer deception or effect on purchasing decision, according to the FTC Act, the decision to bring a case takes into account the number of consumers actually harmed and the extent of that harm. For example, if there were few consumers that would be likely to make a purchasing decision based on the advertising, or if the harm were only of a small monetary nature and if the consumer is likely to determine from actual product use that the claim is deceptive, there is a lower probability that the FTC will initiate action. If, however, the monetary harm is substantial, for example, purchasing a car because of a deceptive advertisement, or there is likely to be physical harm, as from the purchase of an ineffective drug or a hazardous cosmetic, then the FTC is likely to take action.

Adequacy of Corrective Market Forces

This analysis ties into the materiality criterion identified above. If the consumer can determine that the claim is false at a relatively low cost, then the FTC is unlikely to take action. Before initiating an investigation, the FTC also considers whether there are other market forces at work that might correct the deceptive claim, such as labeling on the product, or a competitor's advertising.

Effect on Flow of Truthful Information

The FTC will consider the effects of any action on the flow of information that might be truthful. For example, the Commission is generally careful to assure that any action brought be limited in its scope to the most narrow solution that will stop the deceptive practices, and to guard against over-interpretation of the statute. Some claims may be misleading to a small number of consumers, but provide useful information to the majority. The FTC will often overlook the deceptive nature of a claim in such a case.

Deterrence

There are both positive and negative aspects to the consideration of deterrence. An important factor is whether a litigated order is useful in establishing an industry-wide standard that could be enforced under section 5(m)(1)(B) of the FTC Act. The FTC also considers the significance of the possible relief and the importance and visibility of the product and its advertising in the marketplace as a whole to predict if an enforcement action will have an impact on other members of the industry. Finally, the FTC considers whether the violation is so visible that a failure to act would somehow diminish the Commission's credibility and deterrent effect among other industry members.

Law Enforcement Efficiency

Law enforcement efficiency considerations determine whether the FTC is the most efficient way to ameliorate the problem. The FTC will also look to voluntary industry efforts, and even to private law suits among competitors as alternatives to direct Commission action.

Additional Considerations

Social considerations may play a role in the decisions of the FTC. For example, an action may be brought against an advertiser because the claim made directly affects a vulnerable group, such as children. The FTC's ability to justify the burden it imposes on a company because of such social considerations is to varying degrees guided by the executive and legislative arms of the federal government (the administration and Congress).

Standards of Support for Advertising

The FTC requires that the advertiser have adequate substantiation for a claim at the time the claim is first made to consumers. This doctrine was first established in a case against Pfizer, Inc. in 1972 [31], and has been vigorously upheld since that time.

The level of substantiation required for any given claim depends on the type of claim made. The kind, quantity, and quality of the substantiating information also varies depending on the nature of the claim, the product, and the advertiser [32].

The FTC policy statement regarding advertising substantiation is the bedrock of its law enforcement efforts [33]. Claims are expected to be supported by the level of substantiation they communicate to the consumer. For example, if the claim states that the attribute is supported by clinical tests, there must be clinical tests that support it. Further, if the advertisement implies a higher level of substantiation than it in fact expressly claims, the actual substantiation relied upon must support the higher standard.

For advertisements that do not either expressly or impliedly state a particular level of support, the FTC will require a "reasonable basis" for the claims. Reasonable basis is an analysis that depends on cases established in law. Factors considered include: the type of claim, the type of product, the benefits of a truthful claim, the consequences of a false claim, the cost of developing substantiation for the claim, and the amount of substantiation experts in the field would consider reasonable.

The FTC has also issued a policy statement dealing with comparative advertising [34]. The FTC encourages comparative advertising which names or makes reference to competitors; however, it requires clarity to avoid consumer deception. The FTC noted that one industry "codes of practice" that prohibited or restricted comparative advertising or that imposed a higher standard of substantiation than that necessary for a unilateral claim would be challenged by the Commission.

In the past, there has been little FTC activity in regard to the advertising of traditional beauty and personal appearance claims for the cosmetic industry. In an early case brought against a product claiming to restore youth or the appearance of youth to the skin, the Court of Appeals for the Second Circuit upheld the FTC finding that the advertising was false and misleading [35]. Court cases involving advertising that causes primarily economic injury have also been brought by the FTC against hair restorer products that falsely claimed to prevent or cure baldness [36].

Although there are few FTC cases that have involved cosmetic products, those that do exist have focused on advertising that includes health or safety claims, or on products for which there was an underlying safety concern. Products that are advertised for health or safety purposes can cause economic injury, as well as actual injury, by preventing the consumer from seeking appropriate medical help.

In several cases the FTC required additional warnings in the advertising about the possible consequences of product use. These include cases against ads for products marketed to African-Amercians for the purpose of straightening or relaxing the hair. Because these products contain ingredients that can cause skin and eye irritation and injury, and may cause hair loss if used improperly, the FTC ordered a number of different companies to include warnings and specific directions for use [37]. Another case of a product without adequate warning involved an eyelash dye that the FTC said could cause severe eye pain for a substantial period of time [38]. In that instance, the Commission required the manufacturer to quit advertising and packaging the product unless a warning about the potential problem appeared on the labeling and promotional materials.

Other cases have been brought against advertising for products with claims to safety with which the FTC disagrees. In one case, the FTC moved against a skin peeling product that was advertised as safe [39], and in another case, the FTC challenged the safety claims of a facial depilatory and beard removal product [40].

More recently the FTC has focused on "infomercials" and telephone "900 numbers". In comments presented at Infomercial Teleshopping '93 [41], Christian White, then acting director of the Bureau of Consumer Protection of the FTC, noted the challenges facing advertising regulation in this arena. Mr. White noted that the reputation of the industry "may have been harmed" by the actions of some infomercial advertisers that misled the public. Infomercial advertisers must adhere to the same standards as advertisers in other media.

Lanham Act

Section 43(a) of the Lanham Act allows for private lawsuits to be brought for false advertising or false endorsement. It offers companies a quick, efficacious means of stopping an offending competitor from running misleading advertising or making false claims on packaging, or from using another's trade or service mark. In this section we will outline the elements of a false advertising claim under the Lanham Act, generally discuss cosmetics cases, and consider who has standing to bring an action under the Act.

Elements of a False Advertising Claim

In a false advertising case under the Lanham Act a plaintiff must prove that the defendant made false or misleading statements about his own product or another's, that there is actual deception or at least a tendency to deceive a substantial portion of the intended audience, that the deception is material in that it is likely to influence purchasing decisions, that the advertised goods traveled in interstate commerce, and that there is a likelihood of injury to the plaintiff in terms of declining sales, loss of good will, etc. [42].

A critical difference in the requirements of a case under the Lanham Act versus an FTC action lies in the proof required. For a Lanham Act case, the plaintiff must ordinarily prove that the claim is false or misleading, not merely that it is unsubstantiated,[4] unless the defendant's advertising explicitly refers to studies. In the latter case, the burden of showing that the tests being relied upon are adequate in all respects might fall on the defendant, if the plaintiff can raise enough questions about their adequacy [43]. In general, questions of "puffery" will not be addressed by the courts under the Lanham Act.

Cosmetic Cases Under the Lanham Act

Cosmetic cases under the Lanham Act generally involve fragrances, product performance, and comparative claims. Most of the fragrance cases involve "knock-off" products and the claims made regarding them. Since 1975 the courts have provided guidance that is often contradictory. In general, the courts are sympathetic to knock-offs as long as the claims do not go too far in comparing the knock-off with the original.

Although performance claims in advertising are common for cosmetics, only two cases have been litigated where there was a decision on the merits. Most cases are settled privately prior to trial. By far the most frequent basis for Lanham Act suits is a comparative claim. Here courts are likely to require strict adherence to the requirement for valid, quantifiable data, and to find that there is a need for action.

Standing to Bring a Lanham Act Case

Only companies that are direct competitors that would be damaged by the false advertising or false representations can bring suit under the Lanham act. Consumers do not have standing to bring Lanham Act cases [44], nor do non-competitors [45].

State Laws Regarding Substantiation

Most states have enacted "little" FDA and FTC statutes and consumer protection laws which provide the basis for state prosecution of false and misleading labeling and advertising claims. California, which has actively pursued potentially fraudulent advertising, authorizes the Attorney General or any California District Attorney to request persons making advertising claims in the state to provide the factual, objective or clinical evidence referred to or implied in the advertisement [46]. If the claim is not

---

[4] Id.

substantiated within a reasonable time, the state may seek an immediate termination or modification of the claims as well as monetary penalties.

Typical substantiation deficiencies have involved lack of proper control groups (no use of a placebo, positive, or a negative control), potential bias (studies not blinded), statistical weaknesses and failure to provide raw data, poor measuring techniques (ambiguous directions), use of untried or unaccepted devices or measuring techniques, and use of measurements and tests that cannot substantiate the claim [47].

In the past few years, California has required substantiation of claims for cellulite products, toothpaste (whiteners), and various skin care products represented as anti-aging agents. The evidence necessary to substantiate a claim must be at the level expressed or implied in the claim. Thus, according to Daryl Roberts, Esq., Deputy District Attorney, Consumer Environmental Protection Service, Napa County, California, scientific tests referred to or implied in the advertisement must be conducted by persons expert in the field and evaluated in a disinterested manner using test procedures generally accepted in the profession as accurate and reliable. Valid clinical studies are those that include a control and that are double blinded. Claims that merely state the product works must nevertheless have a reasonable basis, such as tests, research, surveys, samples, or evidence based on the expertise of persons in the field, and this evidence must have been evaluated by procedures accepted as providing accurate and reliable results.

National Advertising Division of the Council of Better Business Bureaus

The National Advertising Division (NAD) of the Council of Better Business Bureaus was established in 1971 by industry trade associations to encourage and sustain high standards of truth and accuracy in national advertising. In this section we will outline the procedures of the NAD and discuss its role in addressing claims substantiation.

Procedures of the NAD

The NAD is a voluntary mechanism for receiving or initiating complaints, evaluating, investigating, and analyzing national advertising, and holding initial negotiations with companies involving the truth or accuracy of their national advertizing [48]. Questions can arise from any source. NAD publishes case reports at least ten times a year, summarizing the matters concluded the previous month. When an NAD preliminary review indicates the possibility that an advertisement promotes an unlawful product or service, or that it is false, misleading, or deceptive, and the advertiser will not participate in the self-regulatory process, NAD prepares a review of the facts and sends this to the appropriate federal or state law enforcement agency.

Complaints

Any person, including the NAD itself, may submit a complaint. NAD reviews the complaint to determine if it is national in character and not the subject of litigation or other court or government agency activity, whether such action was withdrawn permanently prior to the date of the complaint, or whether the complaint is of such a technical nature that the NAD could not conduct a meaningful analysis of the issues or so trivial as to merit no expenditure of resources. If the complaint does not meet the inclusion criteria, the complainant is so notified. The advertiser is notified of the complaint and the complainant's identity.

Parties

The parties are: NAD, acting in the public interest, the advertiser, acting in its own interest, and the complainant.

Information in NAD Proceedings

NAD proceedings will only consider data and materials that have also been submitted to the advertiser. Any studies from the complainant must be sufficiently complete to allow for independent expert evaluation.

A challenged advertiser may submit data to the NAD with the request that the data not be made available to the complainant. The complainant is entitled to receive a summary of the advertiser's principle arguments. Circulation is restricted to those persons directly involved with the inquiry.

Responses and Replies

The advertiser may submit a substantial written response to the complaint to substantiate the challenged advertisement. That response is transmitted to the complainant. The complainant can then respond, as can the advertiser again. A meeting may be scheduled to substitute for the written responses.

Decision and Publication

The NAD will formulate a decision within 15 business days of its receipt of the last of the responses and replies. NAD will then make its decision known to the advertiser and the complainant and make copies available to the public. The advertiser has the right of appeal for any disagreement with NAD. Such an appeal is reviewed by a panel of the National Advertising Review Board. Finally the decision of the NAD will be published in the monthly cases.

NAD Role in Claims Substantiation

The NAD role in claims substantiation is two-fold. First, the publication of decisions of the NAD about controversies regarding national advertising provides some information about the substantiation that exists regarding particular claims. While the complainant and the public do not necessarily know what data existed to qualify a particular claim, there is the knowledge that something considered sufficient exists, and there is information on its general nature. Another function of the NAD procedure is to allow the quick identification of those advertisers that do not have substantive data, and the expeditious removal of the offending advertising or the transfer of their cases to the appropriate enforcement authority for action. This screening process allows a more efficient use of the scarce resources of the FTC.

Other Sources Requiring Claims Substantiation

There are several other sources that may require claims substantiation, depending on the type of claim. These include broadcast and print companies, Federal Mail Fraud Act, and the Tariff Act.

Broadcast and Print Companies

Broadcast and print companies generally have standards for advertising that can require claims substantiation. These standards focus on decency concerns as well as consumer deception. For example, advertising standards and guidelines for Capital Cities/ABC, Inc., March 1992, stated that: "It is the policy of Capital Cities/ABC to present advertising which is truthful and tasteful, and not misleading or deceptive. Claims must be substantiated, and qualifying information about a product must be disclosed when needed to avoid misleading customers". Of some interest is that, while such guidelines may include sections that can generally apply to cosmetics, for example, product demonstrations, research (comparative advertising, perception testing), and endorsements, the guidelines do not directly address cosmetics.

Federal Mail Fraud Act

Federal Mail Fraud Act, which dates back to 1872, prohibits fraud through the use of the mails. This statute has been used over the years to prevent the dissemination of false or misleading promotional materials by the US Postal Service.

The Tariff Act of 1930

The Tariff Act of 1930, administered by the US Customs Service, requires that the country of origin be marked on foreign articles imported into the United States. The FTC Act also addresses the need for accurate country of origin labeling, used to the Tariff Act can be used to address this specific claim at the product's entry into the US.

Summary

In summary, the basis of cosmetic claim substantiation in the United States is extremely complicated. There are federal laws that apply to labeling and others that apply to advertising, laws that are invoked by the Federal government and those invoked by competitors, State laws that mimic the Federal laws, and those that actually provide other avenues of challenge for the advertiser. Then, there are the voluntary standards of the National Advertising Division of the Council of Better Business Bureaus, applied after the fact, and the standards of the broadcast and print media that are applied to the advertising before it is allowed to air. Each of these avenues of challenge for the advertiser addresses proof in a slightly different manner as well. With all of these challenges, however, there is still significant advertising for cosmetics in the US, demonstrating that companies are able to produce adequate substantiation for claims that can address all of the possible pitfalls. Products can be sold with claims that are solely truthful and not misleading, and this is the answer to questions about claims substantiation in the US.

References

1. 21 United States Code (USC) section 301 et seq.
2. 15 USC sections 1451–1461
3. 15 USC sections 42-58
4. 15 USC section 43(a)
5. Mail Fraud Act, 18 USC 1341-1342
6. 21 USC sections 331(a) and 361(a); 21CFR section 1.21
7. 21 USC section 321(m); US v. Kordel, 355 US 345 (1948)
8. 21 USC section 321(n); 21 Code of Federal Regulations (CFR) section 1.21
9. 15 USC sections 45, 52, 55(a)
10. Memorandum of Understanding between the FDA and FTC, 36 Federal Register (Fed Reg) 18,539 (1971)
11. 21 USC section 321(i)
12. 21 USC section 321(g)(1)
13. FDA, Nicotine in cigarettes and smokeless tobacco products is a drug and these products are nicotine delivery devices under the Federal Food, Drug, and Cosmetic Act, 60 Fed Reg 41454, 41482 (August 11, 1995)
14. FDA has issued proposed or final regulations for OTC drug products intended to treat or prevent conditions such as acne (21 CFR 333), chapped skin (21 CFR 347), topical itching and pain (21 CFR 348), tooth decay (21 CFR 355), warts and calluses (21 CFR 358, subpart B), dandruff, sebborhea and psoriasis (21 CFR 358, subpart H), and products such as skin lighteners, [47 Fed Reg 39108–117 (September 3, 1982)], antiperspirants [47 Fed Reg 36492–505 (August 20, 1982)], hair grower and hair loss prevention (21 CFR 310.527) and sunscreens [58 Fed Reg 28/94 May 12, 1993]
15. United States v. An Article ... Line Away, 283 F Supp 107 (D Del 1986), aff'd, 415 F 2d 369 (3rd Cir 1969)
16. United States v. An Article ... Sudden Change, 288 F Supp 29 [EDNY 1968, rev'd, 409 F 2d 734 (2d Cir 1969)]
17. United States v. An Article ... Magic Secret, 331 F Supp 912 (D Md 1971)
18. Line Away, 415 F 2d at 371
19. Letter from John M. Taylor, Associate Commissioner for Regulatory Affairs, to Stuart Friedel, Davis and Gilbert, re: Cosmetic Regulatory Letters, (November 19, 1987)
20. 21 CFR section 701.1(b)
21. Revocation of Certain Regulations Affecting Food, 61 Fed Reg 27771 (June 3, 1996) "Section 700.10 Shampoo preparations containing eggs as one of the ingredients is removed."
22. 39 Fed Reg 7288 (February 25, 1974)
23. Almay v. Joseph A Califano, 569 F 2d 674 (D C Cir)(1977), Revocation of Rule 43 Fed Reg 10559 (March 14, 1978)
24. 21 CFR 310.50(a); see also 54 Fed Reg 40618, 40620 (October 20, 1989) (Proposed Rule on OTC Topical Hormone-Containing Drug Products); 58 Fed Reg 47611, 47613 (September 9, 1993) (Proposed rule on the use of hormones as ingredients in cosmetics); FDA Guide to Inspections of Cosmetic Product Manufacturers (1995), pp 7–8
25. Id., FDA Guide to Inspections of Cosmetic Product Manufacturers (1995), p 8
26. 15 USC section 5
27. 15 USC section 12
28. 15 USC section 15
29. Advertising Age, December 14, 1981, p 6
30. FTC v. Colgate Palmolive Co, 380 US 374 (1965); Resort Rental Car Systems, Inc v. FTC, 518 F 2d 962 (9th Cir 1965)
31. Pfizer, Inc et al., 81 FTC 23 (1972)
32. National Dynamics Corp, et al., 82 FTC 488 (1973), aff'd and remanded on other grounds 492 F 2d 1333 (2d Cir 1973), cert. Denied 419 US 993 (1974), reissued 85 FTC 391 (1976)
33. Federal Register 49 (150) 30999–31001 (August 2, 1984)
34. Federal Register 44 (157) 47378–47329 (August 13, 1979)
35. Charles of the Ritz Dist Corp v. FTC, 143 F 2d 676 (2d Cir 1944)
36. US v. Braswell, Inc, et al., No. C81–55 A (ND Ga September 14, 1983); FTC v. Intra-Medic Formulations, Inc, et al., (S D Fla February 28, 1986)

37. Lustrasilk Corp of America, Inc, et al., 87 FTC 145 (1976); The Perma-Strate Company, et al., 87 FTC 155 (1976); Soft and Sheen Company, Inc, et al., 87 FTC 164 (1976); Johnson Products Company, Inc, et al., 87 FTC 206 (1976); Revlon, Inc, et al., 89 FTC 1 (1977)
38. CEB Products, Inc, et al., 85 FTC 565, 569, 573 (1975)
39. Miriam Mascheck, Inc, et al., 85 FTC 536 (1975)
40. Carson Products Co, et al., 86 FTC 1079 (1975)
41. Remarks of Christian S White, Acting Director, Bureau of Consumer Protection, Federal Trade Commission, Monday, September 13, 1993, Hyatt Carlton Tower, Infomercial Teleshopping '93
42. Johnson and Johnson-Merck Consumer Pharmaceuticals Co v. Rhone Poulenc Rorer Pharmaceuticals, Inc, 19 F 3d 125 (3d Cir 1994)
43. McNeil-PCC, Inc v. Bristol-Myers Squibb Co, 938 F 2d 1544 (2d Cir 1991)
44. Serbin v. Ziebart International Corp, 11 F 3d 1163 (3d Cir 1993); Barros v. Sylvania, 34 USPQ 2d 1859 (9th Cir 1995)
45. Stenfield v. Osborne Industries, Inc, 52 F 3d 867 (10th Cir 1995); Ortho Pharmaceutical Corp v. Cosprophar, Inc, 32 F 3d 690 (2d Cir 1994)
46. California Business and Professional Code § 17508
47. Roberts D (1995) Substantiating cosmetic advertising claims. Society of Cosmetic Chemists Program, December 6, 1995
48. Council of Better Business Bureaus, Inc, National Advertising Division, Childrens Advertising Review Unit and National Advertising Review board Procedures, November 1, 1993

The Contribution of the European Cosmetics Directive Towards International Harmonization: Impact on the Evaluation of Safety and Efficacy

Ph. Masson

Introduction

Historically, the purpose of the cosmetic product, a generic term which embraces personal hygiene products, skin care products, make-up, and perfumery products, was to embellish and modify appearance and odor, stimulate fantasy, and ultimately heighten attraction. The need to seduce, together with the quest for eternal youth, date back to antiquity; they have inspired countless writers, painters, and musicians. They have also stimulated the creativity of cosmetologists throughout the centuries.

Although originally its purpose was essentially to enhance appearance and odor, the cosmetic product has evolved towards a more functional role and progressively acquired the capacity to cleanse, drastically modify, protect, and maintain the appearance in good condition. This evolution has necessitated a re-evaluation regarding the position of the cosmetic product in relation to food and medical products:

- Intended for application on the skin, external mucous membranes, hair, and nails, and to have a local effect, it clearly distinguishes itself from food products in terms of its administration and its purpose; it is not intended to respond to metabolic needs, even if, conversely, some foodstuffs claim an ability to have effects matching those traditionally attributed to cosmetic products.
- Furthermore, it is not the function of the cosmetic product to treat skin disease, nor to prevent effects or organic dysfunction; thus, it does not have to satisfy any benefit:risk ratio specific to medicines, but is expected to respond to the user's needs regarding self-confidence.

The existence and success of a cosmetic product are linked not only to its capacity to fulfill the consumer's expectations in terms of preconceptions and desire for social advancement, but also very concrete expectations regarding effectiveness and safety. The survival of the cosmetic industry is itself linked to its ability to fully satisfy these expectations in the short, medium, and long term.

The need to continually adapt products to evolving market demands also justifies joint deliberations on the part of the industry and the relevant authorities, intended to culminate in the regulatory framework being brought in line with the requirements of modern cosmetology. These are primarily industrial requirements since, as we have seen, in order to hold a long-term market position, the priority of a cosmetic product must be to satisfy safety requirements. It is therefore the industry's responsibility to ensure the safety of products brought onto the market. They are also requirements made of the authority, whose responsibility it is to ensure the conformity of products circulating on the market and to remain vigilant in its efforts to prevent the distribution of products evading the relevant quality controls.

Any evaluation must take all phases of production into consideration:

- The quality of raw materials in terms of safety, physico-chemical properties, and microbiological purity.
- The manufacturing process.
- The quality of the finished product in terms of its physico-chemical stability and its microbiological purity and stability.
- The safety of the finished product in terms of potential irritant, allergic, or toxic effects on contact with skin. This assessment must rely on the ingredients, but may be checked whenever necessary against the finished product.
- The substantiation of claimed effects or action.
- The easy availability to the consumer of all information necessary for the correct and safe use of a product.
- Follow-up of the products progress following its launch on the market.

It is clear that such a series of checks could not be reasonably and effectively carried out by the authority alone unless a preliminary system of authorization were to be set up which, in practice, would prove totally inadequate given the number of products released every year on each country's market. Therefore, in this context, it was logical to move towards a shared responsibility, whereby: (a) The industry sets up a suitable system of inspections to ensure the safety and stability of products at the time of their launch on the market, and (b) the authority verifies a posteriori whether the industry is satisfactorily carrying out the responsibilities which it has been given, and prevails on its capacity, where necessary, to sanction offenders.

The countries which largely import must not be excluded from the equation, since they may have real difficulty in identifying the products circulating on their markets; that being the case, it may be justifiable for them to set up a system of declaration which would provide them with information on the manufacturers, distributors, and importers, as well as those products regularly marketed. In the long term, however, the ever increasing economic exchange between states, and thus the multilateral opening up of markets, do not permit the observance of national techno-regulatory provisions since these would implicitly hinder the free circulation of their own goods and services.

This general trend concerns mainly cosmetic products and perfumes which are, by nature, products of wide international distribution. This fact was universally acknowledged in Florence in April 1998, where the delegates of some 35 countries gathered to work on the subject "Global cosmetic regulatory harmonization: an impetus to the development of export markets" [1]. At this conference, where representatives of both the authorities and the cosmetic industry spoke, a common desire to achieve international harmonization was expressed. Indeed, it was acknowledged that, despite inhomogeneous regulatory mechanisms, a need to adapt in the same direction was felt throughout the world.

The common recommendation for such an adaption proved to be the European Cosmetic Directive since:

- It is in itself the practical demonstration of a capacity for total harmonization made by 15 countries which until 1976 had differing legislation.
- It constitutes the most recent legislative provision.

- The 15 countries in question are those with the highest concentration of cosmetic and perfumery industries.
- It is the part of the world in which the sector is the most innovative.
- The European Cosmetic Directive constitutes as a result the regulatory mechanism which best responds to the needs of the modern cosmetic product and to current safety and consumer awareness requirements.

The Emergence of European Cosmetic Regulations

In 1976, the Council of the European Communities ratified for the first time a text known under the reference 76/768/CEE [2], aimed at bringing the legislation of Member States on cosmetic products in line. In fact, it seemed to make sense to try to harmonize the regulation of cosmetic products, for which some of the nine Member States already had at that time an advanced specific legislation, while others had no regulatory mechanism to refer to. Six successive amendments [3–8] were necessary to arrive at a legislation which was acceptable on the one hand to the originators of this Community initiative, and on the other to the six Member States which came progressively to strengthen the European Union, i.e., Greece (1981), Spain and Portugal (1986), Austria, Finland, and Sweden (1995). The most significant amendments were introduced by Council Directives 88/667/CEE [6] and 93/35/CEE [8].

We must not exclude the future ratification of new amendments aimed in the short term at removing difficulties in application or interpretation which could arise following the implementation of regulatory texts, and aimed in the long term at taking into consideration particular needs which could be introduced by eventual new members of an enlarged European Union. In addition to more fundamental legislative changes, the European cosmetic regulation is regularly up-dated in order to keep abreast of technical progress. This is made official by the adoption of Commission Directives, 23 of which were published in the Official Journal of the European Communities between March 1982 and September 1998.

Thus, the European cosmetic regulation, last modified in 1993, is the final gesture of a desire for harmonization between Member States of the European Union. Although not perfect, this initiative has led to a clarification of the essential ambiguities generated by the recognition of a modern cosmetology. It is intended to respond not only to traditional expectations, but also, due to increasing scientific knowledge of the skin, its properties, and its aging process, to anticipate new consumer demands.

The Contents of the Community Regulation

General Considerations

The European Cosmetic Directive has three essential objectives: (1) To ensure consumer safety, (2) to harmonize legislation between the different Member States of the European Union, and (3) to respond to the consumer's need for information. The Directive is supported on two sides: On the one hand by the industry responsible, which is in a position to assure itself fully of the safety of its products and which is willing to cooperate openly; on the other by the inspection bodies to ensure the efficacy of monitoring once products have been released on the market.

The Directive responds to all the requirements of modern cosmetology with the following:

- A new definition of the cosmetic product, taking all the expectations of the consumer into account, as discussed above (Article 1)
- Clearly outlining the responsibilities of the manufacturer or importer as regards the safety of products put on the market (Articles 2 and 3)
- Clear regulations regarding the conditions under which certain hazardous raw materials are used, or indeed the straightforward banning of such products when the safety margin is insufficient (Articles 4, 5, and 11)
- The compilation of a list of ingredients used by the cosmetic industry and the introduction of a common nomenclature (Article 5b)
- Heightening consumer awareness by means of enforcing regulations on a common labeling policy among all Member States as regards, in particular, identifying all ingredients and, where necessary, stating precautions on the use of the product (Article 6)
- Compiling a list of all the information which must be made available by the industry to the monitoring authorities prior to the launch of a product on the market, demonstrating that the product meets safety requirements (Article 7b)
- Proposing physico-chemical and microbiological methods for analyzing ingredients and finished products capable of guaranteeing their stability over time (Article 8)
- The enforcement of safe-guard clauses enabling the authorities of a Member State to initiate emergency measures if public safety is seen to be at risk (Articles 7, 12, and 13).

To accompany this series of measures, a scientific committee made up of independent experts has been set up on a Community level, linked to the General Direction for Consumer Protection, the purpose of which is to provide technical and scientific advice (article 8b), together with a Committee on the Adaption of Directives to technical progress, composed of Member State representatives (Article 9). The rules governing their function have been set out in Article 10.

An Analysis of Some Specific Points

Some important amendments have been made to Directive 76/768/CEE in order to define its scope and possibly to clarify ambiguities which became apparent following its enforcement; some of these amendments have wrought subtle changes in the behavior of the industry, the authorities concerned, and the consumers themselves. The following sections discuss these amendments in greater detail.

Adjusting the Definition of a Cosmetic Product (Article 1 of Directive 93/35/CEE of June 24, 1993)

The European definition differs slightly from the definitions which previously existed in other countries, in particular Japan and the United States. By the term "cosmetic product" we understand "any substance or preparation intended to come in contact with the various surface areas of the body (epidermis, hair and capillaries, nails, lips, and external genital organs) or with the teeth and buccal mucosae, solely or principally for cleansing, perfuming, or protective purposes in order to maintain them in good condition, modify their appearance, and/or improve body odor, and/or protect or maintain them in good condition".

According to this definition, the cosmetic product is not only capable of cleansing and perfuming, but also henceforth of modifying appearance, improving body odor, and protecting and maintaining the human body in good condition. In addition to this definition, the Directive and subsequent legislation have definitely clarified the ambiguities regarding the status of the cosmetic product. A decree made by the Court of Justice of the European Communities on April 16, 1991 [9] concerning the interpretation of Council Directives 65/65/CEE [10] regarding pharmaceutical specialities and 76/768/CEE regarding cosmetic products specified in particular that a product with no curative properties as regards disease is a medication if it can be administered with a view to restoring, improving, or modifying an organic function. Conversely, a product with no significant effect on the metabolism and which does not modify its functioning is excluded from the definition of "medication"; Annex 1 of the Cosmetic Directive has compiled a general list indicating the products covered by these regulations.

It should also be noted that, according to the Community definition, a cosmetic product is intended to come in contact with various surface areas of the human body or with the teeth and buccal mucosae without any clarification being given as to its end state or degree of possible penetration. It is to be inferred from this that, in order to perform some of the functions claimed, at least part of the ingredients used in a cosmetic formulation must be absorbed by the skin or mucosae.

The Compilation of a List of Ingredients Used in Cosmetic Products and Perfumery Articles (Article 5b introduced by Directive 93/35/CEE of June 14, 1993)

The principal objective of such a list was to promote the setting up of a common nomenclature within the European Union regarding the labeling of cosmetic products in order to facilitate the identification of their ingredients by the monitoring authorities, the medical profession, and possibly also the consumers themselves. The list comprises both raw perfumery and aromatic materials and other substances used in the cosmetic industry.

In contrast to the specific lists given in Directive 76/768/CEE concerning particular categories of ingredients (currently colorants, preservatives, filters), this list is purely declarative and does not in any way constitute a list of authorized substances; that is to say, the use of ingredients given in the list remains the entire and sole responsibility of the manufacturer. The information needed for the addition of a substance to the list is provided by the industry. In practice, the process involves submitting a request to the CTFA (Cosmetic, Toiletry and Fragrance Association, International Nomenclature Committee 1101, 17th Street N.W., Suite 300, Washington 20036, 4702 USA) for the attribution of an INCI (International Nomenclature of Cosmetic Ingredients) name for any new raw material prior to its use in the cosmetic sector. The questionnaire to be completed pertains to the chemical structure, production method, soluble properties, and cosmetic application of the substance in question.

The list is more than simply a catalogue of ingredients since for each entry, in addition to its identity which, where appropriate, is expressed in INCI, European Pharmacopeia, or the Linnée classification terminology, the ingredient's EINECS, IUPAC, CAS and CI (color index) numbers are given where it is mandatory to state the essential function(s) of the ingredient in the finished product, if necessary, restrictions and conditions of use, and warnings on the label, in accordance with the requirements of the various annexes of the Directive.

The list needs to be up-dated periodically. In practice, and in spite of numerous errors and inaccuracies which came to light following publication of the first list in June 1996, no up-date has as yet been made. However, it is reasonable to assume that, given the vast amount of work required for such a revision, the question here is simply one of technical teething problems which will undoubtedly improve in the near future.

Labeling Requirements (Article 6 introduced by Directive 88/667/CEE of December 21, 1988 and supplemented by Directive 93/35/CEE of June 14, 1993)

The European regulations put the manufacturer under the obligation to provide the consumer with as much information as possible at the time of a product's entry on to the market. With the exception of the list of ingredients given on labels essentially for the purpose of providing the consumer with information at the time of purchase, and which thus can only be displayed on external packaging, the following indications must appear on all containers or packaging, whereby the obligatory text sets out in detail:
- Name, corporate name, and address of the manufacturer or distributor, established within the European Community, as well as the particulars of the "primary Community importer"
- Nominal content indicated in weight or volume
- Minimum expiry date if this is within less than 30 months
- Specific precautions for use and, in particular, those clauses which could arise from the incorporation of ingredients subject to restrictions of use
- Batch number or reference enabling identification of manufacturer
- The function of the product.

As regards the list of ingredients, these must be named according to the European nomenclature, as given in the list, and "the ingredients are to be entered in descending order of weight at the time of incorporation". Admittedly, this order is only obligatory for weights in excess of 1% of the final formulation; below this, full licence is given for possible groupings. Particular provisions have been set out regarding:
- Fragrance or aromatic formulations mentioned under the simplifying reference "perfume" or "aroma"
- Decorative products released on the market in a range of varying colors for which all colorants used in the range could be mentioned by adding the words "may contain...", or simply the symbol "+/–".

On the other hand, impurities contained in raw materials used, technical substances used in the course of production but not found in the finished product, as well as substances used as solvents or vectors in fragrant or aromatic formulations, are not considered ingredients and thus need not be given in the list. Specific provisions have been made for those cases relating to commercial confidentiality and to the size, shape, or presentation of certain cosmetic products.

Some difficulties in interpreting the Directive pertain to the language in which information must be given. The amendment introduced in June 1993 [8] clarified this point by suggesting that labeling be made in national or official languages, or in a language easily understandable to the consumer, thus entrusting Member States with the task of fixing their level of requirements at the time of adopting the Directive as national regulations.

Points Raised Regarding the Nature of Information to be Gathered for Inspection Purposes (Article 7b of Directive 93/35/CEE of June 14, 1993)

The industry bears a priori sole responsibility regarding the conformity of its products to safety requirements; thus, prior to releasing any product on the market, it is obliged to put together an information dossier enabling conformity checks to be made a posteriori by the appropriate monitoring authorities of Member States. This information pertains mainly to:
- The identity of the manufacturer or the distributor responsible for releasing a product on the Community market
- The elements which identify the product itself, its formulation, its physico-chemical and microbiological specificities, and its use
- The conditions of its manufacture and, in particular, their conformity to standards of good practice, including information on the credentials of the person responsible for a product's manufacture or initial importation into the European Community
- Safety assessments, with particular mentioning of the identity and credentials of the assessor
- All information regarding the progress of the product following its entry on the market, regarding, in particular, undesirable effects experienced by users
- Where justified, evidence of the product's claimed effect.

Checks are carried out by the competent authority of the Member State in which the product is manufactured or to which its initial importation to the European Community takes place. It is obvious, however, that this list of information is essentially qualitative and does not enable a requirement level for assessors to be set. Thus, the situation calls for Member States to take immediate practical measures regarding the mutual recognition of the inspection process and to set out common criteria in terms of requirements in order to avoid disparities which may prove detrimental to the free circulation of goods. Moreover, there are a number of imprecisions regarding the criteria to be considered when assessing the efficacy and safety of cosmetic products. These points will be dealt with in more detail in the following section.

An Overall Evaluation of the Safety of the Finished Product (Article 7b, point d, of Directive 93/35/CEE of June 14, 1993)

The Directive makes no stipulations regarding the procedure to be followed for evaluating the safety of a finished cosmetic product, thus leaving the qualified evaluator to choose his own evaluation criteria. Long experience in the field leads one to suggest an approach which takes the following points into consideration:

1. Elements directly linked to the positioning of the product itself and, in particular:
   - Its cosmetological category: There are in fact many cosmetic products and these can be more or less aggressive in nature on the skin and mucosae.
   - Its method of use: The potential aggressiveness of a cosmetic product is linked mainly to the conditions of its use; the nature of any risks to be considered differ according to whether the product is intended to be used in pure or diluted form, whether it is intended for occassional or regular use, and whether it is designed to be removed following use or not.
   - Its composition: The nature of raw materials used in a cosmetic formulation, experience of their use in similar formulations, toxicological data on the constituents and their combination are all parameters which must be taken into consideration when evaluating the safety of a product.
   - Its stability and microbiological purity: The quality of any preserving agents used in the formulation, as well as the product's long-term stability under normal and foreseeable storage conditions are also important parameters in any risk analysis.

2. Points directly related to the area of application, in particular:
   - The intended application area: Application to the skin or mucosae and to sensitive or insensitive areas constitutes a determining factor in any toxicological evaluation.
   - The target user: When evaluating risk, it is appropriate to consider the population intended as the main or foreseeable user of a product. Does the population have reactive or atopic skin, normal complexion, oily or dry skin, or is it a young, adult or elderly population?

3. Existing toxicological data or complementary data to be provided.

Taking all the above information into consideration, the evaluator must decide whether or not there is call for further investigation into the finished product prior to authorizing its use on humans. To do this, he must evaluate his degree of knowledge acquired from his own experience and from the information available regarding all possible risks posed by the product under appraisal.

Even if it can be assumed, in a slightly simplistic way, that the systemic risk can be avoided by strengthening toxicological knowledge of raw materials, and that the irritant risk could be completely eliminated since one may be able to surmise that the consumers themselves will be able to eliminate it, allergenicity remains a real potential risk. Moreover, it is a risk which can only increase if effective knowledge of the incidence of interactions between raw materials on the immune system and of the influence of the galenical nature of the finished product is limited to its capacity to penetrate.

The investigator must reach his conclusions on the basis of an overall assessment of the these questions. However, financial, technical, or regulatory constraints imposed upon him or his methods of investigation may prevent him from taking one or more risk parameters into account.

The Safety Inspector's Credentials (Article 7b, point e, of Directive 93/35/CEE of June 14, 1993)

The difficulty inherent in assessing safety fully justifies that reference be made to the suitability of the assessor himself. It was inevitable that, in order for assessors to obtain mutal recognition from inspection authorities, the emphasis initially be put on the requisite qualifications. In practice, however, a university diploma alone, particularly if newly awarded, does not satisfy the practical requirements of safety evaluation which are based essentially on the assessor's actual experience; experience of galenics, experience in the field of experimental and clinical toxicology, as well as experience of pharmacokinetics, have all become essential requirements with the emergence of active cosmetology.

As regards the requisite diplomas, again there are significant differences between the national requirements of Member States based on pre-existing usage or regulations. Thus, a move towards harmonization in the future appears necessary.

Setting Up Safety Clauses (Directive 76/68/CEE of July 27, 1976, supplemented by Directive 88/667/CEE of December 21, 1998)

The formulation of a Community text which, once adopted by all Member States, was given force of law, logically led to the setting out of parallel provisions enabling Member States to avail themselves of safety clauses when a product, although conforming to Directive stipulations, constitutes a health hazard to consumers. In such cases, each Member State is entitled, on the basis of detailed notification, to provisionally ban the release of a product on the market once the other Member States and the Commission have been informed. This must then proceed rapidly to consultation between the Member States concerned and appropriate measures must be taken without delay which then constitute the new rule for all partners.

In order to avoid the abuse of such safety clauses and to discourage, where necessary, any action of a protectionist nature, the European Commission is currently preparing guidelines which define the "Precaution Principle", together with the framework within which it is to be considered.

Residual Ambiguities

As mentioned above, the European Cosmetic Directive 76/768/CEE and its successive amendments are essentially intended to ensure the safety and awareness of the consumer. In this context, it is surprising that current regulations still contain some imprecisions, even notable contradictions specifically regarding the evaluation of the safety of finished products and their effectiveness. It is also surprising to note that Member States undertook specific adjustments on adoption of the modified Directive 76/768/CEE, adding in places national provisions to the Community text which could constitute real barriers to the free circulation of products.

An Evaluation of Safety in the Context of Bans on Animal Testing

Safety requirements are set out in Article 2 of Directive 76/768/CEE: "Cosmetic products released on the market within the Community must have no damaging effect on the health of humans when applied under normal or reasonably foreseeable conditions of use". Parallel to this, and as mentioned above, it states in Article 7b that there are grounds for any safety evaluation of a finished product to take "the toxicological profile of the ingredients, their chemical structure and their general level of exposure" into consideration.

The same regulatory text finally states in Article 4b introduced by Directive 93/35/CEE, that after the deadline set according to progress made in finding alternative methods (currently set for June 30, 2000, by the Commission's 23rd Directive 98/62/CEE), the release on the market of cosmetic products containing ingredients or combinations tested on animals will be forbidden. These provisions serve to clarify ambiguities on both a regulatory and a scientific level.

The Regulatory Level

It may be surprising, in fact, that a text can make provision for a future ban on the marketing of products containing ingredients which had previously been tested on animals. This would lead to a ban on the use of a large majority of raw materials currently available. At the very most, one could envisage in this regard the banning, after a given date, of recourse to animal experimentation to test new ingredients used in cosmetic products. For this, however, it would be necessary to review all the regulatory texts concerning the classification of chemical substances which, at present, stipulate recourse to animal experimentation.

Banning the sale within the European Community of cosmetic products containing ingredients tested on animals would also constitute a substantial obstacle to the rules of international commerce. It is not actually apparent how products containing ingredients tested on animals could possibly be prevented in practical terms from penetrating the Community market when such products are subject to the different regulatory requirements of their country of manufacture. Transferring the ban to finished products tested themselves on animals would not resolve the ambiguity.

The Scientific Level

The essential question is the nature of the hazards a finished cosmetic product can pose. Experience shows that these fall into three categories:
1. Systemic toxicological hazard: This can result from percutaneous penetration of all or part of the constituents of the cosmetic product applied. This hazard depends mainly on the raw materials themselves, although the effect of interactions between ingredients must also be taken into consideration. Thus, the availability of full toxicological data compiled essentially from animal tests is a prerequisite which helps side-step needless research on the finished product.
2. The allergic hazard: This can result from the recognition of an antigen and its activation, which subsequently initiates an immune defense reaction at all new areas on contact with the antigen. This contact hypersensitivity may exist prior to application of the product, but may also be caused by the product itself. The allergic hazard is difficult to define since it corresponds to an individual sensitivity which appears infrequently, generally not well known as regards raw materials, and likely to be due as much to the constituents of the formula as to the finished product its-

elf. Any investigation of this hazard requires extreme caution and, in most cases, should justify that tests be re-done on the finished product itself.

3. The irritative hazard: This results from direct contact between the product and the receptor surface, and can cause a reaction confined to a single site of contact. An irritative reaction may appear following initial contact; it may also appear only after repeated contact as a result of a weakening of the receptor surface or of bioaccumulation of the product. Since the raw materials used in cosmetology are selected on the basis of their non-irritant properties, we must concede that a cosmetic product's potential irritant effect depends essentially on the finished product. Due to the lack of sufficient experience with formulations of the similar type, knowledge of the potential irritant effect of raw materials is generally insufficient to prevent hazard in the finished product. Moreover, the hazard incurred is likely to be unapparent following a single application, but increasingly visible following multiple applications.

This brief overview of the hazards incurred highlights the persistence of two significant anomalies in the current Community text: (1) Information on ingredients enables us to prevent systemic effects, particularly in terms of general cumulative toxicity, but current knowledge does not offer any alternative methods capable of replacing animal experimentation in this field; (2) toxicological data on raw materials is not sufficient to enable an evaluation of all the potential risks of a finished cosmetic product; its galenical form can directly influence its local tolerance, possibly its allergenicity, and alternative models to animal experimentation are at present inadequate to investigate this latter field.

Given these questions which, to date, have defied technical answers, it will fall to the legislator, in the form of new amendments to the regulatory text, to reposition the problem of animal experimentation and to redefine, if necessary, the scope and framework of a ban. Also, if, for non-scientific reasons, it should become necessary, the legislator will need to at least redefine the limit of responsibility of the evaluator, the manufacturer, or the primary importer, and redefine what is in this context a finished cosmetic product and what is a combination of ingredients. To ease the task of the evaluator, guidelines have been set out by the Scientific Committee on Cosmetics and Non-Food Products on a Community level [11], and by the European Cosmetic Toiletry and Perfumery Association (COLIPA) on an industry level [12].

The Lack of Ground Rules for Demonstrating Proof of Efficacy

Article 7b introduced by Directive 93/35/CEE puts the manufacturer or primary importer within the Community under the obligation to make evidence of the claimed effect of a given product available to the competent authorities. There has basically been no new legislation since a Council Directive in 1984, which made provision for the question of misleading advertising [13].

The novelty resides on the one hand in the fact that this document has become an integral part of a technical dossier, on the other in the fact that it can henceforth be used as valid evidence in the event of disagreement between the industry and the inspection authorities, or even the consumer associations. From this point, and even if it is clear that we are leaving the question of safety behind and embarking on the question of the advertising message, there are grounds, in the absence of specific information relating to this point in the Cosmetic Directive, to enquire as to the legal value of such a document and the criteria to be considered for its acceptance.

Another important aspect is that of how the authorities in charge of carrying out inspections (both national authorities and the authorities of other Member States) interpret the document. This raises – besides, of course, the question of mutual recognition of inspections which remains unresolved on a European level – the no less problematic question of inspectors' actual competence to evaluate the quality of an "efficacy dossier". The final act presupposes the resolution of each of these problems, while avoiding as far as possible an increase in both national and Community regulations which, it must be admitted, has proved very tempting, particularly to some Member States, since it appeared – erroneously – to simplify the issue. Two courses of action have been embarked upon to stop this trend:

1. One is intended to provide the competent authorities with guidelines which will make the inspection of dossiers easier.
2. The other is intended to provide points of reference enabling the authorities to evaluate the relevance of results provided.

Significant progress has been made as regards the former due to an initiative taken by France and particularly by a commission of experts attached to the Direction Générale de la Concurrence, de la Consommation et de la Répression des Fraudes (DGCCRF) (General Direction for Competition, Consumption and the Prevention of Fraud). This working group comprising scientists specialized in the field of cosmetic efficacy has worked out a general guide for inspectors attached to their departments, enabling them to: (a) Easily substantiate the veracity of claims; (b) have a uniform approach among inspectors; (c) have a reference document enabling them to enter into discussions with the industries under inspection.

While the working group conceded that the data gathered on raw materials contributes to establishing proof, it very soon became apparent that, in view of the influence of their galenical form on the capacity of active ingredients to penetrate, proof must be established, wherever possible and preferably on the finished product, by tests carried out on human subjects:

- The consumer self-evaluation test, or "usage test", enables the evaluation of the efficacy and acceptability of a finished product under the normal conditions of use intended by the manufacturer/distributor on a population sample which matches the target consumer population. This evaluation is made purely on the basis of a system of scores calculated from the responses of volunteers to a questionnaire.
- Tests carried out by an experimenter are intended to evaluate the efficacy of a product without the use of instrumentation. The test is carried out on volunteers by an experimenter; results are gathered on the basis of visual, tactile, and olfactory findings, as well as the volunteer's answers to the experimenter's questions. The experimenter may also provide information on cutaneous tolerance and cosmetic acceptability of a product, although these last two points do not take priority.
- Tests using instrumentation carried out on volunteers enable the evaluation of an active substance or a finished product when used under conditions as close as possible to those of normal use by potential consumers. An evaluation of efficacy is made essentially on the basis of results of instrument readings.

– Tests on other media: Although unable to provide the same data as tests carried out on human subjects, these provide information about the penetration of an active substance, its mechanism of action, and its efficacy. These tests are also particularly useful when tests cannot be carried out on human subjects.

These guidelines, which furnish inspectors with very concrete information relating to the elements a test report must contain and to sensitive points which need to be considered, have been reiterated by COLIPA in a special document circulated to all concerned [14]. Overall, and in order to ease understanding of the dossiers, it was deemed necessary that all data be included in the information handed over to the authorities; moreover, the purpsose of the information must be clear and the relevance of methods used must be fully substantiated.

However, these guidelines do not solve all the problems, particularly in the field of instrumental methods. While they enable the quality of documentation included in the information dossier on a cosmetic product to be evaluated, they provide no information on the correct practice, advantages, and limitations of methods used. Such information can only be provided by trained scientists, which not all inspectors concerned necessarily are, and which not all Member States have at their disposal. It is important that the opinion of an objective scientific authority can be sought in the event of disagreement over the experimental results of any of the parties concerned. It was for precisely this reason that the European Group for the Efficacy Measurements on Cosmetic and other Topical Products (EEMCO) was set up on a European level in 1994. EEMCO brings together eminent specialists in the field, from both the public and private sectors of various countries in the European Union.

In practical terms, the EEMCO Group analizes each of the various effects likely to be found using clinical and instrumental methods. To this end, and during the initial stage, they need to up-date existing knowledge of the biological parameters at play. During the second stage, they review existing evaluation methods, published or not, and, wherever possible, characterize their relevance, advantages, and limitations in order to provide experimenters and inspectorates with a general guide on how to use them effectively. Anxious not to restrict the freedom of investigators and equipment manufacturers, it is not the wish of the EEMCO group to propose precise protocols or to endorse systems; it restricts its activities to giving its scientific opinion in the fields it is called upon to investigate [14–17].

These two levels of activity provide the evaluator with the necessary references enabling him to tackle unhindered the cosmetic industry's permanent and ever-changing needs for innovation in advertising claims, while at the same time fulfilling the requirements of the European Cosmetic Directive.

Difficulties Arising from the Adoption of the Modifying Directive 93/35/CEE by Member States

Despite a willingness shown for the harmonization of European legislation, we are forced to note that the adoption of Directive 93/35/CEE, which had been finalized prior to December 31, 1997, introduced disparities which could lead to some practical difficulties regarding the free circulation of unique formulas in uniform packaging for the 15 Member States. Some states actually superimposed particular provisions belonging to pre-existing national regulations onto the Community text. Such particularisms relate notably to:

- The preservation of certain national provisions which could constitute obstacles to the Community text
- The obligation imposed by some Member States to declare the manufacturer or importer
- The qualifications required for safety inspectors
- The obligation to make relevant declarations to antipoison authorities
- Bans on animal experimentation for the purposes of safety evaluations.

Conclusion: The European Cosmetic Directive as a Point of Reference for International Harmonization

The enforcement of the European Cosmetic Directive as it is today has only been made possible due to the size and maturity of the cosmetic industry, an industry which can be relied on to put safe products on the market. The demands of the European consumer, accustomed to high-quality products, constitute an added defence against the proliferation of manufactured or imported goods which do not satisfy the required safety criteria. The environment is possibly not the same in other parts of the world where industrial powers are not as strong and where monitoring bodies do not enjoy the same advantages. Most importantly, only a combination of the industry's ability to manufacture or distribute quality products, together with the inspection authorities' ability to monitor a product's progress following its release on the market, can guarantee consumer safety in an effective way.

The following points must also be taken into consideration: (a) The appropriate standards among laboratories and bodies responsible for the inspection of products both before and after they have been marketed; (b) the credentials of inspectors themselves as regards both the release of products and the a posteriori evaluation of information made available.

Experience in the past has shown that imposing stringent mechanisms can actually lower awareness of responsibility and, in some cases, has even resulted in attempts to evade regulations altogether. The Community decision, particularly in terms of safety evaluation, to leave the experimenter, and therefore also the manufacturer, to their own responsibility to a large extent, has resulted in a refinement of the evaluation criteria to be considered and thus resulted in greater consumer safety; moreover, this is achieved, in all likelihood, in a more acceptable economic context. Ensuring consumer safety does not exclude pragmatism and a consideration of the cost of such safety. The economic weight of inspections is without doubt a criteria which must not be dismissed, and which is, in fact, all the more important when the size or area of the market are small.

The Congress of Florence [1] demonstrated that modern commerce requires global regulatory harmonization which goes beyond the European economic area. It in fact made it evident that only the European Union, the USA, and Japan want to unite to improve and harmonize their cosmetic legislation. Representatives from all around the world are seeking to install global regulatory measures in order to guarantee the safety of products and to find common solutions which would enable the authorities to monitor markets fairly. Given that, at present, trade is worldwide and that many companies are setting up manufacturing units in different parts of the world, regulatory harmonization represents a vast mechanism of simplification. It concerns not only the large multinationals which have the means at their disposal to conform to legislation, but also the small and medium-sized businesses which do not always have the necessary resources.

Participants at the congress adopted the following principles, known as the "Florence principles", which could serve as guidelines to improve future cosmetic legislation:

- The universal use of the same definition of a cosmetic product, as clearly distinct from the definition of a pharmaceutical product
- To accept a common regulatory basis whereby the manufacturer is directly responsible for safety and whereby the authorities are responsible for inspecting their market
- To have only one formula per product, for which safety and efficacy are the principal marketing criteria
- To develop "international" packaging for each product, which would prove more profitable in economic terms
- To standardize labeling in order to ensure complete clarity of information.

These principes, closely related to those of the European Cosmetic Directive, should enable the latter to be used as a point of reference in discussions which will necessarily have to take place between governments and the representatives of national industries, country by country and economic zone by economic zone, in order to achieve the necessary international harmonization.

References

1. COLIPA (The European Cosmetic Toiletry and Perfumery Association) (1998) Global cosmetic harmonization: an impetus to the development of export markets. Proceedings of an international cosmetic industry congress, Florence, 22nd and 23rd April. CPL Press
2. Council Directive Nr. 76/768/CEE of 27th July 1976. OJ Nr. L262 of 27th September 1976
3. Council Directive Nr. 79/661/CEE of 24th July 1979. OJ Nr. L192 of 31st July 1979
4. Council Directive Nr. 82/368/CEE of 17th May 1982. OJ Nr. L167 of 15th June 1982
5. Council Directive Nr. 83/574/CEE of 26th October 1983. OJ Nr. L332 of 28th September 1983
6. Council Directive Nr. 88/667/CEE of 21st December 1988. OJ Nr. L382 of 31st December 1988
7. Council Directive Nr. 89/679/CEE of 21st December 1989. OJ Nr. L398 of 30th December 1989
8. Council Directive Nr. 93/35/CEE of 14th June 1993. OJ Nr. L151 of 23rd June 1993
9. Decree of the Court of Justice of the European Communities (1991) Matter C. 112/89 of 16th April
10. Council Directive Nr. 65/65/CEE of 26th January 1965. OJ Nr. L022
11. SCCNFP (1997) Notes of guidance for testing of cosmetic ingredients for their safety evaluation. European Commission DG24
12. COLIPA (The European Cosmetic Toiletry and Perfumery Association) (1997) Guidelines for the safety assessment of a cosmetic product
13. Council Directive 84/450/CEE of 18th July 1984. OJ Nr. L228 of 25th August 1984
14. COLIPA (The European Cosmetic Toiletry and Perfumery Association) (1998) Guidance for the evaluation of the efficacy of a cosmetic product
15. Serup J (1995) EEMCO guidance for the assessment of dry skin (xerosis) and ichtyosis: clinical scoring system. Skin Res Technol 1:109–114
16. Pierard G (1995) EEMCO guidance for the assessment of dry skin (xerosis) and ichtyosis: evaluation by stratum corneum strippings. Skin Res Technol 2:3–11

17. Berardesca E (1997) EEMCO guidance for the assessment of stratum corneum hydration: electrical methods. Skin Res Technol 3:126–132
18. Pierard G (1997) EEMCO guidance for the assessment of skin colour. J Eur Acad Dermatol Venereol 10:1–11

CHAPTER 3

Claim Support in Japan: Legal Aspects

H. Tagami

Introduction

When we compare the laws and regulations governing cosmetics in the United States, European Union and Japan, we notice that the pre-manufacturing approval system of the Ministry of Health and Welfare Japan (MHW) has many unique characteristics. Despite repeated efforts made from outside parties in the past to revise this system in line with the changes recently occurring in other countries, no substantial alterations in the stance of the MHW on efficacy claims of cosmetics have taken place since 1980 when the last drastic amendment of the Pharmaceutical Affairs Law (PAL) was carried out [1, 2]. We will provide here information about the PAL, especially about those regulations related to efficacy claims for cosmetics (We use the term of efficacy simply here; however, it can also denote clinical effectiveness, usefulness and even product claims).

The efficacy profile of cosmetics has remarkably broadened along with recent scientific advances in cosmetology. Thus, it has widened to encompass immunomodulatory, neuro-endocrinological and physio-psychological effects. Some of them are now represented by aromatherapy or anti-aging therapy that includes the prevention of wrinkling, male pattern baldness and gray hair. Moreover, corresponding to the recent demands from consumers for desirable effects in cosmetics, studies searching for such effects in cosmetics have greatly advanced to involve the modulation of skin functions to maintain youthful and healthy conditions of the skin or to soften the effects of aging. Recently, the term "successful aging" has been proposed by a part of the Japanese industry. We expect that the Japanese laws and regulations related to cosmetics will be amended by the MHW in order to take into account such social demands. To attain such a goal, we believe that recent advances in the basic research of the skin and rapid developments in non-invasive biotechnology methods will play important roles in improving the pharmaceutical activities of cosmetics.

Definitions of Cosmetics and Quasi-drugs in Japan's Pharmaceutical Affairs Law

In addition to the unique approval system, the presence of quasi-drugs constitutes another feature of the PAL. Quasi-drugs occupy an intermediate position between drugs and cosmetics and are defined as articles used only for certain purposes that are specifically designated by the MHW. These agents are summarized in Table 1. Since they are defined by their specific indications and effects, the detailed scope and range of their efficacies are listed in Table 1. It should be pointed out that, similar to cosmetics, quasi-drugs are clearly stipulated to be articles whose biological activities are gentle and mild.

Table 1. Scope of indications for or effects of quasi-drugs

Type of quasi-drugs	Scope of purpose of use and principal product forms		Scope of indications
	Purpose of use	Principal product forms	Indications or effects
Mouth refreshers	Oral preps for prevention of nausea or other indispositions	Pill, plate, troche, liquid as a rule	Heartburn, nausea and vomiting, motion sickness, hangover, dizziness, foul breath, choking, indisposition, sunstroke
Body deodorants	External agents to prevent body odor	Liquid or ointment, aerosol, powder, stick	Body odor, perspiration odor suppression of perspiration
Talcum powders	Agents to prevent prickly heat, sores, etc.	Powder for external use as a rule	Prickly heat, diaper rash, sore, hip sores, razor burn
Hair growers (hair nutrients)	External agents to prevent loss of hair and to grow hair	Liquid as a rule	Hair growth, prevention of thinning, itching and falling hair, promotion of hair growth, dandruff, loss of hair after illness or child birth, hair nutrition
Depilatories	External agents for hair removal	Ointment as a rule	Hair removal
Hair dyes (incl. hair color and dye removers)	External agents for dying hair, removing hair or dye colors	Gray hair dye, hair dye, hair bleach. excl. agents for physical hair dying	Hair dying, removal of hair color dye
Bath preparations	External agents to be dissolved, as a rule, in the bath (bath soaps excluded from this category)	Powder, granule, tablet, soft capsule, liquid, etc.	Prickly heat, roughness, ringworm, bruises, stiff shoulder, sprains, neuralgia, eczema, frostbite, hemorrhoids, tinea, chills, athlete's foot, scabies, itch, lumbago, rheumatism, fatigue recovery, protection of the skin, prevention of dry skin chaps, cracks, chills before and after childbirth, acnes

Table 1. Continued

Type of quasi-drugs	Scope of purpose of use and principal product forms		Scope of indications
	Purpose of use	Principal product forms	Indications or effects
Permanent waving agents		For quality standards for ingredients etc., refer to the Standards for Permanent Waving Agents	Creation and preservation of waves in the hair; straightening frizzy, curly or wavy hair, and preserving that condition
Insecticide			
Rodenticides			
Sanitary cotton			
Medicated cosmetics(incl. medicated soaps)	External agents used for cosmetic purposes, in forms resembling cosmetics	Liquid medicated soaps generally resembling cosmetic soaps in view of their ingredients, method of use, etc.	
1. Shampoos	Prevention of dandruff and itching Prevention of perspiration odors in the hair and on the scalp Cleaning of the hair and scalp (a) Keeping the hair and scalp healthy (b) Making the hair supple Choose either (a) or (b)		
2. Rinses	Prevention of dandruff and itching Prevention of perspiration odors in the hair and on the scalp Supplementing and maintaining moisture and fat of the hair (a) Keeping the hair and scalp healthy (b) Making the hair supple Choose either (a) or (b)		
3. Skin lotions	Chapping and roughness of the skin Prevention of prickly heat. frostbite, chaps, cracks, acnes Oily skin Prevention of razor burn Prevention of spots and freckles due to sunburn Burning sensation after sunburn or snow burn Bracing, cleaning and conditioning the skin		

Table 1. Continued

Type of quasi-drugs	Scope of purpose of use and principal product forms		Scope of indications
	Purpose of use	Principal product forms	Indications or effects
	Keeping the skin healthy; supplying the skin with moisture		
4. Creams, milky lotions, hand creams, cosmetic oils	Chapping and roughness of the skin		
	Prevention of prickly heat, frostbite, chaps, cracks, acnes Oily skin Prevention of razor burn Prevention of spots and freckles due to sunburn Burning sensation after sunburn or snow burn Bracing, cleaning and conditioning the skin Keeping the skin healthy; supplying the skin with moisture Protection of the skin; prevention of dry skin		
5. Shaving agents	Prevention of razor burn, protection of the skin for smoother shave		
6. Sunburn prevention agents	Prevention of chapping due to sunburn and snowburn, prevention of sunburn and snowburn, prevention of spots and freckles due to sunburn, protection of the skin		
7. Packs	Chapping and roughness of the skin, prevention of acnes, oily skin, prevention of spots and freckles due to sunburn, burning sensation after sunburn and snowburn, making the skin smooth, cleaning the skin		
8. Medicated (incl. face cleansing) agents	Soaps that are mainly bactericidal: Cleaning, sterilizing and disinfecting the skin, prevention of body odor, perspiration odor and acnes Soaps that are mainly antiinflammatory: Cleaning of the skin, prevention of acnes, razor burn and chapping		

Table 1. Continued

Type of quasi-drugs	Scope of purpose of use and principal product forms		Scope of indications
	Purpose of use	Principal product forms	Indications or effects
9. Medicated dentifrices	External agents to be used for cosmetic purpose in forms resembling ordinary cosmetic dentifrices		Making the teeth white, cleaning and refreshing the mouth, prevention of pyorrhea, prevention of gingivitis, prevention of tartar, prevention of dental caries, prevention of foul breath, removal of tobacco stain

The definition of cosmetics is essentially the same as that in other countries. They are stipulated as articles that are applied to the human body for the purposes of cleansing, beautifying, promoting the attractiveness, improving the appearance or maintaining the skin or hair in a healthy condition without affecting structure or function. Their biological activity on the human body is required to be gentle and mild.

Although the definition of drugs clearly indicates that they are intended to be used for treating diseases or that they affect the structure and function of the body, there are no such direct stipulations in the definition of quasi-drugs or in that of cosmetics. This may be interpreted as that the PAL does not necessarily mean an absolute prohibition of pharmaceutical effects for cosmetics and quasi-drugs as long as their effects are kept gentle and mild. Because drugs are those used for the treatment of diseases, indications for their use are strictly regulated. In contrast, there are no such rigid indication areas for cosmetics or quasi-drugs, permitting their general use. This means, in addition to the mild biological activity, safety is more strongly required for cosmetics and quasi-drugs than for drugs. In a way, we can interpret that absolute safety is required for cosmetics.

The indications of cosmetics approved by the PAL are summarized in Table 2. It may be noted that there is no big difference between the efficacy stipulated for cosmetics and that for quasi-drugs.

The approved effects of cosmetics are that to treat skin rash, chapping and roughness, conditions which are observed in dry skin or in inflamed skin. Although the terms of dry skin and inflamed skin are directly cited in the case of the activity of medicated cosmetics that belong to the category of quasi-drug, in the case of cosmetics a word of "prevention" is further written together with these conditions. A similar conceptional difference can be recognized in the description of the efficacy against dandruff and itching. In contrast to that an expression of "the preventive effect" is used in the case of quasi-drugs, only "a suppressive effect" is stipulated in the case of cosmetics.

Another example is found in the effects for skin spots and freckles. The use of a so-called skin lightening (bleaching or whitening) effect is allowed for cosmetics, whereas this effect is allowed to be used only in association with those words such as "prevention of skin spots and freckles" and "caused by sunburn" in the case of quasi-drugs.

Table 2. Type and scope of indications of cosmetics

Type	Item of product	Scope of indications
Hair cosmetics	1. Hair oils	(1) Supplementing and maintaining moisture and fat of the hair
	2. Hair coloring preparations	(2) Moistening the scalp and the hair
		(3) Keeping the scalp and the hair healthy
	3. Hair combing oils	
	4. Wave set lotions	
	5. Stick pomades	(4) Making the hair supple
	6. Hair fixers	(5) Preventing the hair from splitting and cutting
	7. Hair creams	
	8. Hair tonics	(6) Preventing the hair from electric charge
	9. Liquid hair dressings	(7) Suppressing dandruff and itching
	10. Hair sprays	
	11. Pomades	
	12. Others	
Hair washing preparations	1. Hair washing powders	(1) Cleaning the scalp and the hair
	2. Shampoos	(2) Keeping the scalp and the hair healthy
	3. Others [1]	(3) Making the hair supple
		(4) Removing dandruff and itching
Skin lotions	1. After-shaving lotions	(1) Preventing chapping, conditioning the texture, and preventing sunburn
	2. Ordinary skin lotions	
	3. Eau de Cologne	(2) Astringing and cleaning the skin
	4. Shaving lotions	(3) Moistening the skin
	5. Hand lotions	(4) Keeping the skin healthy
	6. Suntan lotions	(5) Softening the skin
	7. Sunscreening lotions	(6) Conditioning the skin after shaving
	8. Others	(7) Prevention of spots and freckles due to sunburn
Creams and lotions	1. After-shaving creams	(1) Preventing chapping, conditioning the texture, and preventing sunburn
	2. Cleansing creams	(2) Prevention of spots and freckles due to sunburn
	3. Cold creams	(3) Adstringing and cleaning the skin
	4. Shaving creams	(4) Keeping the skin healthy
	5. Milky lotions	(5) Moistening the skin to keep it soft
	6. Vanishing creams	(6) Protection of the skin, prevention of dry skin
	7. Hand creams	(7) Conditioning the skin after shaving
	8. Suntan creams	
	9. Sunscreening creams	
	10. Others	
Packs	1. Cosmetics for packs	(1) Smoothing and cleaning the skin
	2. Others [2]	(2) Moistening the skin
		(3) Conditioning texture
		(4) Making the skin supple
Foundations	1. Creamy foundations	(1) Protection of the skin, prevention of dry skin
	2. Liquid foundations	(2) Prevention of sunburn
	3. Solid foundations	(3) Prevention of spots and freckles due to sunburn
	4. Others	
Face powders and toilet powders	1. Creamy powders	(1) Prevention of sunburn
	2. Pressed face powders	(2) Protection of the skin
	3. Loose face powders	(3) Prevention of spots and freckles due to sunburn
	4. Talcum powders	(4) Prevention of prickly heat (toilet powders)
	5. Paste powders	

Table 2. Continued

Type	Item of product	Scope of indications
	6. Baby powders 7. Body powders 8. Liquid face paints	
Lip colors	1. Lipsticks	(1) Prevention of chapping, and conditioning texture
	2. Lip creams 3. Others	(2) Moistening and smoothing the lips
		(3) Keeping the lips healthy
		(4) Protecting the lips to prevent them from drying
Eyebrow, eye and cheek makeup preparations	1. Eye creams 2. Eye shadows 3. Eye liners 4. Cheek colors 5. Mascaras 6. Eybrow colors	Moistening the skin to keep it healthy
Nail makeup preparations	1. Nail enamels 2. Nail enamel removers	Protecting the nails to keep them healthy
Bath preparations	1. Bath oils 2. Bath salts	Cleaning the skin
Cosmetic oils	1. Cosmetic oils 2. Baby oils 3. Others	(1) Prevention of chapping (2) Moistening the skin to keep it soft (3) Keeping the skin healthy (4) Protecting the skin, and preventing it from drying (5) Prevention of sunburn (6) Prevention of spots and freckles due to sunburn
Face cleansing preparations	1. Face cleansing creams 2. Face cleansing powders 3. Face cleansing foams 4. Others	(1) Prevention of acnes and prickly heat (2) Conditioning the skin (3) Conditioning the texture (4) Cleaning the skin
Soaps	1. Cosmetic soaps 2. Others	(1) Cleaning the skin (2) Conditionin the texture
Dentifrices		(1) Prevention of dental caries, making the teeth white, and removal of tooth plaques (2) Cleaning the mouth (3) Prevention of foul breath and removal of tobacco stain (4) Prevention of tartar deposition

The background for the development of such differences in the stipulation of efficacy of cosmetics and that of quasi-drugs is closely related to the above-mentioned approval system. In this system, cosmetics are simply approved as a mixture of different ingredients. On the other hand, quasi-drugs are required to contain active ingredient(s) that exert the depicted efficacy. Therefore, not only submission of the formulation used but also that of the testing method utilized for the identification and quantification of active ingredients are required in the approval process of quasi-drugs. In addition, stability of the active ingredients in the formulation has to be guaranteed over 3 years at room temperature.

Table 3. Deleted lines of efficacy of cosmetics along with the 1980 Amendment of the Pharmaceutical Affairs Law

Type	Deleted lines of efficacy
Quasi-drugs, medicated cosmetics	Ichthyosis,fine wrinkles, dark skin complexion, allergic reaction, sagged skin, skin nutrition, sore, prevention of skin-aging
Quasi-drugs, medicated dentifrice	Removal of tartar, strengthen the teeth
Cosmetics	Prevention of skin-aging, strengthen the teeth

We want to emphasize here that the efficacy of quasi-drugs is defined in relation with the specific active ingredients, while that of cosmetics is defined as a whole product. In other words, even a humectant which is one of the most important ingredients for skin care products is not required to be specified in a formula of cosmetics.

When we discuss the laws and regulations in Japan relating to cosmetics, the history of the PAL is indispensible. Particularly we cannot skip the review and amendment made regarding the efficacy of cosmetics that were carried out concomitantly with the amendment of the PAL in 1980. In this amendment, an extensive review of the literature was made by the Technical Committee of the Japan Cosmetic Industry Association (JCIA) and the results were submitted to the critical assessment by the Central Scientific Advisory Board (CSAB) of the MHW. After the investigation performed by the CSAB, part of efficacy of cosmetics listed in Table 3 was deleted from the previously approved list on the ground that it was not scientifically substantiated. As clearly seen from Table 3, these deleted lines are those mostly related to the anti-aging effects such as the prevention of skin aging and small wrinkles or the whitening effects on spots and freckles.

However, the notification issued by the Director General of the Pharmaceutical Affairs Bureau indicated at that time that the deleted lines had been inappropriately used for the efficacy of cosmetics or quasi-drugs [3]. It also stated that, whenever there comes out any scientific substantiation for such effects, they would reconsider the possibility of restoring them at the CSAB. This is the most important part in the history of the PAL. Namely, it does not rule out totally or absolutely the deleted portion that was related to the anti-aging effect or skin whitening effects of cosmetics.

Scientific Substantiation of Efficacy of Cosmetics and Its Status in the Pharmaceutical Affairs Law

The pattern of description used for efficacy of cosmetics and that of quasi-drugs are regulated in details by the PAL. Namely it is written that only a determined expression should be used for the product claims without making any alterations. As long as the product claims stay within the limit of the approved effects, the cosmetics will be approved without any further requirements. The PAL does not indicate any specific evaluation methods to prove the described activity of cosmetics. This means that the PAL does not require any scientific substantiation of their efficacy, as long as the active ingredients that have been previously approved by the MHW are formulated in the approved range of concentration. These names of the approved active ingredients and their permitted concentrations have been partially disclosed officially. Examples of such ingredients are vitamins, anti-microbials and anti-inflammatory agents.

On the other hand, when an application is made for an approval of new efficacy for cosmetics or for a new active ingredient for quasi-drugs, the PAL requires a submission of the data substantiating such claims. Table 4 summarizes the data required to be submitted when a filing is made for approval of new cosmetics and quasi-drugs. In the case of cosmetics, they consist mainly of those related to the specification with utilized methods to prove it and the data related to the safety. In the case of quasi-drugs the data showing the effects must be further submitted together with the above mention ones. The required data are mainly the results of an actual use test in humans supplemented with pharmacological data obtained in basic research. Such difference in the requirement of data for filing makes it clear the difference in attitude taken by the MHW toward cosmetics and quasi-drugs.

Table 4. Data required in application for approval of cosmetics and quasi-drugs

Data required	Scope of data	Quasi-drugs	Cosmetics
A. Data on origin, background of discovery, use in foreign countries, etc.	1. Data on origin and details of discovery	R	R
	2. Data on use in foreign countries	R	R
	3. Data on characteristics and comparison with other quasi-drugs or cosmetics	R	R
B. Data on physical and chemical properties, speci fications, testing methods, etc.	1. Data on determination of structure	R	R
	2. Data on physical and chemical properties	R	R
	3. Data on specifications and testing methods	R	R
C. Data on stability	1. Data on long-term storage test	R	
	2. Data on severe test	R	(R)
	3. Data on acceleration test	R	
D. Data on safety	1. Data on acute toxicity	R	R
	2. Data on subacute toxicity	R	(R)
	3. Data on chronic toxicity	(R)	
	4. Data on reproductive effects	(R)	
	5. Data on antigenicity (skin sensitization test, photosensitization test, etc.)	R	R
	6. Data on mutagenicity	R	R
	7. Data on carcinogenicity	(R)	
	8. Data on local irritation(skin irritation test, mucosa irritation test, etc.)	R	R
	9. Data on absorption, distribution, metabolism and excretion	R	R
E. Data on indications or effects	1. Data on fundamental laboratory test supporting indications or effects	R	
	2. Data on use in humans	R	

R: required (R) may be omitted under certain conditions

Despite these requirements made by the MHW, the PAL does not specify any standard testing method for the evaluation of the clinical effects of quasi-drug. Only one stipulation found in it is the performance of a clinical use test in humans conducted under conditions simulating an actual usage situation, which supplies basic data of the assessment of the effects and safety in daily use of such a product. Because active ingredients used in quasi-drugs are legally the same as those in drugs, the requirements for quasi-drugs are greatly influenced by those regulations used for drugs. In the case of drugs, the PAL stipulates information about such requirements and evaluation methods much more in details. Therefore, all the newly approved active ingredients for quasi-drugs in the past 10 years have been approved based on the data obtained in double blind clinical trials carried out in a fashion similar to that used for drugs. They are magnesium ascorbyl phosphate, kojic acid, and arubutin. All of them claim so-called skin whitening effects. At this point, we must indicate that the gentleness and mildness of action required for quasi-drugs somewhat contradict the requirements for clinical testing that is performed to demonstrate effectiveness as well as side effects.

We must also indicate here that not all of the active ingredients previously approved for quasi-drugs have undergone such a clinical test. Most of the ingredients are those having been used before as drugs and they are just formulated for quasi-drugs in concentration lower than that used in drugs to secure gentle and mild action. Therefore, a different approach for approval can be taken in the case of quasi-drugs, because clinical testing that can demonstrate the required gentleness and mildness for quasi-drugs are not easy to find. Instead an approval step can simply be taken by preparing lower concentrations for the ingredients to be formulated. Such an approach seems to be well matched with the definition of quasi-drugs (articles other than drugs).

The PAL clearly stipulates that the results of human data obtained in the tests conducted in countries other than Japan are acceptable, except for those in which an influence of race is expected. As such agents, there are those used for skin lightening that definitely interact with melanin formation, those used for pigmentation after sun exposure or those for permanent waving or hair dyeing.

There is also no detailed stipulation in regard to basic research data except for that they should be obtained by pharmacological studies or that they should clarify the basic mechanisms underlying the effects.

As mentioned above, clinical testing is legally required for quasi-drugs to substantiate their effectiveness produced by the active ingredients. In contrast, no such measures are required to prove efficacy of cosmetics. Only humectants and UV absorbers used in cosmetics are the ones whose clinical effectiveness can be shown together with the ingredients. Although the latter is an active ingredient, in most cases it is considered to be a part of a vehicle, because its action mechanism solely depends on the physico-chemical screening effects rather than the biological effects. However its concentration is regulated by the law. When it is formulated at an extremely low concentration to prevent color fading of the product, the purpose of adding UV absorbers are required to be stated as such.

Recently, the addition of anti-oxidants to cosmetics is also raising a delicate problem because of the great advances made in the biological research of free radicals. They were previously approved to be used to prevent auto-oxidation of oils and fats that are formulated in quasi-drugs. But they may mislead users to think that those agents be used as anti-oxidants for the skin. Thus, when the name of a certain anti-oxidant in the product is described as a part of product claims, it is desirable to describe it as an "anti-oxidant for the product".

Such regulations are also present in the case of advertising. They restrict listing of moisturizing ingredients, reminding the manufacturer that they should not mention any specific name of moisturizers but only list them as humectants. Accordingly, various extracts prepared from plants which are now becoming a focus of public attention cannot be named on the label but be stated only as humectants, unless the active ingredients are approved for quasi-drugs. In other words, it can be interpreted that only one pharmaceutical effect permitted for cosmetics is the maintenance of a good moisture balance in the skin surface [3].

Clinical effectiveness of cosmetics is not approved in relation with specific ingredients. There are some trials searching for new efficacy in cosmetics but such claimed effects will more or less end up with the maintenance of a good moisture balance in the skin surface. A challenge to open a way for new efficacy for cosmetics should not be made by an effort of a single cosmetic manufacturer. There must be joint efforts from the whole industry in Japan. Or scientific substantiation of the efficacy of cosmetics may require a different approach, for instance, by presenting data obtained from an epidemiological study.

Therefore, at present, the existence of the category of quasi-drugs between drugs and cosmetics in Japan is very important because using this category we can expect the development of any new effective cosmetics, the so-called cosmeceuticals. A similar concept may be found in the over-the counter drugs of the United States such as sunscreen, skin lightener (bleaching), hair growth promoter and anti-perspirant. However, in this case they have cosmetic efficacy. Because in general drugs are still regarded to be active agents to treat diseases, the legal positioning of such skin agents in the category of pseudo-drugs appears to be more appropriate.

A New Approach to Substantiation of Clinical Effectiveness of Cosmetics

Activities of the Japan Cosmetic Industry Association

In 1993 the Japan Cosmetic Industry Association (JCIA) established a special ad-hoc subcommittee on efficacy of cosmetics within its Technical Committee to study the present regulations on efficacy of cosmetics, especially trying to revive the above mentioned lines relating the anti-aging effects deleted in the 1980 amendment of the PAL. We cannot give details of the study here, because discussions and negotiations are still going on with the MHW. Several important points proposed by the industry are the end point where the industry will and have to reach.

The first step suggested in the review process has been the utilization of a much more appropriate way to describe the efficacy of cosmetics that is different from that presently approved by the PAL. For example, they are; (i) a description of "preventing skin roughness and rash" used for the effects of creams and emulsified lotions should be depicted as "making the skin soft and smooth," in order to ensure more direct expression for the effects, (ii) a description of "keeping the skin moist" can be expressed as "supplementing moisture, oils, emollients, and humectant to the skin," in order to relate activities of ingredients to the efficacy, and (iii) the description of "preventing skin spots and freckles caused by sunburn," should be written as "preventing skin spots and freckles caused by sunlight or ultraviolet light" in order to clarify the clinical effects against the damage caused by the sunlight, for which there should also be a distinction between suntan and sunburn.

Another step suggested is the revival of the once deleted lines related to the efficacy of cosmetics (Table 3). The typical example is the anti-aging effects which covers the efficacy of basic skin care cosmetics, such as "making fine wrinkles inconspicuous", "relieving skin dullness" and "lightening skin color." Furthermore, it is related to the physio-psychological effects of cosmetics that are represented by aromatherapy such as "feeling active and stable".

Efficacy of cosmetics which has been discussed in this process is thought to reflect the demands of consumers and the efforts of the industry to cope with such demands.

As already mentioned, the PAL does not provide any specific testing methods for assessing the effectiveness of cosmetics. Thus, efforts have been made from the industry in this respect as voluntary measures. Most of them have also been discussed with the MHW, trying to make such methods as semi-official ones. These efforts initiated by the industry are made to employ evaluation methods that allow relatively easy judgment. The first one is an improved testing method for sun protection factor, which was originally developed in the U.S.

The leadership of the industry in Japan in this field can be observed as the development of a testing method for UVA protection factor that was taken up in the second step. The finalized test method [4] was enforced in 1996 to allow attaching a label showing a UVA protecting factor on the finished cosmetic products. This method presents an index based upon immediate and persistent darkening of the skin induced by a UVA exposure.

Because the social demands in Japan have already shifted from the UV light protection to the anti-aging effect, it is desirable to establish a testing method to detect gentle and mild activity of cosmetics for such a purpose. Although joint studies for this project have not started yet among the industry, efforts on an individual basis have become apparent. Hence, it will not be a distant future for the above mentioned industry efforts to become a trigger to lead to an approval of new efficacy for cosmetics.

Development of New Technology for Measuring Various Properties of the Skin

In the above, we have repeatedly emphasized that gentle and mild action has been regarded as an important property of cosmetics as well as quasi-drugs, because they are used daily for a prolonged period of time without any restriction on the amount used as well as on the frequency of usage, which distinguishes them from drugs. However, the requirements for the gentleness and mildness in action of cosmetics and quasi-drugs make it extremely difficult to evaluate their effectiveness. It is necessary to search for evaluation methods that can substantiate such gentle and mild effects on the skin objectively and accurately and that can detect even a minor change which may be invisible clinically. So far there have been coming out various evaluation methods useful for this purpose, some of which are designed even for the acquisition of approval, being proposed as a sort of official testing methods.

Until about 20 years ago, most dermatologists and skin scientists had been mainly concerned with the studies of abnormally looking skin of various dermatoses or damaged skin by injurious agents. They studied properties of such lesional skin histo-logically and biochemically by surgically obtaining skin specimens. Such methods are invasive, always leaving scars to the skin after sampling of the materials. Although the invasive methods could be repeatedly performed in experimental animals to investigate changes of the lesional skin in a time-dependent fashion, it is impossible to perform them several times in the same lesional skin of the patients, not to speak of normal skin in healthy individuals. Moreover in most cases a skin sample obtained from non-lesional areas was utilized only as a control, under a general idea that normal skin was almost the same each other.

However, current product realities have made it difficult to make a clear distinction between drugs that treat diseased skin and cosmetics that promote attractiveness of the skin, making the term of cosmeceuticals legitimate to be used for a product cate-gorg intermediate between them [5]. Cosmetics and quasi-drugs have been proven to have an effect and action as drugs. Even simple applications of moisturizers alter the skin surface structure and function. Furthermore, normal healthy skin has been re-cognized to have a great variation. On the other hand, there is a diseased skin state which may clinically look normal but actually is abnormal if studied meti-culously [6].

It is remarkable that a variety of instrumental bioengineering methods have been developed in the past 20 years [7–9]. They are not only non-invasive but are sensitive enough to detect even a delicate difference of the skin that even expert dermatologists may not be able to discern. Undoubtedly these methods are suitable to demonstrate the efficacy of cosmetics. They are applicable to any part of the skin or to any kinds of skin lesions repeatedly without inflicting any injuries. For example, clinically non-inflam-matory, but somewhat dry and pruritic non-lesional skin of patients with atopic dermatitis, i.e., atopic xerosis, is demonstrated to have numerous abnormalities when studied functionally with a combination of these techniques [10]. Such skin shows the abnormal features consisting of functionally and biochemically defective stratum cor-neum accompanied by metabolically active and subclinically inflammatory tissue changes. Similar mild functional and biochemical abnormalities are found in senile dry skin [11].

As repeatedly mentioned above, whenever we discuss the efficacy of cosmetics, we must always take into account the regulations enforced by the PAL require that cos-metics are mild and gentle in its action accompanied by almost absolute safety. With the advent of these bioengineering techniques it becomes not only possible to detect delicate individual differences in a normal population but also to reveal that there occurs a rather great change in the skin after treatment with efficacious cosmetics. Sometimes the clinical effectiveness of articles that belong to the category of cosme-tics or pseudo-drugs are found to be far superior even to that of a prescription medi-cation [12]. It is because pharmaceutical companies are mainly concerned with the active ingredients in topical agents, whereas cosmetic companies have been always studying delicate formulation of topical agents that can promote the attractive quali-ty of normal skin by formulating various effective ingredients whose safety has been guaranteed. Thus, together with the ongoing progress in the field of non-invasive bioengineering methods and basic skin research, we think that the time will come in the near future when even the MHW cannot ignore any more a wider efficacy profile for cosmetics.

Acknowledgments. The author is indebted greatly to Mr. Tasuku Takamatsu, General Manager of the Safety and Analytical Research Center, Shiseido Co., Ltd. for his kind help, during the preparation of this manuscript, with the collection of a wide range of information on the regulations governing cosmetics.

References

1. The law amending a part of the Pharmaceutical Affairs Law (Law No.145, August 10, 1960): Law No. 56, The Ministry of Health and Welfare, Japan, October 1, 1979
2. Notification No. 1341 from the Director General, Pharmaceutical Affairs Bureau, the Ministry of Health and Welfare, Japan, October 9, 1980
3. Ozawa T, Nishiyama S, Horii I, Kawasaki K, Kumano Y, Nakayama Y(1985) Humectants and their effects on moisturization of skin. Skin Res 27:276–284
4. Naganuma M, Fukuda M, Arai S, Hirose O, Kawai M, Motoyoshi K, Masaki H, Suzuki T, Yoshii T (1996) Standard test methods for classification and labeling of sunscreen having UVA protective efficacy in Japan. Proceedings of the 19th Congress of the International Federation of Societies of Cosmetic Chemists (available only on CD-ROM), Sydney, Australia, October 1996
5. Vermeer BJ, Gilchrest BA (1996) Cosmeceuticals. A proposal for rational definition, evaluation, and regulation. Arch Dermatol 132:337–340
6. Kligman AM (1991) The invisible dermatoses. Arch Dermatol 127:1375–1382
7. Leveque J-L(1989) Cutaneous investigation in health and disease. Noninvasive methods and instrumentation. Marcel Dekker, New York
8. Elsner P, Berardesca E, Maibach HI (1994) Bioengineering of the skin: water and the stratum corneum. CRC Press, Boca Raton
9. Serup J, Jemec GBE (1995) Handbook of non-invasive methods and the skin. CRC Press, Boca Raton
10. Watanabe M, Tagami H, Horii I, Takahashi M, Kligman AM (1991) Functional analyses of the superficial stratum corneum in atopic xerosis. Arch Dermatol 127:1689–1692
11. Hara M, Kikuchi K, Watanabe M, Denda M, Koyama J, Nomura J, Horii I, Tagami H (1993) J Geriatr Dermatol 1:111–120
12. Tagami H (1994) Quantitative measurements of water concentration of the stratum corneum in vivo by high-frequency current. Acta Derm Venereol (Stockh) Suppl 185: 29–330

CHAPTER 4

Claim Support: Ethical Aspects for Conducting Human Studies

V. Zuang

Claim Support: Ethical Aspects for Conducting Human Studies: Why Are Human Volunteers Used in Cosmetics Testing?

The EU Cosmetics Directive requires that: "A cosmetic product put on the market within the Community must not cause damage to human health when applied under normal or reasonably foreseeable conditions of use, taking account, in particular, of the product's presentation, its labelling, any instructions for its use and disposal as well as any other indication or information provided by the manufacturer or his authorized agent or by any other person responsible for placing the product on the Community market" [1].

This requirement reflects the general expectation of the consumer population concerning the safety of cosmetic products. Most cosmetic ingredients are tested according to regulations for industrial chemicals, apart from certain preservatives, UV filters and colourants, which need to be specifically approved by the Scientific Committee on Cosmetic and Non-Food Products intended for consumers, an expert advisory group to the European Commission. There are standard in vivo animal toxicity tests outlined in the Organisation for Economic Co-operation and Development (OECD) guidelines for chemicals [2], and in Annex V of the EU Directive 92/69/EEC [3]. However, in order to avoid unnecessary animal testing, various testing strategies have been recently suggested for skin corrosivity, irritation and sensitisation testing [4–6]. In vivo animal studies cannot wholly predict human responses due to species differences. In particular, the well-known Draize rabbit skin and eye irritation tests are unable to differentiate between the absence of irritation potential, and the presence of mild or slight irritation potential, under practical use conditions [7]. The assessment of subjective reactions such as itching, stinging and burning specifically requires in vivo human investigation.

In general, cosmetic products are assessed for safety on the basis of their component ingredients, and their intended use. Human volunteers have been used in the evaluation of skin irritation for many years. Recently, a human 4-h patch test has been developed for acute dermal irritation testing of chemicals. The test was specifically designed to address the issue of the classification and labelling (irritant/non-irritant) of pure chemicals and preparations [8]. It was shown that, if the chemical or preparation is not corrosive (as demonstrated in a validated in vitro skin corrosivity test, such as the rat skin transcutaneous electrical resistance (TER) or Episkin™ (EPISKIN, Chaponost, France) assays) and is free from other toxicologically unacceptable hazards, it is possible to conduct a human test, performed to the highest ethical standards, which is similar to the Draize rabbit skin irritation test, but is designed to limit the intensity of any skin reactions [9].

Once the ingredients of a formulation have been tested, additional testing of the finished product in in vivo animal toxicity tests is now rarely performed in the EU. On the contrary, cosmetics manufacturer prefer to have in vivo human data available to confirm the compatibility and tolerance of their finished products in the intended consumer population. Also, is it more reasonable to release a finished cosmetic product to carefully monitored groups of human subjects first, before exposing larger populations, where monitoring, or the possibility to register adverse effects, is difficult or unfeasible [10]. Ultimately, user trials which reflect the real use conditions of the products as well as problems with misuse due to badly designed or defective packaging, are of significant value for a detailed description of the finished product's safety.

Neither animal tests nor alternative non-animal test methods can confirm product efficacy accurately. For product efficacy testing, the only valuable and appropriate model is the human in vivo model. However, an in vitro approach based on physico-chemical or biological endpoints such as, for example, ceramide metabolism in human skin pieces [11], may be used at different stages of product development in order to formulate efficient products. All these situations have resulted in an increasing use of human volunteers in cosmetics testing to provide assurance of tolerance to topical exposure of the finished product and to confirm product efficacy.

Ethical Aspects

The ethical requirements differ depending on whether the study has been designed to assess the safety or the efficacy of a cosmetic product. A cosmetic product should have been cleared for safety before its efficacy is being evaluated. Efficacy testing is performed to support marketing claims and can only be carried out ethically when there is evidence that the product does not cause local or systemic adverse responses. Evaluation of safety and efficacy in the same test can be considered as unethical. However, if an adverse reaction has been generated unintentionally in an efficacy trial, it should be recorded and treated as complementary information for the safety profile of the product prior to its release on the market.

Several existing codes of practice and guidelines related to ethics and human testing are essential for the ethical rationale [12–18]. The basic provisions to guide investigators are set out in the Declaration of Helsinki of 1964 and its subsequent amendments, the latest one being in 1989 [16]. The current revision of the Declaration of Helsinki is the accepted basis for clinical trial ethics, and it has been advocated that all engaged in research on human beings should follow these recommendations [17]. The Declaration of Helsinki presents a fundamental set of guidelines covering human experimentation. It states that non-therapeutic biomedical research involving human subjects is ethically acceptable only under certain conditions. Basically, biomedical research involving human subjects cannot legitimately be carried out, unless the inherent risk to the subject is in proportion to the expected benefit for the volunteer, or for society as a whole. For that reason, every human volunteer study should be preceded by a careful assessment of the predictable risk to each subject, which is usually the task of an ethical review committee (ERC). The function of such a committee has been described in relation to the UK [19]. The primary purpose of such an ethical review is to ensure the protection of the welfare and rights of human subjects. The ethics committee should also ensure that the investigation is adequately supervised and conforms to good clinical practice guidelines. The independence of an ethical review committee cannot be guaranteed with company employees present on a committee. This is also true for hospital ethics committees reviewing proposals for contract testing within their clinics, by their employees. However, without expert advice from company members, the ability of a committee to judge proposals can be limited. This is particularly true for the clinical evaluation of non-therapeutic agents like cosmetics, where the benefit to humans is not directly apparent. It has been recommended that ERCs should have relevant members of the company available to provide the necessary explanations and advice, but that these individuals should not be granted full membership of the committee, or voting rights [20].

The scientific rationale for undertaking a study with human subjects has to be correct, i.e., before human testing is undertaken, some essential questions have to be answered. The first question is whether the work is not unnecessarily repeating work already performed elsewhere, and if the study has been adequately planned and appropriately designed to give a valid answer. The second one is whether the knowledge gained from exposing volunteers is important enough to justify using volunteers and cannot be gained in other ways. The third question concerns the extent of the risk to the volunteer [21]. The risk to the volunteer of coming to harm as a participant in the study should be minimal. The concept of "minimal risk" has been described by the Royal College of Physicians [15] and by the US Food and Drug Administration (FDA) [13]. The term "minimal risk" has been used by the Royal College of Physicians to cover two situations. The first is when there is a small chance of a reaction which is itself trivial, e.g., a mild headache or feeling of lethargy. The second is where there is a very remote chance of serious injury or death, comparable to the risk of flying as a passenger on a scheduled aircraft. According to the FDA in the United States, "minimal risk means that the risks of harm anticipated in the proposed research are not greater, considering probability and magnitude, than those ordinarily encountered in daily life or during the performance of routine physical or psychological examinations or tests".

Individual countries differ in their approaches to the use of humans in biomedical research, with varying legal requirements concerning clinical research. However, the fundamental principles tend to be common, with expectations that clinical research must be conducted in accordance with good clinical research principles. At the European Union level, there is virtually no legislation addressing human experimentation. However, the protection of trial subjects, provision for ethics review, informed consent and other aspects of experiments on human subjects are comprehensively defined in the EEC Note for Guidance on Good Clinical Practice for Trials on Medicinal Products in the European Community, prepared by the EU Committee for Proprietary Medicinal Products in 1990 [17]. This document is directed primarily towards the pharmaceutical industry, but in substantial parts it, also applies to trials on non-medicinal products. Specifically, this is true with regard to the requirements for the privacy, integrity, and well-being of volunteers subjected to research, and for fully informing them about the risks and benefits potentially associated with the use of a test product.

The objectives of clinical safety testing should be to define the limits of local toxicity and the potential to generate adverse reactions in the intended consumer population.

When cosmetics are tested for compatibility on human subjects in vivo, the endpoints measured are usually non-permanent dermatological conditions such as varying degrees of erythema, oedema and dryness. In sensitisation trials, however, it can happen that a healthy human volunteer with no history of previous sensitisation is sensitised. Therefore, in some countries, testing laboratories do not consider it ethical to wilfully sensitise healthy volunteers. The risk imposed on the human volunteer, namely to generate a permanent adverse health effect, is considered too high. On the other hand, in certain other countries, predictive allergic patch testing on human beings is considered as an important means of detecting allergens and eliminating them from formulations, and the risk of inducing a sensitisation reaction in a healthy volunteer is considered very remote when compared to the benefit that ensues for the whole consumer population from such a study. A typical example of such a predictive sensitisation test is the human repeated insult patch test, which is performed in many testing laboratories. From an ethical point of view, if the well-being of the test subject should be the primary concern in human testing, the risk of generating an allergic response, including its photodynamic variants and cross-allergies, in a non-sensitised human volunteer, cannot be outweighed by the information derived from conducting such a test.

The evaluation of a product's safety in a human volunteer must be justified on a case-by-case basis; no general rule exists. Some basic criteria, however, have to be fulfilled and can be summarised as follows: an ethically performed human test should comply with the ethical recommendations included in the Declaration of Helsinki and its subsequent revisions. The volunteers should be selected in accordance with a well-designed study protocol and with the inclusion/exclusion criteria defined in the protocol. Only fully informed human volunteers, signing a written informed consent form prior to the study, should participate in the study. The informed consent form should explain the purpose and nature of the study, as well as any foreseeable risk or benefit which may result from participation in the study. Relevant safety information on the test material is necessary before the test starts. Previous experience with the test formulation and its individual ingredients, as well as the quality of the toxicological data available, will determine the eventual risk to which the subjects will be exposed. The test should be conducted by a trained and qualified investigator. The study should be submitted to an Ethical Review Committee if unusual risks to participants are involved. Appropriate medical cover in the event of unexpected/adverse reactions should have been foreseen; and, finally, the human volunteers should be compensated for their time and inconvenience, but the reward must not be so large as to incite them to participate in the study.

Conclusion

A properly designed and well-conducted efficacy trial for claim support does not generate particular ethical problems, since the products' safety should have been established beforehand. For product safety testing, a thorough analysis between the minimal risk imposed to the subject and the benefit of the outcome of the study for the subject and for society, should be made. However, the interests of science and society should never preside over considerations related to the well-being of the subject [16].

At the moment, too many ethical and legislative differences exist within individual Member States of the European Union, and between the EU, United States and Japan, with respect to human volunteer testing. Many of these problems are based on differences in national ethical points of view. A risk assessment process of new cosmetic ingredients or formulations, based on non-animal alternatives, followed by confirmatory human testing, without any animal in vivo data, would be unacceptable within certain Member States. Without some consensus across the EU on this issue, advancement and acceptance of this type of risk assessment cannot occur.

References

1. Anon (1993) Council Directive 93/35/EEC of 14 June 1993 amending for the sixth time Directive 76/768/EEC on the approximation of the laws of the Member States relating to cosmetic products. Off J Eur Commun L151:32–36
2. OECD (Organisation for Economic Co-operation and Development) (1993) OECD guidelines for testing of chemicals: health effects. Paris, OECD, vol 2, section 4
3. Anon (1992) Annex V to Commision Directive 92/69/EEC adapting to technical progress for the seventeenth time Council Directive 67/548/EEC on the approximation of laws, regulations and administrative provisions relating to the classification, packaging and labelling of dangerous substances. Off J Eur Commun L383 A:124–139
4. Botham PA, Earl LK, Fentem JH, Roguet R, van de Sandt JJM (1998) Alternative methods for skin irritation testing: the current status. ECVAM skin irritation task force report 1. ATLA 26, 195–211
5. Balls M, Basketter D, Berardesca E, Edwards C, Elsner P, Ennen J, Lévêque JL, Loden M, Masson P, Parra J, Paye M, Piérard G, Rodrigues L, Rogiers V, Salter D, Schaefer H, Zuang V (1998) Non-invasive measurements in human volunteers and their potential use in the safety assessment of cosmetics. ECVAM workshop report. ATLA, in preparation.
6. de Silva O, Basketter DA, Barratt MD, Corsini E, Cronin MTD, Das PK, Degwert J, Enk A, Garrigue JL, Hauser C, Kimber I, Lepoittevin JP, Peguet J, Ponec M (1996) Alternative methods for skin sensitisation testing. ECVAM workshop report 19. ATLA 24:683–705
7. Schlatter C, Reinhardt CA (1985) Acute irritation tests in risk assessment. Food Chem Toxicol 23:45–148
8. Basketter DA, Whittle E, Chamberlain M (1994) Identification of irritation and corrosion hazards to skin: an alternative strategy to animal testing. Food Chem Toxicol 32:539–542
9. Basketter DA, Chamberlain M, Griffiths HA, Rowson M, Whittle E, York M (1997) The classification of skin irritants by human patch test. Food Chem Toxicol 35:845–852
10. DHSS (Department of Health and Social Security, UK) (1982) Report No. 27 on health and social subjects. Guidelines for the testing of chemicals for toxicity, pp 1–57
11. Garcia C, Chesne C (1996) In vitro approaches for cosmetic product development and claim substantiation. Cosmetics and Toiletries Manufacture Worldwide, p. 267–268
12. Annas JG (1992). Regulation of human experimentation. The changing landscape of human experimentation: Nuremberg, Helsinki, and beyond. J Law Med 2:119–140
13. Federal Register (FDA) (1981) Protection of human subjects: informed consent. Standards for institutional review boards for clinical investigations, vol 46, No. 17, pp 8942–8980
14. World Health Organisation (1982) Proposed international guidelines for biomedical research involving human subjects. Council for International Organizations of Medical Sciences, Geneva, pp 1–45
15. Royal College of Physicians (1986) Research on healthy volunteers. J R Coll Physicians Lond 20:243–257
16. World Medical Association (1989) World Medical Association Declaration of Helsinki: recommendations guiding physicians in biomedical research involving human subjects. 41st World Medical Assembly, Hong Kong, September 1989
17. CPMP Working Party on Efficacy of Medicinal Products (1990) EEC note for guidance: good clinical practice for trials on medicinal products in the European Community. Pharmacol Toxicol 67:361–72
18. COLIPA/SCAAT (1996) The Colipa position paper on human testing for skin compatibility of products or skin tolerance of potentially irritant cosmetic ingredients. Doc 96/304
19. Royal College of Physicians (1986) Guidelines on the practice of ethics committees in medical research involving human subjects. The Royal College of Physicians of London, pp 1–43. 2nd edn 1990
20. Ward R, Clothier R (1997) The use of human volunteers in cosmetic efficacy and safety testing. ECVAM contract report. In press.
21. Gompertz D (1994) Of mice or men? Hum Exp Toxicol 13:381–382 (editorial)

Efficacy

In Vivo Evaluation of the Hydration State of the Skin: Measurements and Methods for Claim Support

A. O. Barel, P. Clarys, B. Gabard

Introduction

The presence of an adequate amount of water in the stratum corneum is important for the following properties of the skin: general appearance of a soft, smooth, flexible and healthy skin and presence of an intact barrier function allowing a slow rate of transepidermal water loss (TEWL) under dry external conditions, which are often encountered [1–4].

Clinically, dry skin is defined as a dry, less flexible, scaly and rough aspect of the upper layers of the epidermis [1, 4, 5]. Itch may accompany these symptoms. In more severe cases of dryness (a condition described by dermatologists as xerosis) and in pathological conditions fissuring, scaling and cracking may occur [6–9]. There is no universally accepted definition of the concept of dry skin [10]. Some authors consider dry skin as being more related to disorders of corneocyte adhesion (rough and scaly surface), to a deficiency in epidermal lipids, or to disorders of the water retaining properties of the horny layer [3,4]. The perception of a dry skin state by the patient himself also may be different from the diagnosis of the clinician.

There is currently no data confirming or infirming that dry skin is actually linked to a diminution of the water content of the horny layer. Only the positive pharmacological effect of moisture applied to the skin surface to relieve the conditions of dry skin has been repeatedly confirmed. This does not prove a water deficiency. Nevertheless, given the fact that the presence of an adequate amount of water is an essential prerequisite for the maintenance of the normal structure and function of the stratum corneum, research has been directed at the evaluation of the water content of this tissue. This water content is influenced by several factors:

- Water diffusing from the deeper viable layers of the epidermis. This water is normally retained by the barrier function of the lipid bilayers in the stratum corneum.
- Water present in the horny layer. This water is fixed among other elements by the natural moisturizing factors (NMF) containing amino acids, lactic acid, pyrrolidone carboxylic acid, urea and various other components.
- Equilibrium between water in the upper layers of the horny layer and the external ambient humidity of air. Depending on the value of the external relative humidity, the upper layers of the stratum corneum may take over or release water.
- Treatment of the skin surface with a moisturizer. Moisturizers are hydrating products used to combat the signs and symptoms of dry skin [11]. They may hydrate the skin along different manners either by reducing the loss of water due to the occlusive effect of oils and fats contained in the formulation on the skin surface, by adding water to the stratum corneum and fixing it with the help of humectants, or by a combination of both [1–4, 12].

As a consequence, the in vivo determination of the degree of hydration of the horny layer is important for the characterization of normal and pathological skin conditions, such an actinically aged or irritated skin, and, finally, for the assessment of the effetiveness of various moisturizing products.

The use of such dermato-cosmetic products in order to restore softness, smoothness and moisture to dry skin is widely practised. Clinically, moisturizers are also considered to be extremely important treatment adjuncts [13]. This chapter is concerned with the clinical evaluation and with the non-invasive bioengineering measurements of the hydration state of the skin. A critical overview of the different available bioengineering methods will be given in order to carry out hydration measurements on normal, well hydrated skin and on (very) dry skin, and to quantitatively assess the efficacy of moisturizers.

As has been described earlier, reliable and reproducible hydration measurements are only obtained if the in vivo experiments on humans are carried out under well controlled standardized conditions [2-4, 14-18]. A description of the influence of intrinsic and extrinsic factors which could influence the hydration measurements will be given. Some general recommendations will be made in order to substantiate the claims of cosmetic products manufacturers. Finally, some typical applications of the assessment of skin hydration will be described and discussed.

Methods for Evaluating the Hydration State of the Skin Surface

Clinical Evaluations

The clinical assessment of symptoms of dryness can be performed either by an expert evaluator or by the subject him(her)self [8, 19-21].

The appearance and feeling of a dry skin surface can be clinically evaluated by trained experienced researchers (physician, dermatologist or other persons) based on well defined objective criteria. For example, visual evaluations of dryness and roughness may be carried out using numerical scales for rating (a score of 0-10 or 0-4). The participation of several independent examinators is usually advantageous. This procedure is called objective clinical rating. The absolute rating of dryness and roughness may differ for each examinator but the relative comparative ratings are accurate, reproducible and sensitive. Generally good correlations are found between the visual clinical evaluations of dryness and the bioengineering methods [8, 19, 20].

This is not true for the subjective perception of the subjects themself about their skin condition (feeling of discomfort, stiffening and itching). Using the same numerical scales for dryness of the skin as in the objective ratings, some interesting comparisons can be obtained. The correlations of the subjective perceptions with the clinical ratings and bioengineering measurements are variable: sometimes very good or sometimes very poor since great discrepancies may be observed [8, 19-21].

Bioengineering Methods

The clinical symptoms of dryness are numerous: dryness, scaling, roughness and diminution of flexibility. A large variety of bioengineering methods are available to evaluate directly or indirectly a dryness of the skin [1–4, 16–18]. Here follows an overview of these different non-invasive methods.

In contrast to the rather simple experimental approach of measuring quantitatively the water content of the stratum corneum in vitro, it is very difficult to assess in vivo non-invasively the hydration state of the upper layers of the epidermis [22]. Different bioengineering techniques have been developed to measure skin properties which are influenced in some way by the water content of the horny layer. These techniques include measurements of electrical properties, spectroscopic methods such as infrared absorption spectroscopy and emission, evaluation of the barrier integrity (TEWL), mechanical properties, nuclear magnetic resonance imaging, skin surface topography and scaling of the skin surface [3, 4, 23].

For each technique the following aspects will be described: principle and measuring method, experimental laboratory or commercially available instrument, calibration, if possible accuracy and sensitivity range, facility of use for routine hydration measurements, and if available, some typical practical applications.

Measuring the Electrical Properties of the Upper Layers of the Epidermis

It has been known for a long time that the electrical properties of the skin are related to the water content of the horny layer [1, 24]. Therefore the measurement of the impedance of the skin, the total electrical resistance of the skin to an alternating current of frequency F, has been studied extensively and is the most widely used technique to assess the hydration state of the skin surface. The impedance (Z) depends on two components, a resistance (R) and a capacitance (C) in agreement with a simple theoretical model where the skin was modelled as a resistance in parallel with a capacitor [1].

The outcome of the measurements is influenced by numerous factors that may be roughly separated in biological and physical ones. Dry stratum corneum is a typical medium of weak electrical conduction (medium of low permittivity). When this medium is hydrated, great changes in its electrical properties occur. Among biological factors, many proteins and other chemicals are involved in these electrical properties which are related to hydration [1–3, 22, 24]. Proteins such as keratins and other matrix proteins present in the corneocytes are dipolar molecules and are more or less hydrated. Various ions are contained in the intracellular polar space of the corneocytes and in the intercellular hydrophilic space of the multilamellar lipid structures located between the corneocytes. Hydrogen-bonded dipolar structures of the water molecules are also involved. That means that not only the electrical impedance of the horny layer depends on the water content but that it can be further influenced by other compounds than water (ions, glycerine etc.) and also sweat gland activity. Thus, as pointed out by many authors, the complex electrical impedance properties of the horny layer are dependent from a variety of factors [3, 4, 16–18, 25–26].

Among physical factors, frequency of the electrical current used (single or multiple frequency), type of electrode applied on the skin surface, design of the oscillating electronic circuit, external temperature and temperature of the skin, external humidity, contact between electrode and the skin surface, pressure of application of the electrode etc., all these play an important role. There are actually different electrical commercially available instruments for assessing skin hydration based on the conductance (reciprocal of resistance) or capacitance working either at a single high frequency or at different frequencies.

Corneometer CM 825

The most recent version of this well known device, the Corneometer CM 825 based on the capacitance method operates at a mean frequency of 1 MHz (varying from 1.15 MHz for a dry medium to 0.95 MHz for a hydrated medium [26–29]). The measuring probe (surface 0.64 cm², 0.7×0.7 cm) consists of an interdigital grid of gold-covered electrodes with interdigital spacing of 75 μm. The interdigital electrode is covered by a low dielectric vitrified material of 20 μm thickness. As a consequence there is no direct galvanic contact between the electrode and the skin surface. A spring system is built in the probe ensuring a constant application pressure of 1.6 N/m². The electrical field present in the upper parts of the epidermis is a function of the dielectric material covering the electrodes and the capacitance of the skin in contact with the surface of the electrode. The whole system works as a variable capacitor, the total capacitance is influenced by changes in the dielectric constant of the skin surface. The changes in total capacitance as recorded by this type of instrument are expressed in arbitrary capacitance units (A.C.U.) or Corneometer units ranging from 0 to 120; the units are related to the hydration of the upper parts of the epidermis.

In vitro calibration of the instrument at respectively low (20 A.C.U.) and high values (120 A.C.U.) is possible with cellulose filter discs impregnated with physiological saline. A relationship was established in vitro between the Corneometer units and the amount of water present in the cellulose filters on one side, and with the dielectric constant of the solvent impregnating the filter papers on the other [28].

Different ways of measuring with this instrument are possible: after 1.5 s (up to ten consecutive measurements are possible with display of the mean value and of the range) and continuous measurements (respective total duration of 3 s, 70 s and 7 min).

The new instrument measures over the total depth of the stratum corneum and some upper layers of the vital epidermis. The penetration depth of the electrical field is of the order of magnitude of 20–40 μm. The range of measurements is rather large: from values of 30–40 A.C.U. for very dry skin to 120 A.C.U. for very hydrated skin. The instrument is very sensitive for measuring low levels of hydration but clearly lacks sensitivity at very high levels of hydration of the skin (plateau values of 105–110–115 A.C.U.).

The repeatability of this instrument is very good: coefficient of variation ranging from 3% to 11%. The reproducibility is also good: coefficient of variation ranging from 3% to 11%. A high correlation was found in vivo respectively with the Skicon (r = 0.89) and with the DPM 9003 (r = 0.97; 22).

Nova Dermal Phase Meter, DPM 9003

The DPM is a pocket size commercial device which works at variable selected frequencies up to 1 MHz [30–32]. This instrument features a standard circular surface probe of two concentric brass ring electrodes separated by a dielectric material with respective external diameters of 8.76 and 4.34 mm. The surface of the standard electrode is 0.98 cm². There is a direct galvanic contact between the electrodes and the skin surface. The probe is applied with a constant pressure of maximum 0.6 N/m² by means of a spring system. Other smaller measuring probes are available with respectively 2-, 4- and 6-mm external diameter.

The DPM measures the impedance-based capacitance properties of the skin (imaginary part of the impedance called capacitance reactance) at variable selected frequencies. The final readout is given in arbitrary capacitance-reactance units ranging from 90 to 999 DPM units. The DPM units are directly related through an empirical equation to capacitance units [30, 32]. The capacitance-reactance units are related to the hydration of the horny layer. When starting, the instrument is automatically calibrated by an internal device.

There are different ways of measuring: immediate measurements, after 5 s application of the probe and continuous measurements.

The DPM measures the superficial part of the stratum corneum. Large ranges of measuring values of 90–100 DPM units for dry skin and of 110–350 DPM units for very hydrated skin are usual. The instrument is very sensitive for grading a normal or elevated hydration state of the horny layer and less sensitive for situations of very dry skin.

The repeatability of this instrument is very good: coefficient of variation ranging from 3% to 6%. The reproducibility is also rather good: coefficient of variation ranging from 10% to 25%. A high correlation was found in vivo with the Skicon (r = 0.96) and with the Corneometer (r = 0.97; [26]).

Skin Surface Hygrometer, Skicon-200
The Skin Surface Hygrometer, Skicon-200, is a single frequency instrument which measures the conductance of the skin [1, 2, 18, 29]. This instrument features a standard circular surface probe of two concentric gold covered ring electrodes separated by a dielectric material with respective external diameters of 2.0 and 6.0 mm. The surface of the electrode is 0.28 cm². There is a direct galvanic contact between the electrodes and the skin surface. The probe is applied with a constant pressure of maximum 1.04 N/m² with a graduated spring system. The instrument measures at 3.5 MHz the electrical conductance (reciprocal of resistance) of the skin in µSiemens ranging from 0 to 1999 µS. This instrument gives conductance units which are related to the hydration of the horny layer. There is a standard external calibration device of 300 µS to calibrate the equipment.

The Skicon measures automatically the conductance after 3 s application of the probe on the skin surface. There is no continuous measurement possible. Besides the standard electrode there are larger sizes of probes available. The Skicon measures the very superficial part of the stratum corneum: the penetration depth in the skin of the Skicon is of the order of magnitude of less than 20 µm.

The range of measurement values in vivo is very large (10–15 µS for very dry skin to more than 500 µS for very hydrated skin). However at low levels of hydration of the horny layer the conductance method lacks sensitivity (plateau values ranging from 0 to 10–15 µS). On the contrary the sensitivity at high levels of hydration is very good. High intra-individual coefficients of variations (repeatability) were observed in vivo: from 16% to 25%. The reproducibility is not very good: coefficients of variation ranging from 30% to 50% are currently noticed. This is a major drawback of this very sensitive instrument. When small increases in hydration of the skin are observed with this instrument, these small effects are generally not significant due to the very high inter-individual coefficient of variations.

A Multifrequency Electrical Impedance Instrument

The use of multifrequency instruments for investigation of electrical skin properties related to hydration is limited to non commercially available laboratory-built equipments. However, recently a multifrequency instrument has been developed at the Karolinska Institute, Huddinge, Sweden and will soon become commercially available [34]. This instrument measures the magnitude and the phase angle of skin impedance at different frequencies from 1 KHz to 1 MHz. The hydration of the skin is indirectly estimated from a magnitude index ratio and from a phase angle index. At the present time only very limited information is available for this type of instrument.

Two Recent Commercial Instruments

These instruments operate at a single frequency and are based respectively on impedance measurements, Dermolab, Cortex Technology [35] and on capacitance measurements, Dermanalyser 3F, Robinson Electronic Limited [36]. The principle of the moisture reading Dermanalyser 3F is a capacitance measurement similar to the principle of the Corneometer. Since no scientific published information is presently available concerning the use of these instruments, only technical data can be obtained from the manufacturers.

In conclusion, as mentioned by many authors [2–4, 15–18], one must bear in mind that the electric measurements are not water-specific, and that any polar material present in the horny layer may in principle influence the recordings. However, the methods have in practice proven to be very useful for recording skin hydration. The recorded electric units are generally arbitrary units indirectly related to skin hydration. These devices are simple low cost electrical instruments easy to use and hence particularly suited for routine measurements.

Infrared Spectroscopy

Different infrared absorption bands in the 4000–650 cm^{-1} wavenumber range are characteriscic of the absorption of water. The absorption at these wavelengths is directly related to the water content of the upper layers of the horny layer [37–39].

Fourier-transformed infrared spectroscopy of the skin surface can be made using an attenuated total reflection unit (ZnSe crystal) as a special device to a normal Fourier Transform Absorption Spectrometer. Single (short time effect) and repetitive (long time effect) applications of hydration products on the skin surface are accompanied by changes in absorption bands at specific wavenumbers [40]. The increase in absorption is directly related to the water content of the horny layer. However, interference of other infrared absorbing compounds present in the horny layer is possible and must be taken in account. This instrument measures absorption of water only at the upper layers of the horny layer (a few microns). It is an expensive commercial laboratory apparatus for fundamental research not suited for routine hydration measurements.

Opto Thermal Emission Spectroscopy

At present, infrared opto thermal emission spectroscopy is an experimental noninvasive laboratory technique [41, 42]. The skin surface is illuminated with a strong pulsed infrared laser light ($\lambda = 2.94$ μm). The thermal emission of the superficial layers of the epidermis is analyzed at infrared wavelenghts with strong water absorption bands (λ of 6.05 or 13 µm). From the obtained thermal emission curves an empirical hydration index of the stratum corneum can be computed. At present time the analysis of the thermal emission decay curves is complex and the obtained hydration index is an arbitrary unit not directly related to the water content of the horny layer. It is an expensive experimental laboratory apparatus for fundamental research not suited for routine hydration measurements.

Transepidermal Water Loss (TEWL)

The measurement of the rate of evaporation of water through the stratum corneum is an indication of the integrity of the barrier function of the skin. There are several commercial instruments available. Among these, two are mostly used: the Evaporimeter EP1 and new EP2 (ServoMed, Kinna, Sweden) and the Tewameter 210 (Courage and Khazaka, Cologne, Germany). Both instruments are accurate and have a broad range of sensitivity. A high correlation was found (r=0.97) between the two over a wide range of in vivo TEWL values [46]. Guidelines have been published about proper measurements of TEWL [44–46].

The relation between the flux of water through the horny layer and the water content in this layer is complex [39]. Normal values of TEWL are observed in healthy skin showing a large range of hydration values as evaluated by electrical methods. Increased values of TEWL may be noticed in conditions such as atopic dermatitis, ichthyosis and psoriasis, but at the same time a decrease of the horny layer hydration is not necessarily observed [6]. An increase of TEWL may also be observed immediately after application of a moisturizing product. This skin surface water loss is due to the evaporation of the water present in the product which has been applied on the skin surface and is related to the content of water in the moisturizer and not to the real water content of the stratum corneum [3, 12]. An increase of TEWL is also observed immediately after alteration of the stratum corneum with chemical agents (detergents, acids, bases and strong oxidators) or physical agents (stripping). Only in these cases a positive correlation may be observed between the increase of TEWL and a higher content of water in the upper layers of the epidermis.

A decrease of TEWL may be observed when the skin surface is occluded with oils, fats, lipogels or suitable emulsions. This decrease in TEWL is generally accompanied by a corresponding slow increase in skin hydration [3, 4]. The efficacy of an occlusive hydration product can be indirectly followed by the reduction of the TEWL at the skin surface. Such measurements have been used to describe the short time effects of emollients and W/O moisturizers on the skin [12].

Visco-elastic Properties of the Upper Layers of the Epidermis

Unaltered mechanical properties are important for the normal physiological functions of of the skin. Symptoms of a very dry skin such as cracking and scaling can be related to the visco-elastic properties of the different layers of the skin. These mechanical properties have been studied noninvasively by a number of methods using stretching, torsion, indentation or suction [47–51]. Few instruments are commercially available at the present time, based on the torsion method (Dermal Torque Meter, Dia-Stron Limited,

Andover, UK), on uniaxial extensibility (Extensometer, Dermotronics Limited, Cardiff, UK) or on the suction method (Dermaflex A, and DermaLab from Cortex Technology, Hadsund, Denmark and Cutometer SEM 575 from Courage and Khazaka Electronic, Cologne, Germany) [47–53].

These instruments generally measure the mechanical properties of the combined layers epidermis-dermis when large deformation forces are applied on the skin. However when exerting small forces (torque or suction) and when the opening of the suction probe is small (2-mm diameter probe), the observed skin deformations are more related to the visco-elastic properties of the upper layers of the epidermis with a major contribution from the horny layer. Short time effects of emollients on the skin and stripping of the horny layer have thus consequences on the pure elastic and viscoelastic properties of the upper layers of the epidermis. No significant differences in the elastic properties as evaluated by the elasticity parameter Ur/Uf were observed after application of glycerine and paraffin oil. On the contrary, the viscoelastic deformation ratios were significantly increased after the topical treatments [51,52]. An intensive treatment of the skin such as 40 strippings which corresponds to removing most of the horny layer, will provoke a small decrease in elasticity (Ur/Uf) but a large increase in the viscoelastic parameter (Uv/Ue; [52]). Long time application of emollients will lead to an increase in elasticity factors [54]. However it is difficult to explain the alterations of the classical purely elastic and viscoelastic parameters of the upper layers of the epidermis (with a substantial contribution from the horny layer) in function of solely the water content in this layer. One must also take into account other skin properties such as plasticity and emolliency when applying moisturizers with hydrating properties [2, 3].

Nuclear Magnetic Resonance Imaging, NMR Imaging

High resolution in vivo magnetic resonance images of epidermis can be obtained nowadays with special skin surface coils and high magnetic fields [55, 56]. However the spatial resolution (presently 50 μm) is insufficient for detailed studies in the epidermis. Furthermore the specially designed NMR surface coils are presently only available in a few research laboratories. NMR imaging has presently only be used for the determination of the hydration of a very thick stratum corneum such as in the foot heel [55,56]. A short time effect of moisturizing of the startum corneum, with a buildup and desorption of water was visualized. But again there is no simple relation between the obtained NMR spectra and the quantitation of water. This very promising technique needs further technical improvement both in spatial resolution and sensitivity for routine measurement. Finally it is a very expensive experimental laboratory apparatus for fundamental research which is presently not suited for routine hydration measurements.

Topography of the Skin Surface

Skin surface topography may be examined using high resolution soft silicone replicas and analyzing these replicas by shadows produced by lateral illumination, laser optical profilometry and mechanical profilometry [57–60]. Lateral illumination of the skin replicas under well-defined conditions creates shadows due to the furrows and wrinkles of the replica that can be evaluated by image analysis [58]. Laser focusing technique is a technique using an optical laser profilometer with automatic autofocus of the laser beam [59]. In the mechanical profilometry a fine stylus follows the variations of the relief and the topography of the skin surface is characterized by classical parameters used in metallurgy [57].

Recently an new technique was developed by measuring the thickness of a translucent replica [60]. Here too, the topography of the skin surface is characterized by the parameters used in metallurgy. Application of moisturizers to the skin produces a smoothening effect of the skin of short duration [2]. Comparative image analysis of the skin replicas shows a flattening of the skin. This flattening is due to the emollient effect of the lipids present in the cream, to the swelling of the corneocytes and to the filling of the intercellular spaces between the corneocytes. After this short time effect (maximum 2–3 h) the original skin roughness returns to the start values. It is important to clean the skin after topical application of an emollient in order to remove any excess of lipids and fats before taking the replica. The skin flattening may be due to the filling of the skin irregularities with products left on the skin surface. Long time treatment of the skin located at the face, forearms, lower legs during several weeks with a moisturizing cream will give a finer texture of the skin surface [54]. This smoothening of the skin surface is not directly related to the water content of the horny layer.

Scaling of the Skin Surface

Roughness and scaling of the skin is to a certain extent attributed to dryness and may be evaluated using adhesive tape which removes the superficial layers of the horny layer. Commercially available adhesive tapes can be used to sample these superficial cells [61, 62]. The sampling device is a transparent adhesive coated disc. Upon application of the disc on the skin surface with standardized constant pressure, the adhesive removes superficial corneocytes. The disc is then removed from the skin and placed on a black storage card for futher examination. The obtained scale patterns can be evaluated qualitatively by visual examination and/or quantitatively by image analysis, colorimetry and by optical transmission [63–65]. D-Squames discs, from CuDerm Corporation Texas, USA, are generally used for scaling evaluation. Assessment of leg dryness and dryness on the back of the hands can be made using image analysis of D-Squames [61, 62, 65–67].

Conclusions of Bioengineering Measurements

Noninvasive bioengineering methods provide thus possibilities for demonstrating the effects of cosmetic products aiming at the alleviation of dry skin symptoms and could be used to substantiate the claims of the cosmetic manufacturers. However, most of these biophysical methods give readings which are only in some way related to the hydration state of the skin and not directly related to the amount of water in the horny layer. The results of the instrumental readings are given either in physical units (roughness in μm, TEWL in g/hm^2), or most frequently in arbitrary instrument units (Corneometer or Nova DPM units).

New experimental interesting techniques have been developed in many laboratories to characterize some properties in relation with the hydration state of the horny layer:

near infrared spectroscopy, multifrequence electrical impedance, nuclear magnetic resonance, etc. But the use of these new techniques remains experimental (not suited for routine), and they are very expensive. As a consequence, the electrical methods for measuring hydration remain at the present moment the most basic and most widely used technologies.

General Guidelines for Hydration Studies

Objective assessment of the hydration state of the horny layer and evaluation of the efficacy of moisturizers may be readily done with simple instruments based on electrical methods, provided that these instruments are used in an appropriate manner. Irrespective of the instrument used, practical guidelines have been published and should be followed in order to perform accurate and reproducible measurements [1–4, 14–18]. These guidelines provide the frame for the recommendations given here and the reader should report to the corresponding publications for more details.

Environmental Temperature, Relative Humidity and Season

Environmental temperature and relative humidity should best be kept constant at 20±2°C and 45%±5%, respectively. Consequently the measurements should be carried out in a climatised experimental room. A linear relationship has been reported between external relative humidity and hydration of the horny layer [14, 68]. Similarly, increasing environmental temperature results in an increase in stratum corneum hydration (above 22°C an invisible sweating occurs). Subjects should be relaxed and an acclimatization time of at least 15 min is necessary ensuring that the skin sites to be studied are exposed and in equilibrium with the environmental conditions.

It is well known that during the winter, a dry, rough, sometimes scaly skin may be present in older people or other sensitive persons at the lower legs and other anatomic skin sites (winter xerosis). This clinical picture is ideal for evaluating a moisturization effect. In contrast the skin is optimally hydrated in summer due to the generally high external humidity. This situation is not suited to demonstrate the favourable effect of moisturizing products. Seasonal variations of temperature and humidity have to be taken in account when doing long time hydration studies. Due to possible large climatic variations in the summer period, testing should be avoided in the months of June, July and August in north-western countries.

Age and Gender

There are no differences in the hydration of the stratum corneum between women and men [69]. The hydration level diminishes with age above 50 with the gradual appearance of a typical very dry stratum corneum in the elderly persons (e.g. xerosis of the lower legs). For optimal skin hydration studies it is important to select the subjects as belonging to an homogeneous group (same age, similar skin type, similar phototype, only caucasian, Asian or African as ethnic group). Depending on the protocol, we generally select in our studies women or men with either normal or dry or very dry skin, with normal or oily skin and with phototype II and III. Male and female subjects may be included in a hydration study, but it advisable not to select males with very hairy skin sites (see "Skin Sites"). History of the potential volunteers and final selection of the subjects are carried out with great precaution in order to obtain a homogeneous group ensuring mean baseline hydration values within a narrow range before any cosmetic treatment and thus an interindividual coefficient of variation as low as possible.

Number of Subjects

The number of volunteers participating in a hydration study should be sufficient in order to permit statistical analysis of the data and in order to observe statistically significant changes of the hydration values of the horny layer after a cosmetic treatment. The adequate number of participants is best evaluated before starting the study by classical power calculation [70]. Generally, a minimum of 12–15 subjects is needed for valid statistical analysis of the data.

Skin Sites

The choice of the anatomical skin site for hydration studies is important. According to many authors, variations in stratum corneum thickness, sweat glands number and activity, and amount of skin surface lipids (epidermal lipids and sebum) are encountered among different skin sites. Generally higher hydration values are observed at the forehead, cheeks and the palms and lower values at the lower legs, ankles and abdomen [69].

The skin at the volar forearm, a skin site frequently used for hydration studies, has no constant hydration state [14, 18]. Corresponding skin sites on the left and right side of the forearm, lateral part of the forehead and of the back and the legs do not show any significant differences in their level of hydration. This is very practical for contralateral comparisons: active hydrating cream versus placebo (vehicle cream) or versus untreated site as control. When all test sites are located on the forearms (left and right), randomization of the sites must be done. Avoid skin sites which are too hairy. The presence of coarse hair prevents a good contact betwen the skin and the measuring probe [7, 8]. If such hairy skin sites must be examined, hair should be removed using an electrical shaving apparatus at least a few days before measurements [2, 3].

Cleansing of the Skin Site

A standard cleansing procedure of the skin before starting measurements is necessary [2, 3, 14, 18]. A non-aggressive cleansing procedure should be used in order to perturb as little as possible the skin physiology. Non-alcoholic lotions or cleansing milks with non-ionic emulgators should be used for this purpose. But even this very soft procedure may significantly modify the hydration state of the upper layers of the epidermis. One must allow sufficient time in order to restore the original skin state (2–3 h are minimal).

Application of the Moisturizing Products

A constant well defined quantity of moisturizing product should be applied on the test areas. A concentration of 1–3 mg or μl/cm^2 is generally used. The product is gently rubbed into the skin with a finger covered with a latex glove. The eventual excess of product is removed and the skin surface is blotted dry with a cellulose tissue. Alternatively, the test product may be evenly distributed on the skin with a pre-weighed glass rod. Thereafter, the glass rod is weighed again and the weight difference used to estimate the exact quantity of product applied.

A reference moisturizer should always be used as control when testing different moisturizing products. For this purpose, we use in our laboratory O/W or W/O lotions containing 2% or 4% urea as humectant. A well standardized and universally accepted reference moisturizer is strongly needed in order to allow meaningful interlaboratory comparison of efficacy results.

Number of Independent Measurements

It is advisable to perform at least three (ideally between 5 and 10) measurements at sites close together in order to get mean values used for further calculations. Conducting measurements several times are advisable in order to eliminate very low or very high readings [7, 8]. However, if several measurements are carried out on the same skin site at the same time, a moisture accumulation due to occlusion may occur and may lead to higher hydration values. For repeated measurements at identical skin sites a waiting period of 5–10 s should be considered between measurements [18].

Application of the Probe on the Skin Surface

The physical contact of the probe with the skin surface is important. If the skin surface is rough and the physical and electrical contact is poor, low values not representative of the hydration state of the skin surface will be recorded [7, 8]. The pressure of the probe on the skin surface must be kept constant during the measurements. Consequently, the probe of most of the instruments includes a spring mechanism ensuring a constant application pressure [17, 18]. The measuring probe has to be placed vertically on the test sites.

Evaluation of the Results

The efficacy of the moisturizers can be evaluated by comparing the increase in hydration values at individual time periods or better by calculating the whole area under the hydration versus time curve [18]. When testing the efficacy of different moisturizers only a rank order of efficacy can be established (product A >product B >product C). Since the electric parameters are not related in a simple direct way to the water content of the stratum corneum, an increase in electric hydration units (e.g. 20%) is not strictly proportional to the increase in water content in the horny layer. Therefore, we do not recommend the use of this kind of presentation of the results.

Description of Some Hydration Experiments for Claim Support in Cosmetology

Moisturizing Products

Short Time Hydrating Effect or Single Application Test

In this test, the time course of the hydration state of the skin is followed during a few hours after a single application of a moisturizer [1–4, 18, 71–72]. The different products are usually applied on the volar side of both forearms to well delimited skin areas (2×3 or 3×4 cm) at a well defined concentration (1–3 mg/cm²). The products are gently rubbed in the skin with a gloved finger. An untreated skin area is always considered as a control site. A reference area is treated with a reference moisturizer of the same emulsion type as the tested products. Baseline hydration measurements are made before application and at well defined time points post application during 2–5 h on each area.

Figure 1 shows the results of a typical experiment with two different O/W moisturizers using the conductance method. Figure 2 shows the short time hydrating effect of an O/W milk and of a cream as measured with the capacitance method. Shortly after application of the products, an increase in the hydration of the horny layer was measured by both methods. This is followed by a plateau value and a slow decrease of the measured values toward baseline, according to the efficacy of the cosmetic product. The plateau value or slow decrease is the result of the combined effect of the lipids contained in the formulation and left on the skin surface after the evaporation of water and/or of the humectants enhancing the binding of water in the superficial horny layer.

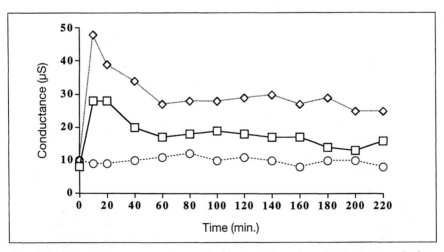

Fig. 1. Effect on skin hydration (ventral part of the forearms) of a single application (2 mg/cm²) of two O/W hydrating products. O/W emulsion with NMF as humectants (*squares*), O/W emulsion with 2% urea as humectant (*diamonds*) and untreated control (*circles*). Fourteen female volunteers, age 39±6 years. Conductance units (µS, Skicon 200)

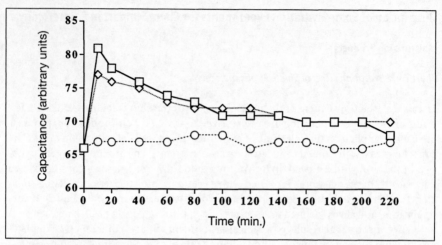

Fig. 2. Effect on skin hydration (ventral part of the forearms) of a single application (2 mg/cm²) of two hydrating products. O/W hydrating cream (*diamonds*), O/W hydrating milk containing NMF as humectants (*squares*) and untreated control (*circles*). Fourteen female volunteers, age 39±6 years. Arbitrary capacitance units (Corneometer CM 820)

After the application of a W/O emulsion, lipogel or an occlusive oil on the skin surface the hydration versus time curve is generally different (see Figs. 3 and 4). There is a gradual increase in hydration until a plateau is reached due to accumulation of water in the horny layer due to the occlusive effect. After a certain time, the hydration of the treated skin areas return very slowly to the baseline values.

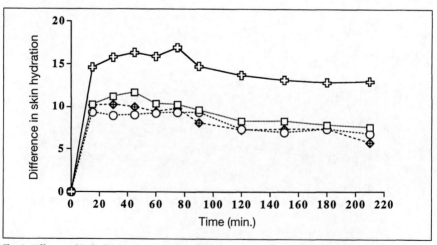

Fig. 3. Effect on skin hydration (ventral part of the forearms) of a single application (2 mg/cm²) of 5% thyme in a W/O vehicle (*crossed diamonds*), W/O vehicle alone (*circles*), W/O emulsion with 2% urea as humectant (*crosses*) and W/O emulsion as vehicle alone (*squares*). Fifteen female volunteers, age 24±4 years. Difference in arbitrary capacitance hydration units (Corneometer CM 820). Taken from [81]

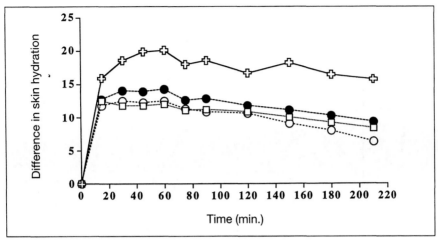

Fig. 4. Effect on skin hydration (ventral part of the forearms) of a single application (2 mg/cm²) of 5% sage in wheat germ oil (*filled circles*), wheat germ oil as vehicle alone (*clear circles*), W/O emulsion with 2% urea as humectant (*clear crosses*) and W/O emulsion as vehicle alone (*clear squares*). Twelve female volunteers, age 27±5 years. Difference in arbitrary capacitance hydration units (Corneometer CM 820). Taken from [81]

Long Time Hydrating Effect or Multiple Application Test

This is a more realistic test where repeated applications of hydrating products (generally twice a day) are carried out in order to evaluate the changes in skin condition after a few weeks [3, 17, 18, 73]. The long term effects of moisturizers are assessed in subjects with dry or very dry skin located at the volar forearm or on the lower legs. The

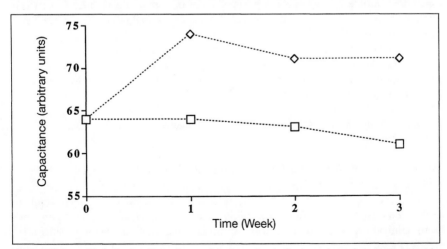

Fig. 5. Effect on skin hydration (frontal part of the lower legs) of a three-times-daily application of a liposomal hydration product (*diamonds*) over 3 weeks. Untreated control (*squares*). Twenty female volunteers, age 52±8 years. Arbitrary capacitance hydration units (Corneometer CM 820)

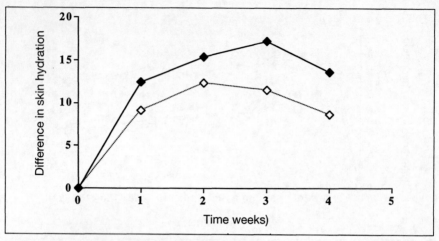

Fig. 6. Effect on skin hydration (frontal part of the lower legs) of a two-times-daily application of 5% sage in W/O emulsion (*filled diamonds*) and W/O emulsion as vehicle alone (*clear diamonds*) over 3 weeks and 1 week after the end of treatment. Fifteen female volunteers, age 36±7 years with typical winter dryness of the skin at the lower legs. Arbitrary capacitance hydration units (Corneometer CM 825). Taken from [81]

selected skin areas are treated twice daily at home over a period of 2, 3 or 4 weeks. In this study generally a simple left right contralateral comparison design study is made for simplicity. The subjects are instructed about the evaluation of the quantity of product to be applied on the test area. Hydration measurements are carried before (baseline) and respectively after 1, 2, 3 or 4 weeks. Last measurements are made at least 8–12 h after the last application. Figure 5 shows a typical long term hydration curve after treatment with a liposomal O/W moisturizer. Figure 6 shows respectively the hydrating and/or emollient effect of wheat germ oil alone or containing 5% sage. In-between visits are necessary to control the amount of moisturizer applied on the test areas and the compliance of the subjects.

Variable environmental factors (temperature and humidity) might influence the results of the hydration study, particularly during a long-term experiment. In order to minimize these factors enrolling a larger number of subjects and conduction of the measurements in a climatised room are advisable.

Use of Hydration Measurements for Studying the Cutaneous Tolerance of Different Cosmetic Products

Many testing procedures exist for comparing the relative cutaneous tolerance of cosmetic products such as cleansing products for example. They include occlusive or semi-open patch test, exaggerated washing procedures, exaggerated soaking procedures and normal use tests [19]. Several possibilities exist to assess and express skin reactions: clinical evaluation of skin dryness and erythema and instrumental measurements [74–76].

When an irritant surfactant interacts with skin surface, it partially or totally removes the hydrolipidic film, disorganizes the barrier function of the horny layer and also extracts some NMF components altering the mechanism of maintaining the normal hydration state of the skin surface [19]. Such an alteration can be evaluated with the use of electrical hydration measurements. In addition, the irritancy potential of cleansing products can also be assessed by other noninvasive techniques such as superficial blood flow, integrity of the barrier function (TEWL), skin colour, viscoelastic properties, skin surface roughness and scaling [19, 20].

Occlusive Patch Testing

A popular test for comparing the irritation potential of various products is the Frosch-Kligman soap chamber test [77] and a largely used, shorter variant soap chamber test, described by Simion et al. [78]. It consists of two successive occlusive application of the potential irritant during 24 h. Irritation is determined after patch removal by visual and instrumental assessments. Mainly with irritant chemicals, skin dryness slowly develops after the patching period and can be quantified by electrical hydration measurements [19, 20]. High correlations are generally observed between the visual scoring of dryness and the capacitance readings 3–5 days after patch removal.

Table 1 shows results of hydration measurements before and at different times in the soap chamber procedure. The irritancy/mildness properties of respectively an irritant surfactant, sodium laureth sulfate with two ethoxylations (Texapon N28) and two milder surfactants, sodium laureth sulfate with seven ethoxylations (Texapon ASV) and lauryl polyglycoside (Plantaren) were examined in the patch test procedure using different bioengineering techniques [79]. The capacitance values decreased after repetitive application of the different test solutions. The dehydration effect is most pronounced 48 h after removal of the second set of patches. At this last time point, the lowest hydration values were noticed for the surfactant N28. No significant differences were observed between the dehydration kinetics of the two milder products but significant ones were observed between the kinetics of the test products and of the water control.

Exaggerated Use Tests

The soap chamber tests does not simulate the normal usage of the test materials for evaluating an irritation potential. As a consequence other tests closer to realistic use conditions of the products by the consumer were developed [19, 20, 65, 66]. The ex-

Table 1. Hydration measurement (capacitance arbitrary units) measured before and at different time intervals in the soap chamber procedure. The irritancy/mildness properties of an irritant surfactant, sodium laureth sulfate with 2 ethoxylations (Texapon N28) and two milder surfactants, sodium laureth sulfate with 7 ethoxylations (Texapon ASV) and lauryl polyglycoside (Plantaren), respectively, was examined in this procedure. Taken from [79]

Time (d)	Water	N28	ASV	Plantaren
0	64±8	64±9	66±9	65±9
1	58±10	60±11	55±8	53±6
2	59±7	61±10	55±13	49±6
3	62±7	57±11	61±10	56±5
4	64±5	35±15	54±8	53±11
Manova		s.	s.	s.

Table 2. Dehydration effect of a conventional irritant dishwashing product with anionic surfactants (product 2) and a softer non-ionic product (product 1), respectively, in the hand/forearm immersion test at 37 and 40°C. Capacitance hydration measurements measured before (im=0) and 24 h after the second (im=2) and fourth immersion (im=4). * $p < 0.05$ Taken from [80]

| | Hand | | | | Forearm | | | |
| | Prod 1 | | Prod 2 | | Prod 1 | | Prod 2 | |
im	37°C	40°C	37°C	40°C	37°C	40°C	37°C	40°C
0	65±9	57±11	64±9	57±9	65±6	57±9	65±8	60±8
2	63±10	58±10	60±8	53±5	66±6	57±5	65±7	50±8*
4	63±7	50±6	60±6	42±9*	67±7	56±10	60±6	52±12*

aggerated use tests combine the application of the product to its normal mode of use but still in an exaggerated way. In the hand/ forearm immersion test the hands and forearms are soaked in product solutions at 37–40 °C for 30 min, one immersion a day for 4 consecutive days (24 h interval [65, 66, 80]). Bioengineering measurements are carried out before and 24 h after the second and the fourth immersion.

Table 2 shows the dehydration effect of respectively a conventional irritant dishwashing product with anionic surfactants (product 2) and a softer non-ionic product (product 1) in the hand/forearm immersion test at 37 and 40°C. The skin parameter used to quantify the irritation (capacitance hydration readings) is sensitive enough to discriminate between the irritation/mildness properties of the two dishwashing products after four consecutive immersions at 40°C.

The Use of Hydration Measurements in Normal "In Use" Testing of Cleansing and Cosmetic Products

The above-mentioned tests featuring extreme application conditions have been designed in order to predict with good confidence the cutaneous tolerance of the investigated product. However, an extended study with people using daily the product under normal conditions is also necessary. Such studies are called "in use" tests or "home use" tests [19, 21, 67]. The product is used at home, on the body area for which it is intended and for a minimum duration of a few weeks. Any unwanted cutaneous reaction is recorded by clinical evaluations and by bioengineering measurements. It is important to check if the cosmetic product does not lead to a dehydration the upper layers of the epidermis, or if any changes of the skin surface occur during use (increased roughness or scaling). The consumer perception of these possible skin changes are also noticed.

As an example, a double blind study of the use at home during 10 consecutive weeks of respectively a classical alkaline soap bar and a more neutral syndet bar was carried out on two identical groups of each 25 healthy female subjects [21]. Possible skin changes on different anatomical sites were evaluated respectively by objective clinical visual evaluations and by bioengineering measurements (skin colour, hydration, surface pH and integrity of barrier function) before the start and every two weeks during the 10 weeks treatment. The objective evaluations were compared with the more subjective perceptions of the consumers (dryness, tightness and irritation). Using the bioengineering measurements and the objective clinical observations, it was impossible to detect any changes on the skin during the ten weeks daily treatment with the two products. Figure 7 shows the hydration measurements (arbitrary capacitance units) of the skin located at the legs and at the hands during the testing. No significant differences in hydration and also in other bioengineering measurements were observed between the daily washing with either the syndet or the soap. These objective measurements

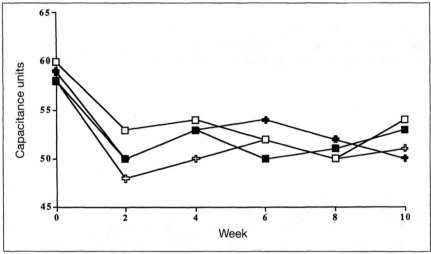

Fig. 7. Hydration measurements of the skin located at the hand and the leg in the in-use test. Measurements were carried out before and every 2 weeks during the 10 weeks of normal daily usage. Usage of the syndet [hand (*filled squares*) and leg (*filled crosses*)] and usage of the alkaline soap [hand (*clear squares*) and leg (*clear crosses*)]. Arbitrary capacitance hydration units (Corneometer CM 825)

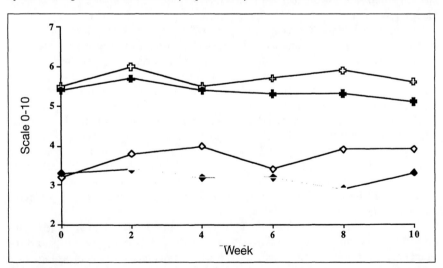

Fig. 8. Subjective consumers perception of skin dryness located at the forearm and the leg before the in use test and every 2 weeks during the 10 weeks of normal daily usage. Scoring by the consumers on a linear dryness scale going from 0 (well hydrated) to 10 (very dry). Usage of the syndet [forearm (*filled crosses*) and leg (*filled diamonds*)] and usage of the alkaline soap [forearm (*clear crosses*) and leg (*clear diamonds*)]

were not confirmed by the perception of the consumers. As shown in Figure 8, the subjective perception of feeling and of dryness of the skin clearly indicated a general trend towards more changes in the skin at all sites induced by the soap compared to the syndet. On the other hand, results from a former soap chamber test with these two cleansing bars clearly pointed out the alkaline soap as being more irritant than the syndet. This showed that skin irritation induced by cosmetic products in an exaggerated application test was not necessarily predictive of an irritation likely to occur in normal use conditions. It also shows that it is difficult to correlate subjective observations of dryness of the skin (looking and feeling of dryness, tightness, etc.) as perceived by the consumers with bioengineering electrical measurements.

General Conclusions

Evaluation of the efficacy of most moisturizers requires the use of several experimental approaches in order to characterize different aspects of skin hydration changes. For instance, application of a W/O moisturizer cream on the skin will reduce dryness by an occlusive effect and reduce the roughness, scaling and feeling of tightness of the skin by an emollient effect of the lipids present in the preparation. As a consequence it is advisable to base cosmetic claims not solely on the results of a single type of instrumental test (for example only an electric determination of horny layer hydration) but rather on a combination of results from clinical evaluations and from different experimental assessments. As far as the efficacy of the W/O moisturizer cream is concerned, the long term hydration effect could be substantiated by the following combined experimental approach: hydration of the horny layer with the conductance or capacitance method, occlusive effect with TEWL and smoothing with scaling or surface topography analysis.

This approach is also valid concerning the safety of cosmetic products and/or the irritation potential of surfactants and emulgators in normal or in exaggerated use tests. Interaction of an irritant product with the skin surface induces among others effects a dehydration of the horny layer. This dehydration will be accompanied by other symptoms such as an increase in the desquamation rate of the corneocytes, modifications of the skin relief and of the viscoelastic properties of the epidermis. Electrical measurements are generally used for the evaluation of the dehydration effect of the products. In addition, other instrumental measurements are carried out in order to objectively and quantitatively characterize skin alterations: skin color, skin surface blood flow and integrity of skin barrier function. Again, a combination of several parameters based on clinical evaluations and different experimental assessments should be used in substantiating claim supports of mildness of cosmetic cleansing products.

This review demonstrates that bioengineering methods make it possible to determine the hydration state of the skin and to measure the hydrating and dehydrating effect of various cosmetic treatments. Routine instrumental hydration measurements appear to be rather simple to carry out, but in order to substantiate claims with these experimental techniques it is necessary to emphasize the importance of standardization and calibration of the measurements conducted under well controlled conditions.

References

1. Tagami H (1989) Impedance measurements for evaluation of the hydration state of the skin surface. In: Lévêque JL (ed) Cutaneous investigation in health and disease, non-invasive methods and instrumentation. Marcel Dekker, New York, pp 79–111
2. Tagami H (1995) Measurement of electrical conductance and impedance. In: Serup J, Jemec GBE (eds) Handbook of non-invasive methods and the skin. CRC Press, Boca Raton, pp 159–164
3. Loden M, Lindeberg M (1994) Product testing of moisturizers. In: Elsner P, Berardesca E, Maibach HI (eds) Bioengineering of the skin: water and stratum corneum. CRC Press, Boca Raton, pp 275–289
4. Loden M (1995) Biophysical methods of providing objective documentation of the effects of moisturizing creams. Skin Res Tech 1:101–108
5. Van de Kerkhof PCM (1997) What are dry skin conditions? J Dermatol Treatment 8 [Suppl 1]: S3-S5
6. Edwards C, Marks R (1994) Hydration and atopic dermatitis. In: Elsner P, Berardesca E, Maibach HI (eds) Bioengineering and the skin: water and stratum corneum. CRC Press, Boca Raton, pp 235–242
7. Serup J (1994) Hydration in psoriasis and eczema: the dry surface-high evaporative water loss paradox. In: Elsner P, Berardesca E, Maibach HI (eds) Bioengineering and the skin: water and stratum corneum. CRC Press, Boca Raton, pp 243–249
8. Serup J (1995) EEMCO guidance for the assessment of dry skin (xerosis) and ichtyosis: clinical scoring systems. Skin Res Tech 1:109–114
9. Berardesca E, Fideli D, Borroni G, Rabbiosi G, Maibach HI (1990) In vivo hydration and water retention capacity of stratum corneum in clinically uninvolved skin in atopic and psoriatic patients. Acta Dermatol Venereol (Stockholm) 70:400–404
10. Piérard GE (1987) What does "dry skin" mean? Int J Dermatol 26:167–168
11. Kligman AM (1978) Regression method for assessing the efficacy of moisturizers. Cosmet Toilet 93:27–35
12. Gabard B (1994) Testing the efficacy of moisturizers. In: Elsner P, Berardesca E, Maibach HI (eds) Bioengineering and the skin: water and stratum corneum. CRC Press, Boca Raton, pp 147–170
13. Marks R (1997) How to measure the efects of emollients. J Dermatol Treatment 8 [Suppl 1]:S15–S18
14. Rogiers V, Derde MP, Verleye G, Roseeuw D (1990) Standardized conditions needed for skin surface hydration measurements. Cosmet Toilet 105:73–82
15. Barel AO, Clarys P (1995) Measurement of epidermal capacitance. In: Serup J, Jemec GBE (eds) Handbook of non-invasive methods and the skin. CRC Press, Boca Raton, pp 165–170
16. Salter D (1996) Non-invasive cosmetic efficacy testing in human volunteers: some general principles. Skin Res Tech 2:59–63
17. Berardesca E (1997) EEMCO guidance for the assessment of stratum corneum hydration: electrical measurements. Skin Res Tech 3:12–20
18. Wilhelm KP (1998) Possible pitfalls in hydration measurements. In: Elsner P, Barel AO, Berardesca E, Gabard B, Serup J (eds) Current problems in dermatology, vol 26. Skin bioengineering, techniques and applications in dermatology and cosmetology. Karger, Basel, pp 223–235
19. Paye M (1999) Models for studying surfactant interactions with the skin. In: Broze G (ed) Handbook of detergents, vol 2. Properties. Marcel Dekker, New York, in press
20. Paye M, Morrison Jr BM, Wilhelm KP (1995) Skin irritancy classification of body cleansing products. Comparison of two test methodologies. Skin Res Tech 1:30–35
21. Barel AO, Lambrecht R, Clarys P, Morrison BM Jr, Paye M (1999) Comparative study of the effect on the skin of two soap bars (a classical soap and a syndet) in normal use conditions and in the soap chamber test. Proceedings of the 3rd International symposium on irritant contact dermatitis, Rome, Italy, in press
22. Tagami H (1994) Hardware and measuring principle: skin conductance. In: Elsner P, Berardesca E, Maibach HI (eds) Bioengineering of the skin: water and stratum corneum. CRC Press, Boca Raton, pp 197–203
23. Salter D (1994) Further hardware and measurement approaches for studying water in the startum corneum. In: Elsner P, Berardesca E, Maibach HI (eds) Bioengineering and the skin: water and stratum corneum. CRC Press, Boca Raton, pp 205–215
24. Lévêque JL, De Rigal J (1983) Impedance methods for studying moisturization. J Soc Cosmet Chem 34:419–428
25. Van Neste D (1991) Comparative study of normal and rough human skin hydration in vivo: evaluation with four instruments. J Dermatol Sci 2:119–124
26. Clarys P, Barel AO, Gabard B (1999) Non invasive electrical measurements for the evaluation of the hydration state of the skin: comparison between three usual equipments, the Corneometer, the Skicon and the Nova DPM. Skin Res Tech 5:14–20

27. Courage W (1994) Hardware and measuring principle: Corneometer. In: Elsner P, Berardesca E, Maibach HI (eds) Bioengineering and the skin: water and stratum corneum. CRC Press, Boca Raton, pp 171–175
28. Barel AO, Clarys P (1997) In vitro calibration of the capacitance method (Corneometer CM 825) and conductance method (Skicon-200) for the evaluation of the hydration state of the skin. Skin Res Tech 3:107–113
29. Instruction manuel of the Corneometer CM 825 (1998). Courage-Khazaka Electronic, Cologne, Germany
30. Gabard B, Treffel P (1994) Hardware and measuring principle: the Nova DPM 9003. In: Elsner P, Berardesca E, Maibach HI (eds) Bioengineering and the skin: water and stratum corneum. CRC Press, Boca Raton, pp 177–196
31. Instruction manual of the Nova Dermal Phase Meter DPM 9003 (1998), Portsmouth, USA
32. Murray BC, Wickett RR (1996) Sensitivity of cutometer data to stratum corneum hydration level. Skin Res Tech 2:167–172
33. Instruction manual of the Skin Surface Hygrometer, Skicon -200 (1998), IBS Co, Tokyo, Japan
34. Nicander I, Ollmar S, Rozell BL, Emtestan (1997) Allergic contact reactions in the skin assessed by electrical impedance-a pilot study. Skin Res Tech 3:121–125
35. Instruction manual of the DermolabR (1998), Cortex Technology, Hadsund, Denmark
36. Instruction manual of the DermanalyserR 3F (1998), Robinson Electronic, Marsa, Malta
37. Potts RO, Guzek DB, Harris RR, McKie JE (1985) A non invasive, in vivo technique to quantitatively measure water concentration of the stratum corneum using attenuated total reflectance infrared spectroscopy. Arch Dermatol Res 277:489–495
38. Potts RO (1986) Stratum corneum hydration: experimental techniques and interpretations of results. J Soc Cosmet Chem 37:9–33
39. Lévêque JL (1993) Near infrared spectroscopy: a new approach to the characterization of dry skin. J Soc Cosmet Chem 44:197-
40. Lucassen GW, Van Veen GNA, Jansen JAJ (1998) Band analysis of hydrated human skin stratum corneum ATR-FTIR spectra in vivo. J Biomed Optics 3:267–280
41. Bindra RMS, Imhof RE, Andrew JJ, Cummins PG, Eccleston GM (1995) Opto-thermal measurement for the non-invasive non occlusive monitoring of in vivo skin conditions. Int J Cosmet Sci 17: 105–117
42. Xiao P, Imhof RE (1998) Optothermal measurement of water distribution within stratum corneum. In: Elsner P, Barel AO, Berardesca E, Gabard B, Serup J (eds) Current problems in dermatology, vol 26. Skin bioengineering, techniques and applications in dermatology and cosmetology. Karger, Basel, pp 48–60
43. Piérard G (1995) Relevance, comparison, and validation of techniques. In: Serup J, Jemec GBE (eds) Handbook of non-invasive methods and the skin. CRC Press, Boca Raton, pp 9–14
44. Pinnagoda J, Tupker RA, Agner T, Serup J (1990) Guidelines for trans epidermal water loss (TEWL) measurements. Contact Dermatitis 22:164
45. Pinnagoda J, Tupker RA (1995) Measurement of the transepidermal water loss. In: Serup J, Jemec GBE (eds) Handbook of non-invasive methods and the skin. CRC Press, Boca Raton, pp 173–178
46. Barel, AO, Clarys P (1995) Comparison of methods for measurement of transepidermal water loss. In: Serup J, Jemec GBE (eds) Handbook of non-invasive methods and the skin. CRC Press, Boca Raton, pp 179–184
47. Piérard G (1989) A critical approach to in vivo mechanical testing of the skin. In: Lévêque JL (ed) Cutaneous investigation in health and disease, non-invasive methods and instrumentation. Marcel Dekker, New York, pp 215–240
48. Agache PG (1995) Twistometry measurement of skin elasticity. In: Serup J, Jemec GBE (eds) Handbook of non-invasive methods and the skin. CRC Press, Boca Raton, pp 319–328
49. Gniadecka M, Serup J (1995) Suction chamber method for measurement of skin mechanical properties: The Dermaflex. In: Serup J, Jemec GBE (eds) Handbook of non-invasive methods and the skin. CRC Press, Boca Raton, pp 329–334
50. Barel AO, Courage W, Clarys P (1995) Suction method for measurements of skin mechanical properties: The Cutometer In: Serup J, Jemec GBE (eds) Handbook of non-invasive methods and the skin. CRC Press, Boca Raton, pp 335–341
51. Olsen Lo, Jemec GBE (1993) The influence of water, glycerin, paraffin oil and ethanol on skin mechanics. Acta Dermatol Venereol (Stockholm) 73:404–406
52. Barel AO, Lambrecht R, Clarys P (1998) Mechanical function of the skin: State of the art. In: Elsner P, Barel AO, Berardesca E, Gabard B, Serup J (eds) Current problems in dermatology, vol 26. Skin bioengineering, techniques and applications in dermatology and cosmetology. Karger, Basel, pp 223–235

53. Quan MB, Edwards C, Marks R (1997) Non-invasive in vivo techniques to differentiate photo-damage and ageing in human skin. Acta Dermatol Venereol (Stockholm) 77:416–419
54. Vilaplana J, Coll J, Trullas C, Azon A, Pelejero C (1992) Clinical and non invasive evaluation of 12% ammonium lactate emulsion for the treatment of dry skin in atopic and non atopic subjects. Acad Dermatol Venereol (Stockholm) 72:28–33
55. Querleux B (1995) Nuclear magnetic resonance (NMR). Examination of the epidermis in vivo. In: Serup J, Jemec GBE (eds) Handbook of non-invasive methods and the skin. CRC Press, Boca Raton, pp 33–139
56. Querleux B, Jolivet O, Bittoun J (1998) In vivo proton magnetic resonance spectroscopy in human skin. In: Elsner P, Barel AO, Berardesca E, Gabard B, Serup J (eds) Current problems in dermatology, vol 26. Skin bioengineering, techniques and applications in dermatology and cosmetology. Karger, Basel, pp 223–235
57. Gasmueller J, Kecskes A, Jahn P (1995) Stylus method for skin surface contour measurement. In: Serup J, Jemec GBE (eds) Handbook of non-invasive methods and the skin. CRC Press, Boca Raton, pp 83–88
58. Corcuff P, Lévêque JL (1995) Skin surface replica image analysis of furrows and wrinkles. In: Serup J, Jemec GBE (eds) Handbook of non-invasive methods and the skin. CRC Press, Boca Raton, pp 89–96
59. Efsen J, Hansen HN, Christiansen S, Keiding J (1995) Laser profilometry. In: Serup J, Jemec GBE (eds) Handbook of non-invasive methods and the skin. CRC Press, Boca Raton, pp 97–105
60. Mignot J (1997) Measurement of the microrelief of the skin. In: Barel AO, Rogiers V, Roseeuw D (eds) Intensive course in dermato-cosmetic sciences. VUB Press, Brussels, pp 316–343
61. Miller (1995) Sticky slides and tape techniques to harvest stratum corneum material. In: Serup J, Jemec GBE (eds) Handbook of non-invasive methods and the skin. CRC Press, Boca Raton, pp 149–151
62. Schatz H, Altmeyer P, Kligman AM (1995) Dry skin and scaling evaluated by D-Squames and im age analysis. In: Serup J, Jemec GBE (eds) Handbook of non-invasive methods and the skin. CRC Press, Boca Raton, pp 153–157
63. Serup J, Winther A, Blichman C (1989) A simple method for the study of scale pattern and effect of a moisturizer. Qualitative and quantitative evaluation bt D-Squame tape in comparison with parameters of epidermal hydration. Clin Exp Dermatol 14:277
64. Piérard GE, Piérard-Franchimont C, Saint Léger D, Kligman AM (1992) Squamometry: the assessment of xerosis by colorimetryof D-Squame adhesive discs. J Soc Cosmet Chem 47:298–305
65. Barel AO, Van de Straat R, Clarys P, Wessels B (1991) Quantitative biophysical measurements of the mildness properties of cleaning and detergent products in the hand immersion trest. Proceedings of the International Symposium on irritant Contact Dermatitis, Groningen, The Netherlands, p 76
66. Clarys P, Van de Straat R, Boon A, Barel AO (1992) The use of the hand forearm immersion test for evaluating skin irritation by various detergent solutions. Proceedings of the European Society of Contact Dermatitis, Brussels, Belgium, p 130
67. Clarys P, Eeckhout C, Taeymans J, Gross P, Barel AO (1992) Influence of short daily exposure to thermal water on th hydration state of the skin. In: Marks R, Plewig G (eds) The environmental threat to the skin. Martin Dunitz, London, pp 333–337
68. Barel AO, Clarys P, Wessels B, de Romsée A (1991) Non-invasive electrical measurements for evaluating the water content of the horny layer: comparison between capacitance and conductance measurement. In: Scott RC, Guy RH, Hadgraft J, Boddé HE (eds) Prediction of percutaneous penetration-methods, measurements, modelling. IBC Technical Services, London, pp 238–247
69. Cua AB, Wilhelm KP, Maibach HI (1990) Frictional properties of human skin: relation to age, sex and anatomical region, startum corneum hydration and trans epidermal water loss. Br J Dermatol 123:473–479
70. Bland M (1987) An introduction to medical statistics. Oxford University Press, Oxford, pp 1-365
71. Blichman CW, Serup J, Winter A (1989) Effects of a single application of a moisturizer: evaporation of emulsion water, electrical capacitance and skin surface (emulsion) lipids. Acta Dermatol Venereol (Stockholm) 69:327–330
72. Borroni G, Zaccone C, Vignati G, Vignoli GP, Berardesca E, Rabiosi G (1994) Dynamic measurements: sorption-desorption test. In: Elsner P, Berardesca E, Maibach HI (eds) Bioengineering and the skin: water and stratum corneum. CRC Press, Boca Raton, pp 217–222
73. Moss J (1996) The effect of 3 moisturizers on skin hydration, Electrical conductance (Skicon-200), capacitance (Corneometer CM420), and transepidermal water loss (TEWL). Skin Res Tech 2:32–36
74. Van Neste D (1994) Skin hydration in detergent-induced irritant dermatitis. In: Elsner P, Berardesca E, Maibach HI (eds) Bioengineering and the skin: water and stratum corneum. CRC Press, Boca Raton, pp 223–233

75. Wilhelm KP, Wolff HH, Maibach HI (1994) Effects of surfactants on skin hydration. In: Elsner P, Berardesca E, Maibach HI (eds) Bioengineering and the skin: water and stratum corneum. CRC Press, Boca Raton, pp 257–273

76. Paye M, Van De Gaer D, Morrison Jr BM (1995) Corneometry measurements to evaluate skin dryness in the modified soap chamber test. Skin Res Tech 1:123–127

77. Frosch PJ, Kligman AM (1979) The soap chamber test. A new method for assessing the irritancy of soaps. J Am Acad Dermatol 1:35–41

78. Simion FA, Rhein LD, Grove GL, Wotjotski JM, Cagan RH, Scala DS (1991) Sequential order of skin responses to surfactants during a soap chamber test. Contact Dermatitis 25:242–249

79 Clarys P, Barel AO (1997) Comparison of three detergents using the patch test and the hand:forearm immersion test as measurements of irritancy. J Soc Cosmet Chem 48:141–149

80. Clarys P, Manou I, Barel AO (1997) Influence of temperature on irritation in the hand/forearm immersion test. Contact Dermatitis 36:240–243

81. Manou I (1998) Evaluation of the dermatocosmetic properties of essential oils from aromatic plants by means of skin bioengineering methods. Ph D Thesis, Free University of Brussels (VUB), Brussels

CHAPTER 6

Oily Skin: Claim Support Strategies

R.L. Rizer

Introduction

Oily skin is perceived by many to be a serious cosmetic and medical problem, and it often provokes much concern for people who have it. The skin appears greasy and shiny, sometimes breaks-out (acne), and is often accompanied by large pores on the cheeks, nose, chin and forehead, mainly on the cheeks and nose. Skin with large pores is sometimes referred to as "orange peel" skin, and tends to be prone to break-outs with blackheads particularly common on the nose. People with oily facial skin tend to have trouble applying make-up, since the skin surface is greasy, and often is roughened due to large pores. Make-up often does not apply evenly, and its wearability is diminished by oil break-through, and settling into the pores.

Oily skin results from large quantities of sebum being produced by the sebaceous glands, filling the follicular reservoir, and spewing onto the skin surface. Sebum, or skin surface oil, is comprised largely of neutral lipids, and, consequently, is of little value in hydrating or conditioning the skin. The sebaceous follicles (facial pores) also provide an anaerobic environment for the bacterium *Propionibacterium acnes (P.acnes)*, an organism known to derive its energy source from the triglycerides in sebum, and contribute to the acne process. Impacted follicles are also susceptible to infestation of the Demodex mite, a saprophytic multicellular organism. Demodex mites appear to be more prevalent in rosacea and rosaceiform eruptions, and may play a role in the pathogenesis of rosacea [1].

Sebum functions primarily as an emollient, and has little or no contribution to the skin's epidermal barrier function. The common notion in the cosmetic industry and in the lay press that active oil production is healthy for dry skin is false. Sebum has no moisturizing properties. The degree of oiliness on the face was shown to be independent of skin moisture [2]. Moreover, the opposite of oily skin is not dry skin, but non-oily skin. Oily skin and dry skin can be found together on the face. People with oily skin rarely appear to have dry skin flaking, because if dry skin is present, the oil (sebum) flattens the opaque flakes and renders them transparent. Washing the skin with a cleanser or defatting the skin with hexane or ether will readily expose the flakes, if present. Skin dryness in African Americans is typically manifested as ashiness due to the opaqueness of the fine flakes against dark skin on the arms and legs where there are few sebaceous glands. However, ashiness is rarely observed on the face due to the presence of sebum. Skin flakiness may be present, but the sebum renders them invisible to the unaided eye. The transformation of opaqueness to transparency is the principle used to quantify sebum using the Sebumeter (Courage & Khazaka).

The rate at which sebum flows to the skin surface, the sebum excretion rate (SER), is dependent on the production rate of sebum by the sebaceous glands, the movement through the follicular reservoir, and the rate of sebum flow onto the skin surface from the reservoir. The degree of oiliness is dependent on genetic, endocrine and environmental factors [3]. Children of parents with very oily skin and large pores are likely to have oily skin and large pores as adults. Males tend to have oilier skin than females, since sebaceous gland activity is stimulated by testicular androgens. Females have a broad range of oiliness, and their sebaceous glands are primarily stimulated by adrenal and ovarian androgens. Children have little to no skin oiliness, but begin to exhibit slight oiliness and some acne as early as 7 years of age due to adrenarche, the period of development when the adrenal cortex begins to secrete pre-cursor androgens such as dehydroepiandrosterone and dehydroepiandrosterone sulfate. Adolescents have a surge of skin oiliness and acne when gonadal activity kicks in. Adults have a slow decline in sebum output with age, but the size of the sebaceous follicles (pores) often remain the same or become larger with age. This is highly unsettling to most adult women, and the condition of large pores has opened up a tremendous opportunity for some clever skin scientist or product development formulation chemist to find a way to minimize their appearance. Skin temperature can produce a 10% change in sebum output per 1°C [4]. Sebum output appears to be greatest in the mid-morning, and minimal during the late evening and early morning hours [5].

Five-Pronged Approach to Support Oily Skin Product Performance Claims

Why Is a Multi-pronged Approach Necessary?

Repeat purchase of products in a product category such as "oil control" is partially driven by the quality of the product, which is supported by the credibility of the *performance* and safety claims. Some examples of oil control claims are "helps adsorb excess oil: where needed; throughout the day; without disturbing moisture balance"; "lasting shine control"; and "rinses away surface oils." A self-assessment questionnaire fielded to a large number of trial consumers, or a biophysical method used in a clinical setting could be used to substantiate any of these examples. However, such a uni-dimensional approach is rarely sufficient to characterize a product's benefit, which could lead to a weak claim, and even more problematic, weak sales! A multidimensional approach provides greater power to a claim, since it reveals a broader information base regarding the product's complex interaction with the skin.

One of the most challenging tasks in supporting a claim is providing credible supporting data. One must understand the anatomy and physiology of the skin and the tools available to measure product effects at the level they are occurring. Moreover, it is important to leverage information directly extracted from the panelist's experience while using the product. Lastly, one must choose the best method of analysis and presentation of the data to draw conclusions that provide credible substantiation of a product claim.

Multi-Pronged Approach to Credible Product Performance Claim Support

The following approaches should be considered when developing claims to support product performance benefits.

Panelist Selection

The success of a clinical trial is dependent upon the recruitment of qualified subjects that are appropriate for the design and the purpose of the study. Examples of criteria that need to be considered include age range of the panel, gender, and whether a certain skin profile is required. For instance, consider a study where the goal is to evaluate the efficacy of an astringent toner targeted to women with oily skin and large pores, and designed to cleanse the skin of excess oil, and minimize facial pores. The first goal of recruiting would be to eliminate males from selection, and to recruit an age range of female panelists for which the test astringent toner has been targeted. In addition, women should be targeted having skin oiliness concerns and moderately large pores. A qualifying facial skin exam may be necessary. Moreover, the target population for your product may be of a specific ethnicity, such as Asian, or Hispanic women. The biological and cultural influences may be central determinants when formulating the product. Ethnic sensitivity may be manifested in many subtle ways [6], and formulating the astringent toner to address this issue may determine the success or failure in a foreign market. Pre-marketing testing with such ethnic populations can be crucial in assuring success in challenging foreign markets. Other more subtle, but important considerations for eligibility criteria are excluding individuals who have a recent history of using oil control astringent toners, and excluding medications that may interact with the active ingredients or may mask adverse reactions resulting from test product usage such as anti-inflammatory drugs, or medications that render the skin hypersensitive to sunlight.

Human Perception of Product Benefit

The panelists' perception of how a test product performs may be the most relevant dimension in evaluating our Astringent Toner example. Frequently the subjects' perception of product benefit gives the evaluator more than that which is captured by clinical grading or biophysical measurements. Certainly if the prospective consumer is unable to perceive the benefit that is claimed, they are unlikely to repeat the purchase, and the product is likely to be a failure. We obtain information from subjects regarding their perception of test products via questionnaires and post-study focus group interviews. *Written questionnaires* can be administered to subjects at intervals throughout the course of a study and/or at the conclusion of product use. They are useful in capturing not only information about product benefit, but may also be used to inquire about cosmetic preferences, intent to purchase, comparison to their regular brand, or product packaging and delivery attributes. Responses to questionnaires may also provide useful information for selecting the most desirable participants for inclusion in a focus group. Properly designed questionnaires are balanced so that the responder of a given question must choose from one or more positive responses, a neutral response, and one or more negative responses (the number of positive and negative choices must balance). "Top Box" analyses where there are two or more positive responses and one negative response are unreliable, and lead to false positive findings. Some questions require a "yes" or "no" answer, or a short open-ended narrative description.

Focus groups provide a unique forum for capturing feedback about subjects' thoughts and feelings regarding their experience using a test product. A moderator serves to initiate and guide the topics for discussion. The ensuing interactive group discussion about the subjects' experiences while using the product provides a wealth of dynamic information that cannot be obtained from written questionnaires alone.

One of the most important aspects of conducting a successful focus group is the selection of panelists. The selection process is dependent on the specific information desired about the test products. For instance, if broad feedback is desired, then the selection process might be a random one where the focus group population is representative of the study population. However, one might prefer to restrict the group to individuals who responded to the post-usage questionnaires in a certain way. For instance, if some of the subjects expressed displeasure with some aspect of the product or the way in which it was used or dispensed from the container, then a session with these individuals could be used to learn more about the nature of the specific problem. Focus group panels can also be chosen based on demographics, such as age, skin type or ethnicity.

Each focus group session is designed to last approximately 1 h and usually takes place with a group of about ten test subjects. The number of subjects interviewed in a session is kept low to encourage each member's participation in the discussion. Multiple groups can be interviewed in succession if a large number of participants is desired. To optimize interactions between subjects and the moderator, sessions are held in a large conference room where participants can sit facing one another. The facility is also equipped with a separate, candid viewing room where sessions can be privately monitored and videotaped. While the information obtained from focus groups is dynamic, it is generally not quantitative, since group sizes are too small. The information obtained is qualitative, and therefore not statistically significant. Nevertheless, this information can be some of the most valuable information one can obtain.

Clinical Assessment and Photodocumentation

Clinical assessment involves careful inspection of the skin, usually under magnification and blue daylight lighting, by a technician or physician trained to grade the full range of a skin attribute. Clinical grading can be particularly beneficial for assessing skin attributes that are not easily measured with bioinstrumentation. Examples of such attributes in the range of skin conditions associated with oily skin are pore size on the cheeks or nose. Clinical grading is especially powerful when combined with high quality clinical documentation photography. The old saying that a picture is worth a thousand words holds especially true with the skin.

A product that effectively controls skin oiliness or minimizes pores will produce changes in characteristics that can be perceived and graded by sight or touch. Severity of intensity or degree of improvement can be assessed using a 10 cm analog scale (10 cm line scale) so that changes in an attribute can be quantified and percent changes from baseline calculated. For instance, the clinical score at baseline or pre-treatment (V_0) is compared to the clinical score at a time after treatment has begun (V_n). The following relationship then enables one to calculate the percent change in the attribute as a function of treatment:

$$\frac{V_0 - V_n}{V_0} \times 100 = \% \text{ change in attribute}$$

Table 1. Oily skin conditions which occur typically on the head, chest, or back, and which can be clinically graded

---

Casual sebum/seborrhea
Large pores[a]
Acne (including blackheads)[a]
Rosacea[a]
Dandruff
Greasy hair
Skin clarity
Sallowness
Tactile roughness
Blemishes[a]
Irritation responses[a]

---

[a] Those conditions best suited for support with clinical documentation photography.

This method of clinical assessment of a product benefit can support claims like "reduces pore size by 30%". Clinical grading can be a simple ranking of an attribute as "mild", "moderate" or "severe". A common application of this method is for assessing potential product irritation such as erythema (redness), edema (swelling), and dryness/scaling, or sub-clinical irritation, such as burning, stinging, itching, tightness or tingling. For instance, stinging, tightness and tingling are typical symptoms associated with astringent toner use.

Table 1 shows the oily skin conditions which, typically occurring on the head, chest or back, can be clinically graded.

Clinical documentation photography lends credibility to the results obtained from clinical grading of certain skin attributes (see items above marked with an asterisk). Photographs taken prior to product use and at subsequent study visits provide a visual illustration of the gradual benefits that a test product provides over time of usage. A variety of photographic options are available for capturing the benefits of a test product. The choice of method should best reflect the skin parameter that the product is targeting. Examples of how some photographic methods accentuate different skin characteristics are illustrated herein. The photographic methods that are used most often are visible light photography, black light fluorescence photography, and cross-polarized light photography.

Visible Light Photography. Visible light photography, usually color photos are best, relies heavily on lighting and shadows to document textural facial features such as pores and blemishes/acne (Fig. 1a/b). Fuji Professional NPS 160 film is particularly effective in capturing the skin tones.

Black Light Fluorescence Photography. This type of photography effectively illustrates the presence of P.acnes in the sebaceous follicles by visualizing the fluorescence associated with the bacteria's porphyrin. Figure 2 shows the effectiveness of Pore Strips (Bioré) in removing the follicular impaction and P.acnes from the nose.

Cross-Polarized Light Photography. Cross-polarized light photography, usually color photos are best, reduces reflection of light from the surface of the skin thereby eliminating the shiny appearance and/or glare that can accompany visible light photogra-

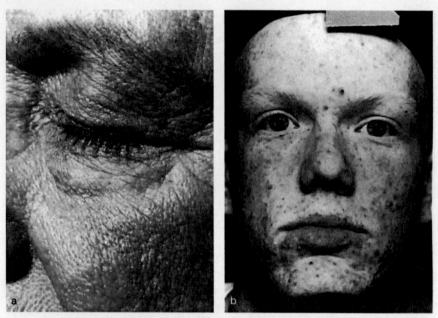

Fig. 1a, b. The photographs illustrate the ability to document textural features such as pores (a) and acne (b). The acne is illustrated here using cross-polarized light photography, which enhances the inflammatory aspect of the condition

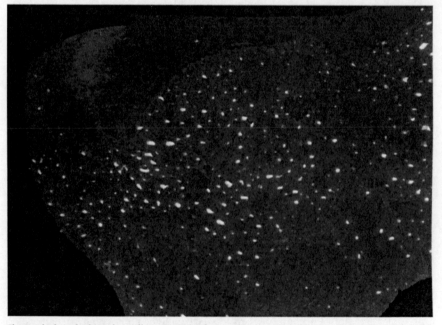

Fig. 2. Black and white photo illustrating the fluorescence associated with P.acnes taken with black-light photography. Each bright dot represents a follicular impaction removed from the nose with a commercial pore strip (Bioré)

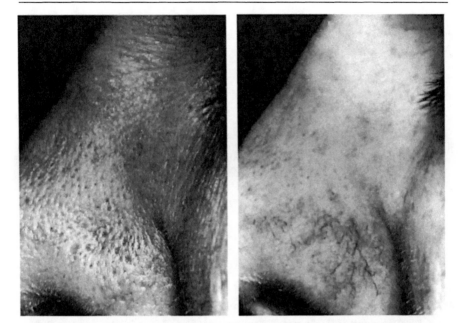

Fig. 3a, b. Black and white photo illustrating the effectiveness of a cross-polarizing filter in capturing pore impactions (a) and telangiectasia (b) of the nose. Skin surface features are eliminated by cross-polarized filter

phy. This technique is particularly helpful in accentuating the inflammatory nature of acne lesions, and teleangiectasia, which is red, finely branching skin capillaries typically found on the nose, cheeks and chin associated with rosacea, and showing the greasy, oily appearance of the skin as well as accentuating the presence of follicular impactions. Figure 3a/b illustrates the effectiveness of this method. Fuji Professional NPS 160 film is recommended.

Biophysical Methods

An integral part of claim substantiation is the ability to support clinical grading and panelists' perception of product benefit with objective biophysical measurements. Such measurements provide technical support for the more subjectively based results obtained with clinical grading. A brief description of selected biophysical methods and instrumentation is discussed below.

Parallel and Cross Polarized Light Video Imaging System [7]. The Zeiss DermaVision System illustrated in Figure 4 allows images of skin characteristics to be taken at a magnification that exceeds conventional photographic methods. The video camera, interfaced to a SV11 Zeiss Stereomicroscope, is connected to a Sony still video recorder (MVR-5300) and a Sony color video printer (UP-5200MD). Images are captured on magnetic disks for subsequent analog to digital conversion and image analysis. A polarized light illuminator (Schott KL1500) with a second polarizing filter (analyzer) allows the operator to visualize the skin surface features of the pores in the parallel polarized

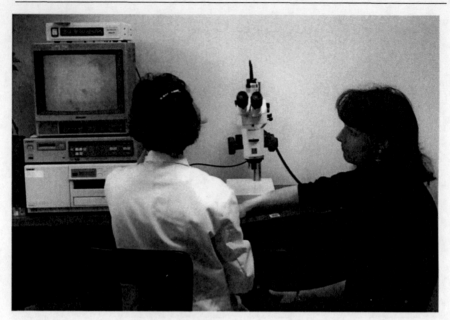

Fig. 4. Zeiss DermaVision Video Imaging System

mode, and the subsurface features of the impactions in the cross polarized mode. Magnified images of features such as facial pores can be digitized for image analysis of the number, and size of pores, and the number and size of impactions.

Sebum Measurements. Sebutape Patches [8] illustrated in Figure 5a/b are devices used to measure the rate of sebum excretion and/or the distribution of active sebaceous follicles. Estimates of these parameters are derived from image analysis of the transparent patterns left by facial oils deposited into the pores of the micro-porous, opaque tape. The sebum filled pores in the tape are no longer capable of scattering light so they appear transparent compared to the air-filled pores of the surrounding tape. Simple visual evaluations of these unique patches can be done by comparing them to reference patterns (Fig. 6). Much work has been done with these patches, and they have been found to be simple to use, and very effective in helping to objectively define "skin type" as well as quantifying sebum excretion rate [9,10]. Astringents, toners, and drugs which modulate sebotropic activity (e.g. antiandrogens) can be effectively evaluated using these patches.

The Sebumeter 810 PC [11] illustrated in Figure 7 is a device that measures the amount of sebum absorbed onto opaque tape. A cassette holds an opaque plastic tape that can be wound to expose new sections. When the cassette is pressed against the skin, the tape becomes transparent due to the absorbed sebum. The cassette is inserted into the device where the degree of transparency is measured by an optical method. The device is best suited for quantifying the "casual sebum" levels, and has been used to characterize skin type as well as evaluate the effects of cosmetics and drugs on skin surface lipids. The instrument has been successfully used to assess scalp sebum levels

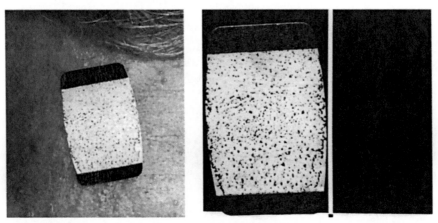

Fig. 5a,b. Sebutape Patches applied to the forehead (a), and then placed against a black background (b) for later image analysis of active follicles and amount of sebum collected

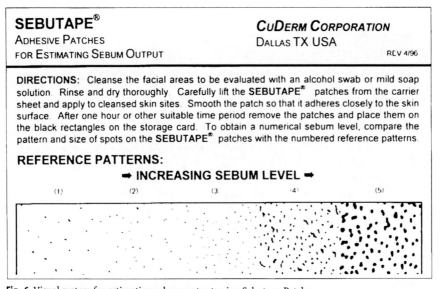

Fig. 6. Visual system for estimating sebum output using Sebutape Patches

by pressing the device onto the scalp. It thus has an advantage over the Sebutape method on hair bearing surfaces.

A Practical Example of Supporting Claims: Controlled Use Test

Skin Oiliness Control Studies

These studies are conducted to evaluate the effects of topically applied cosmetics designed to absorb sebum without drying the skin. Products like toners and clarifying

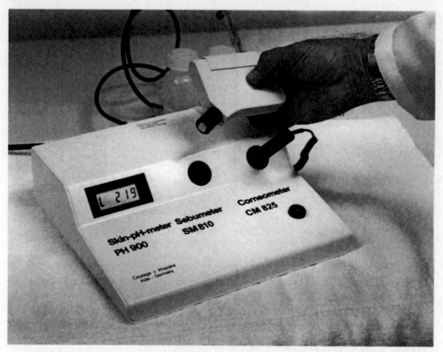

Fig. 7. Sebumeter 810 PC for measuring sebum output

lotions can help to keep the skin surface oil-free, and effectively reduce the amount of sebum in the sebaceous follicle, but their action is typically short lived, since seboge-nesis is a powerful process. The follicular reservoir can refill and begin spewing sebum onto the skin surface within a few hours after treatment. Therefore, products have been developed containing sebum adsorbers to help control skin shining, oil break-through and feathering problems. Product categories using this technology include foundations, loose and pressed powders, cleansers, sticks and oil control treatments. Technologies include Microsponge and Polytrap Transport Systems (Advanced Poly-mer Systems). Microsponge Skin Oil Adsorber 5640 Powder (Dow Corning Corporation) is a highly cross-linked polymethacrylate copolymer (CTFA Designation: Acrylates Copolymer) that selectively adsorbes sebum.

Studies designed to evaluate the properties of products designed to control skin oi-liness typically incorporate a combination of clinical, photographic and biophysical methods. At baseline, volunteer subjects with moderate to severe skin oiliness are qua-lified by determining their casual sebum levels using the Sebumeter. Prospective sub-jects report to the clinic at least 3 h after having cleansed their faces. Alternatively, sub-ject's foreheads or cheeks are cleansed with a mild liquid cleanser, defatted with hexa-ne, and then wear Sebutape patches for 30 min or 45 min to collect sebum. Sebutape samples from each individual are graded against a reference standard for low, mode-rate or high sebum levels. Individuals with moderate to high sebum levels are usually selected for enrollment provided they have met all other eligibility criteria. Factors such as age, gender, and endocrine status of prospective subjects may affect measurements. Consequently, control of these variables will benefit the outcome of these studies.

Degree of skin oiliness and shine can also be assessed by a trained clinical grader, and parallel polarized light photography can document the degree of shine. Test products are administered to the study population to use according to label instructions for varying periods of time, depending on the nature of the products, and the study design. At each subsequent clinic visit, measurements are taken as described above, and compared with baseline values to determine if the test product treatment had a desirable effect, in this case, on the condition of skin oiliness and skin shine. Properly designed and balanced self-assessment questionnaires are also administered in order to determine if the panel perceives a product benefit on these skin properties.

Sometimes its important to assess properties of a test product that are only evident during the first several hours. Foundations, for instance, can be assessed for wearability, oil breakthrough, settling, and other attributes. Careful clinical assessment with good color documentation photography and self-assessment questionnaires are the order of the day.

In conclusion, oily skin and large pores is a cosmetic frontier needing novel and effective products to control oiliness, and minimize the appearance of greasy skin or large pores. I have reviewed the essentials of a multi-pronged approach to support oily skin product performance claims, and included descriptions and illustrations of each. It is hoped that this approach will help validate effective products so desperately needed to address these cosmetic and medical conditions.

Acknowledgements. Special thanks are given to Robert Goodman, professional photographer, Dallas, TX, for assistance with clinical photodocumentation procedures.

References

1. Bonnar E, Eustace P, Powell FC (1993) The Demodex mite population in rosacea. J Am Acad Dermatol 28:443
2. Fisher LB (1998) Exploring the relationship between facial sebum level and moisture content. J Cosmet Science 49:53
3. Pochi PE, Strauss JS (1974) Endocrinologic control of the development and activity of the human sebaceous gland. J Invest Dermatol 62:191
4. Cunliffe WJ, Burton JL, Shuster S (1970) Effect of local temperature variations on sebum excretion. Br J Dermatol 83:650
5. Burton JL, Cunliffe WJ, Shuster S (1970) Circadian rhythm in sebum excretion. Br J Dermatol 82:497
6. Stephens TJ, Oresajo C (1994) Ethnic sensitive skin. Cosmet Toilet 109:75
7. Dorogi PL, Jackson EM (1994) In vivo video microscopy of human skin using polarized light. J Toxicol Cut & Ocular Toxicol 13:97
8. Miller DL (1996) Application of objective skin type kits in research and marketing. In: Cosmetics and toiletries manufacture world wide (1996 Annual). Aston Publishing, Hertfordshire, p 233
9. Nordstrum KM, Schmus HG, McGinley KJ, Leyden JJ (1986) Measurement of sebum output using a lipid absorbent tape. J Invest Dermatol 87:260
10. Piérard G, Piérard-Franchimont C (1992) The Sebutape technique for monitoring androgen dependent disorders. European J Med 1:109
11. Schäfer H, Kuhn-Bussius H (1970) Methodik zur quantitativen Bestimmung der menschlichen Talgsekretion. Arch Klin Exp Dermatol 238: 429

CHAPTER 7

On the Problems of In Vivo Cleansing of the Human Skin

K. Schrader

Main Problems

Cleansers for the human skin are characterized by their delipidizing, dehydrating and protein-influencing effects.

Whereas the dehydrating effect can be tested – albeit in an indirect way only – via skin resistance and natural frequency measurements, it is difficult to record in vivo protein-influencing effects owing to the variety of nitrogenous compounds. The cleansing and delipidizing effect, however, can be determined in a manner that is directly reproducible.

The dehydrating effect on the stratum corneum is preceded by hydration initially. One minute after washing with sodium lauryl sulfate, for instance, the degree of hydration increases as a function of the duration of washing. Initial hydration after application of sodium lauryl sulfate solutions is much greater than after washing with water.

An interesting question that arises is the extent to which this phenomenon is linked to the compatibility of the cleanser. Tests on this issue were carried out at Henkel [1] on the basis of the swelling of pig's skin.

Hydration comes to an end almost immediately after the washing process, and dehydration sets in after about 30 minutes. This dehydration depends on the type of surfactants used. Gloor et al. [2] found that sodium lauryl sulfate, in a concentration that achieved the same washing effect as other surfactants tested, resulted in much greater dehydration [3].

A pH-dependency of the surfactants has also been discovered. The more alkaline the washing effect, the greater the dehydration was found to be [4]. Accordingly, a washing solution always leads to a dehydration effect but this does not necessarily parallel the washing effect. The effect of surfactants on the barrier was examined [5]. Sodium lauryl sulfate was applied to lipid liposomes of the stratum corneum. It was found that the surfactant was deposited in the liposomes, with the structure of the membranes remaining completely stable. However, this did result in increased permeability through the liposome membrane.

These results demonstrate that the barrier function can be changed solely by depositing surfactants without destruction of the barrier. If surfactants exercise a strong action on the skin, this can cause lipids to emulsify out and thus damage the barrier function. Each wash process on the skin destroys the hydrolipid mantle.

According to Gloor [2], repetitive washing causes the moisture level of the stratum corneum to fall, leading to persistent impairment of the water-binding capability of the stratum corneum [6]. Cleansing of the skin is meant to be mild yet thorough. It is important for the cleanser to be adapted to the type and scale of dirt. This is particularly necessary with regard to commercial cleansers. There will always be some sort of trade-off between cleansing effect and skin compatibility. Longer, more intensive cleansing procedures generally entail some loss in skin compatibility.

As far as general personal cleansing is concerned, it is not really washing power that is at issue, because too much wash-active substance is frequently applied to the skin, with the result that most of it goes down the drain unused. In this case there is a chance for product development activities to aim for greater skin compatibility. Evidently the problem cannot be solved by means of conventional refatting agents [7]. Cetiol HE and isopropyl palmitate have not brought a solution according to Gloor [8]. The focus of a good product should therefore always be to incorporate less wash-active substance, and milder surfactants instead. This often makes up for the financial drawbacks. As far as the use of cleansing products is concerned, attention should be paid to differentiation to cater for various skin types.

Consumers frequently rate the "effect" of a cleansing product by its lather. In contrast to modern washing machine detergents, industry has – so far – been unable to relate less lather to unchanged, not entailed other qualities or to furnish an explaination of this.

A commercial skin cleanser generally consists of the following raw material categories:

Various surfactants	For all dirt, fat-/oil-soluble and pigments
Abrasives	For stubborn dirt, e.g. grease, soot, metal particles
Special solvents	For heavy dirt, e.g. adhesives, resins, fats, oils
Reductives	For special dirt, e.g. dyes

All that is needed for a body cleanser is a balanced, mild surfactant system which may be coupled with an abrasive to remove dead skin cells. Polyethylene, finely ground almond meal and finely ground walnut shell meal frequently come into question here.

We recently examined two so-called ultracleansers with regard to their cleansing effect and their potential side-effects on the stratum corneum barrier. We have also carried out experiments on various basic surfactants under the above-mentioned aspects.

Table 1 shows cleansers B and C, and the associated INCI declaration. Comparing the two preparations shows that they differ in the two abrasives: lactose and walnut shell meal. Whereas lactose dissolves in the aqueous cleansing procedure, the walnut shell meal remains undissolved. These two abrasives are almost identical as far as their grain size is concerned and ensure, not least because of their rounded grain shape, that cleansing does not cause any injury. The solvents are identical but the surfactants are different. This is why these two preparations were compared.

A wide range of surfactants are used in the formulation of cosmetic cleansers. Some selected washing raw materials were examined, and are shown in Table 2. The results are intended to help developers of cosmetic cleansers to make choices easier with regard to effects and side-effects of these basic surfactants.

Surfactants have repeatedly been the subject of various skin-physiological tests in the past [9]. Here, too, an optimum preparation entails a benefit/risk assessment, and it is frequently necessary to compromise, for reasons of cost in particular. Application parameters, i.e. visual rating characteristics such as lather, stickiness on the skin, rinsability, fragrance and the like, have to be optimized in a well-formulated preparation.

Table 1. Cleansers B and C and the associated INCI declaration. Two ultracleanser compounds are compared

Raw material	Product B	Product C[a]
Mineral Oil	+	-
Talloweth-15	+	-
Lactose	+	-
Juglans regia	-	+
Trideceth-8	+	
C12–18 Pareth-5	-	+
Silica	+	+
Quaternium-18 bentonite	-	+
Laureth-3	+	-
Beeswax	+	
Cellulose acetate butyrate	-	+
Perfume	-	+
Propylene carbonate	-	+
CJ 77891	-	+
Dimethyl glutarate	+	+
Dimethyl adipate	+	+
Dimethyl succinate	+	+
Sodium polyacrylate	-	+
Octyl stearate	-	+

[a] Samples were provided courtesy of Stockhausen

Table 2. Examination of some selected washing raw materials

INCI name	Abbreviation	Molar mass	Active content	% Content of 0.05% molar mass	pH of 0.05% molar solution
Sodium lauryl sulfate	SLS	289	90%	1.445	7.3
Sodium laureth sulfate	SLES	282	28%	1.910	7.2
Decyl glucoside	DG	809	Approx. 50%	4.405	7.0
Disodium laureth sulfosuccinate	DSLS	542	38–42%	2.710	6.6

As far as personal cleansers are concerned, the focus is not so much on determining their cleansing effect because sufficient surfactant concentrations are available. However, other skin-physiological parameters – such as effect on the surface of the skin, changes to transepidermal loss of water, improvement of compatibility with the skin and mucous membranes, and the sensation of the skin – should be self-evident, objective criteria for good products.

To achieve this, it is necessary to consider a variety of human skin irritation factors to be tested (Table 3).

To determine the washing effect of surfactants or cleansing products, it is advisable to carry out a washing test knowing the compatibility of the surfactants and their mixtures. In designing the test it must be ensured that the concentration of the wash-active substances is not too high (0.1–0.3%) as this would make it impossible to evaluate the differences between the effects.

Table 3. Variety of human skin irritation factors

Roughness of the skin	Various methods	Objective
Elasticity of the skin	No reproducible method	–
	Various methods known so far	Objective
Sebum content	Various methods	Objective
Water content	Various methods	Objective
Skin picture (erythema, peeling, cracks)		Subjective
Subjective sensations (stinging, itchiness, tautness)		Subjective
pH value		Objective
Alkali neutralization time and resistance		Objective
Blood flow	Various methods	Objective

There are various ways of ascertaining washing power. A common in vitro method of testing the defatting effect of surfactants is based on the defatting of wool yarn. However, this gravimetric process only records the lipophile part of the dirt [14]. According to Würbach [15], the skin lipids are extracted on the backs of the volunteers and determined before and after washing using a device called a washing dome.

Also in this case only the skin lipids are recorded. Gehring [7] operates with a foam roller – similar to a paint roller – which, with its weight of 200 g, is moved to and fro on the forearm. Model dirt is rubbed into the forearm beforehand. The colour of the forearm is measured by means of a chromameter in the L*a*b* system before and after washing, the difference is determined and the washing power is calculated from this. This test can also be repeated without model dirt. Then, squalene is eluted as an indicator for the sebaceous gland lipids, and detected by means of HPLC directly from the skin.

Tronnier dealt with the measuring of washing power at an early stage [16]. He developed the model dirt which is shown above and which, according to our experience, represents a good cross-section of all types of dirt that occur. The basis for this is a water-in-oil emulsion (Table 4).

We developed a skin washing machine of our own because we felt the methods outlined did not reflect real life accurately enough (Fig. 1). The model dirt described above is needed to carry out a standard test of the cleansing effect. It replaces the most important noxae for the cleanser in the shape of one standard noxa. The model dirt F (see below), which was provided courtesy of Stockhausen, was used for commercial cleansers, and the model dirt as described above for detergency of other surfactants.

Table 4. Formulation of model dirt

Raw material	%	Supplier
Sicomet-Red F (CI12150)	4	BASF, Ludwigshafen
Sicovit-Cochenille Red (CI16255)	4	BASF, Ludwigshafen
Sicomet-Red P (CI12490)	4	BASF, Ludwigshafen
Protegin	17	Goldschmidt, Essen
Tegin O spec.	2.5	Goldschmidt, Essen
Lanolin, anhydricum	5.5	
Perl. paraffin oil	6.5	
Vaseline	10.0	
Demineralized water	46.5	

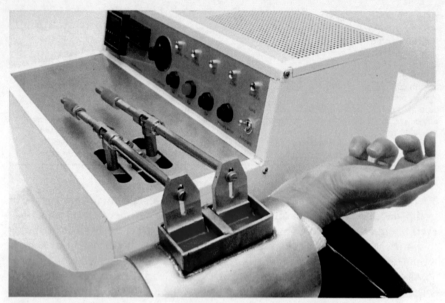

Fig. 1. Skin washing machine

Table 5. Composition of model dirt

Castrol	15 g
Vaseline	5 g
Adeps Lanae	5 g
Graphite	1 g
Flame soot	1.5 g
Iron oxide (Fe_2O_3)	0.2 g

Model dirt F has the composition shown in Table 5. This is mixed one-to-one with a commercially available green lacquer.

The experiments were carried out with the skin washing machine shown above [17]. This machine simulates the process of washing by moving the washing arms to and fro over the skin in an ideal way.

Skin Washing Machine: Description of the Device

Two parallel, excentrically driven washing arms, which have needle-punched felt on them, are applied at constant pressure to the skin of the forearm and moved to and fro at a defined speed.

An inflatable cuff in the washing unit presses the forearm onto the two parallel surfactant containers, thus causing the skin to form a natural seal. A defined quantity and concentration of the cleansers to be tested is filled into these containers, and the washing arm heads are inserted.

Table 6. Conditions for the skin washing machine

Size of the test areas	4×4 cm
Model dirt compositions:	See tables 4 and 5
Quantity of model dirt applied:	20 ml / skin area
Time for model dirt to dry:	10 minutes at room temperature
Water to moisten (if necessary):	0.1 ml
Temperature of test solution:	22° C
Volume of test chambers:	24 ml
Type of felt:	Needle-punched felt
Weight (on the washing arms):	16 g
Angle (of the washing arms on skin):	90°
Speed:	48 movements/minute
Washing time:	60 s

Conditions for the skin washing machine are shown in Table 6. The cleansing effect is rated with the aid of a chromameter (Figure 2) according to the L*a*b* colour system [18]:

$$\frac{\text{Washing effect measurement} - \text{Dirt effect measurement}}{\text{Skin colour measurement} - \text{Dirt effect measurement}}$$

Unwanted effects on the skin were recorded by means of non-invasive skin physiology techniques [19, 20].

Before and after washing, replicas of the skin were taken of the washing area and the skin profiles of these were examined using laser profilometry. Any barrier damage was ascertained by measuring transepidermal water loss with the Tewameter DM 210 from Courage and Khazaka.

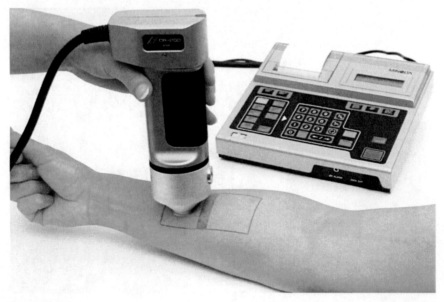

Fig. 2. Chromameter

Irritative effects were determined by the patch test or the flex wash test, and compatibility with the mucous membrane was examined with an in vitro method.

Flex Wash Test

The flex wash test is a standard method of testing surface-acting agents and surfactant end products. It is carried out on 20 volunteers with healthy skin. The product is applied to the flex twice a day for 5 days. At each application, the bend of the elbow is lathered with the first test sample, and then washed by hand for two minutes. After rinsing, there is another two-minute wash, and then the area is rinsed and dabbed dry. The washing procedure is carried out nine times in all. To determine any unwanted reactions induced by the test products, the volunteers are asked, at the end of the test, about any reactions that occurred directly after washing and the test manager records any visible signs [30, 32].

Laser-scanned data can be used to quantify the differences between various surfactants or cleansers in respect of their properties that affect the structure of the skin surface in an in use test [21, 22]. A robotic device with an optical autofocus sensor is employed for touch-free scanning of the skin replica [30]. The silicon replicas are fed into the laser scanner automatically by means of a robot system and measured (Fig. 3). The change to the profile of the skin is quantified on the basis of various DIN parameters. A paired Wilcoxon test is carried out to verify changes that are found between the untreated and treated states.

Laser profilometry permits greater resolution than mechanical profilometry [23] (Fig. 3).

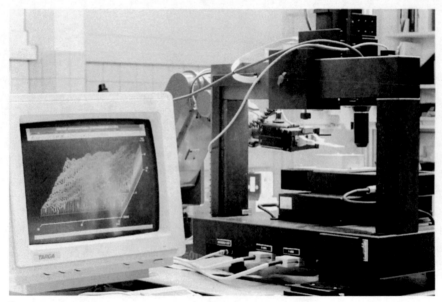

Fig. 3. Laser scanner

Patch Test

The patch test is regularly used to examine the compatibility of surfactants. In our opinion, it is suitable for screening at best, or as a supplement to other examinations, because the occlusive nature of this test is too far removed from actual practice.

This test can be quantified by measuring transepidermal water loss in parallel [24]. The TEWL value is incorporated because of the observation that every disorder of the stratum corneum induced by a surfactant leads to an increase in transepidermal water loss. This method is particularly suitable for comparative tests.

Figure 8 shows an example of the percentage change of TEWL measured over time after treatment with a 5% surfactant [25]. In vitro tests have tended to be of a guiding nature only so far because they are often not precise enough.

Red Blood Cell Test

The red blood cell test according to Pape and Hoppe [26] (Fig. 4) characterizes the typical irritative interrelationships of surfactants with intact cell structures and the destruction of blood cells and the oxyhaemoglobin that is released. Photometry is applied to the process of haemolysis to determine the concentration of the surfactant in µl/ml of wash-active substance which destroys 50% of the erythrocytes in isotonic buffer solution.

The denaturation of the haemoglobin by a 1% surfactant solution is also determined photometrically. Irritation is calculated from the obtained values according to the Mean Indices of Ocular Irritations equation:

$$\text{MIO I} = \frac{189}{\sqrt{H/D}} + 0.054$$

Fig. 4. Red blood cell test

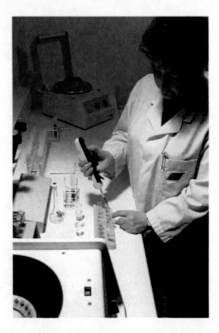

Application of Wash Tests in the Assessment of Model Cleansers (Table 1)

The following experiments are carried out with the orienting hand washing test (Table 7) [28] and our skin washing machine. One hand each is washed in the morning and evening with one product each.

Table 7. Orienting hand washing test

1. 0.5 g of model dirt is spread over the palms and backs of the hands, and then rubbed in for 45 s
2. The model dirt is left to dry for 1.5 min
3. 1.2 g of the test product is applied and rubbed in
4. 1 ml of water is added, and washing takes place for 30 s
5. Again, 1 ml of water is added, and washing takes place for 30 s
6. The washed areas are rinsed with cold flowing water[a]

[a] Rating of the cleansing effect on a 6-point scale (average ascertained by 2 test managers and the volunteers): 0 = clean, 1 = slight amount of residual dirt, 2 = medium amount of residual dirt, 3 = large amount of residual dirt, 4 = very large amount of residual dirt, 5 = no cleansing effect at all

Hand Washing Test (Subjective Rating, n = 20)

Figure 5 shows the residual dirt on the palm and back of the hands. Here, preparation B is distinctly superior to preparation C as far as washing power is concerned.

The tests that were carried out with the skin washing machine on the same volunteers returned the results according to Figure 6.

The cleansing effect of sodium lauryl sulfate was defined as the standard (=100%) and was plotted against the products. Furthermore water was rated as a negative standard and a 2% sodium lauryl sulfate solution as a positive standard.

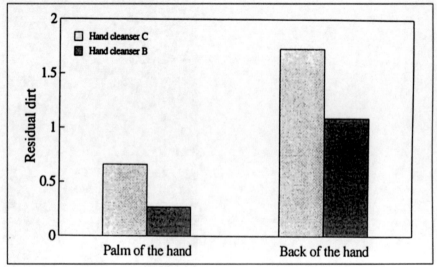

Fig. 5. Hand washing test

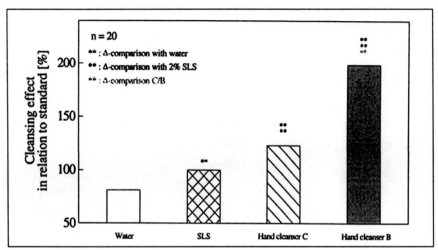

Fig. 6. Washing tests with model dirt

Skin Washing Machine Test

The advantage of the skin washing machine over the subjective hand washing test is that two products can be tested under the same conditions.

Figure 6 shows a comparison of preparations B and C.

Whereas product B again demonstrates washing power that is twice that of sodium lauryl sulfate, C only achieves 60% greater washing power than sodium lauryl sulfate. The results of the washing tests therefore have a similar tendency.

Profilometry

Laser profilometry was used to compare skin replicas 5 and 24 hours after the last wash with the initial values [33]. The rating was based on DIN parameters (DIN 4762) in the material testing technology. The parameters have the following meaning: Ra = mean roughness index, Rz (DIN) = mean peak-to-valley height from five successive measuring distances

Products B and C are compared in Figure 7. Whereas B demonstrates distinct smoothing values for both parameters (Ra and Rz DIN) after five hours and lower values after 24 hours, product C hardly changes the surface of the skin in this test.

Transepidermal Water Loss

The TEWL results after 5 and 24 hours (Fig. 8) in this test series indicate that the barrier function has been damaged by the cleansing procedure, which is expressed more or less in increased TEWL figures. As earlier results showed [29], an increase in TEWL implies less skin compatibility.

The difference to the initial value after 5 hours indicates an increase in transepidermal water loss for both preparations. After 24 hours, transepidermal water loss tends to fall with preparation B, whereas it is still rising with preparation C.

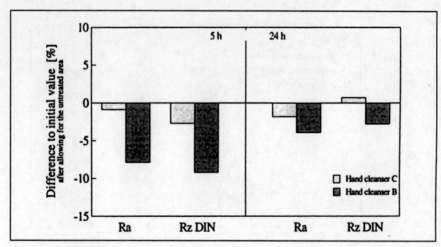

Fig. 7. Laser profilometry

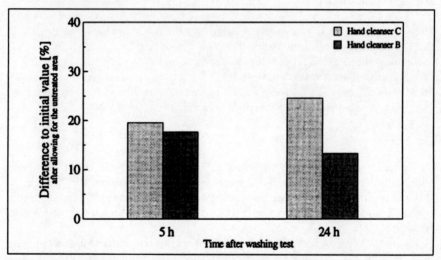

Fig. 8. TEWL measurement

Comparing the results of the skin-physiological parameters for the tested ultra-cleansers reveals that hand cleansing can be accompanied by unwanted effects. The type of side-effects and their severity, however, can be influenced by means of skilful galenic formulations. The selection, and thus the composition, of commercial cleansers should always be based on the principle of better compatibility. A milder skin cleansing may inevitably be connected to spending more time. However, this is in favour of better compatibility.

Results of Basic Surfactants

The cleansing results (in relation to the standard 100% = sodium lauryl sulfate 1/20 molar) on the basis of the model dirt described on p. 95 are shown in descending order. Whereas sodium laureth sulfate achieves a cleansing value that is close to that of sodium lauryl sulfate, disodium laureth sulfosuccinate falls below that and decyl

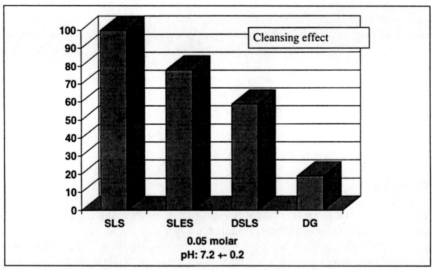

Fig. 9. Cleansing effect in vivo

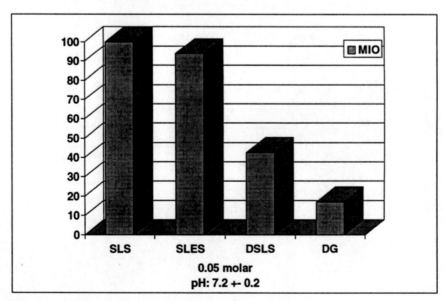

Fig. 10. Compatibility with the eye mucous membrane in vitro

glucoside is particularly weak. This result can be due to the molar concentration used, but this does not have any direct practical significance for skin with a normal level of dirt (Fig. 9).

Figure 10 shows the in vitro results for various surfactants in relation to sodium lauryl sulfate as the standard. Practically no difference was recorded between SLS and SLES. DSLS caused much less irritation, and DG caused even less.

A variety of methods have been suggested to test the irritation potential on human beings. Basically, each method can only cover some partial aspects. It is, therefore, expedient and necessary to combine the results of different methods and to evaluate them simultaneously. Using different methods is generally more meaningful than, for instance, increasing the number of volunteers on the panel, and involves the same amount of effort.

Despite the many discussions that have been held about the patch test, it is still frequently used to test the compatibility of surfactants [29]. This test can be quantified by parallel measurements of the transepidermal water loss (Fig. 11). This figure shows the percentage change of TEWL measured over time after treatment with surfactants. It is given in relation to sodium lauryl sulfate as the standard (= 100%). The results that have been analysed are well below those of the reference surfactant.

Flex Wash Test

The flex wash test is another test approach to characterize mild surfactants. In this case, the test/reference surfactants are rated in a half-side test by the volunteers.

The volunteers apply the samples in manual washes to the bend of the elbow, which is a sensitive area, under qualified control conditions twice a day for two weeks.

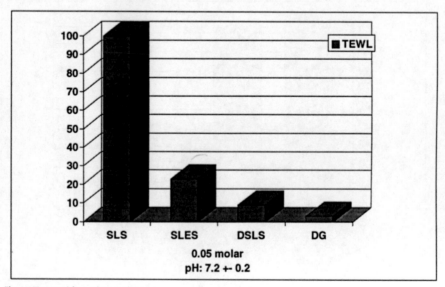

Fig. 11. Transepidermal water loss

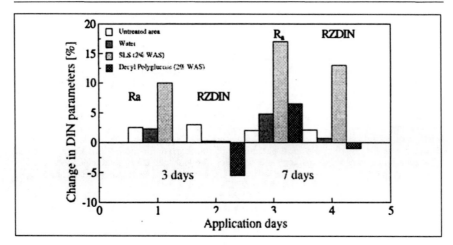

Fig. 12. Percentage change in Ra and RzDIN parameters

Subjective findings such as itching, tingling, stinging and tautness are rated in addition to visible signs such as reddening and desquamation. An irritation score is ascertained in this test from individual ratings for each surfactant in respect of various criteria. Here, too, sodium lauryl sulfate can act as the reference substance.

Laser-scanned data can be used to quantify the difference between surfactants with regard to their effects on skin structure in an in use test. Test design: 20 volunteers, forearms.

Generally, silicon replicas are taken and analysed before the test and 14 days after it (12 hours after the final application). Figure 12 shows an extract of the test results. Here, however, a skin replica was taken and measured after 3 and 7 days of application of the surfactants.

Distinct structure changes induced by the tested surfactants can be seen in respect of the DIN parameters which have been transferred to an area basis. In comparison, the untreated and water-treated areas show hardly any changes.

The tests discussed here are intended to show chemists developing cosmetic cleansers that it is possible to achieve a highly compatible end product by allowing for various skin-physiological criteria when choosing surfactants. In doing so multiple parameters should always be considered.

The prime objective must be to compare the obtained values with results achieved in practice. They should be reconstructable. It is therefore advisable to carry out an additional dermatologically controlled in use test for the end product in addition.

Summary

The results of the tests show that skin-physiological methods can be additionally applied when testing the washing power both of commercial cleansers and of basic surfactants. The aim is to optimize the benefit/risk ratio. It is possible to draw upon the above-mentioned in vitro skin-physiological ratings, although these may not yet be recognized officially, as well as on in vivo ratings. Multiple test parameters corroborate the scientific evidence.

References

1. Osberghaus R, Gloxhuber C, van Raay HG, Braig S (1978) Hydagen: Ein neuer Feuchtigkeitsregulator – Methoden und Ergebnisse des Wirkungsnachweises. I. Soc. Cosmet. Chem. 29:133-146
2. Gloor M (1994)Hornschichtbarriere und ihre Modulation. H+G Band 69, Heft 10:656-661
3. Gehring W, Geier J, Gloor M (1991) Untersuchungen über die austrocknende Wirkung verschiedener Tenside. Dermatol Monatsschr 177:257-264
4. Gehring W, Gehse M, Zimmerman, V, Gloor M (1991) Effects of pH changes in a specific detergent multicomponent emulsion on the water content of stratum corneum. J Soc Cosm Chem 42:327-333
5. Downing DT, Abraham W, Wegner BK, Willman KW, Marshall JL (1993) Partition of sodium dodecyl sulfate into stratum corneum lipid liposomes. Arch Dermatol Res 255:151-157
6. Berardesca E (1993) Physiological parameters of skin barrier function. Third Congress of the European Academy of Dermatology and Venerology Kopenhagen 26–30 September 1993
7. Gehring W, Kemter K, Nissen H.-P., Gottfreund J, Gloor M (1995) Vergleichende Untersuchungen zum entfettenden Einfluß einer Waschlösung. H+G Band 70, Heft 9:643-648
8. Molls W, Schrader K (1986) Vergleichende Lipidmessung an der menschlichen Haut. FSA 194–196
9. Bielfeld S (1990) Vergleich hautphysiologischer Methoden zur Ermittlung des Einflusses von Tensiden auf die menschliche Haut. parfümerie und Kosmetik, 71 Jahrgang, Nr. 5:312-318
10. Schrader K (1990) Praxisbezogene hautphysiologische Untersuchungskriterien mit Seifen und Syndets. P&K, 10:686
11. Schrader K (1992) Meßmethoden zur Prüfung von Kosmetika. SÖFW 118:1411
12. Frosch P (1985) Hautirritationen und empfindliche Haut. (Grosse Scripta 7) Grosse, Berlin
13. Braun-Falco O, Korting HC Gollhausen R (eds) (1990) Griesbach Konferenz, Hautreinigung mit Syndets. Springer, Berlin Heidelberg New York
14. Modde H, Schuster G, Tronnier H (1965) Experimentelle Untersuchungen zum Problem der Hautverträglichkeit anionaktiver Tenside in der Arbeitsmedizin. Tenside 2:368-373
15. Würbach G (1981) Entfettung der Hautoberfläche durch Tenside in Abhängigkeit von Konzentration und Konstitution, Kosmetiksymposium, Halle
16. Tronnier H (1965) Zur Standardisierung von Waschversuchen an der menschlichen Haut FSA 67:7
17. Schrader K (1990) Reinigungswirkung von Syndet-Zubereitungen: Methodische Grundlagen ihrer Erfassung. In: Braun-Falco O, Korting HC (eds) Hautreinigung mit Syndets. Springer, Berlin Heidelberg New York, p 151
18. Schrader K (1990) Reinigungswirkung von Syndet-Zubereitungen: Methodische Grundlagen ihrer Erfassung. P&K 71/10:151-161
19. Elsner P (1995) Reinigungswirkung von Syndet-Zubereitungen: Methodische Grundlagen ihrer Erfassung. In: Tebbe B, Goerdt S, Orfanos CE (eds) Dermatologie. Thieme, Stuttgart, p 28
20. Hevert F et al (1989) Arbeitsmedizin, Sozialmedizin, Präventivmedizin 10:235-237
21. Fiedler M, Müller U (1993) Strukturen der Hautoberfläche TW Dermatologie 23:331-339
22. Rohr M, Schrader K (1994) Surfactant-induced skin roughness. Euro Cosmetics 8:24-28
23. Wolff, KH, et al (1993) The psoriasis plaque test and topical corticosteroids evaluation by computerized laser profilometry. Curr Probl Dermatol 21:107-113
24. Zienicke H (1990) Hautfeuchtigkeit (transepidermaler Wasserverlust): Meßmethoden und Abhängigkeit von Waschverfahren. In: Braun-Falco O, Korting HC (eds) Hautreinigung mit Syndets. Springer, Berlin Heidelberg New York, pp137–145
25. Schrader K, Rohr M (1994) Tenside – Ihre Beurteilung hinsichtlich Wirkung und Nebenwirkungen. Euro Cosmetics 1–2:18–23
26. Richtler HJ, Knaut J (1988) World prospects for surfactants. 2nd World Surfactants Congress, "Surfactants in our word – today und tomorrow", Paris, 24-27 May, Vol IV, pp 414–428
27. Kalweit S, Gerner I, Spielmann M (1987) Validation Project of Alternatives for the Draize Eye Test. Mol Toxicol 1:579-603
28. Komp et al (1989) Haut und Beruf. In: Tronnier H, Kresken J, Jablonski K, Komp B (eds). Grosse, Berlin, p 101
29. Frosch PJ (1982) Irritancy of soaps and detergent bar 5. In: Frost P, Horwitz SN (eds) Principles of cosmetics for the dermatologist. Mosby, St. Louis Toronto London
30. Rohr M, Schrader K (1995) Hautphysiologische in vivo Untersuchungen verschiedener Tenside. Skin Care Forum 12:12
31. Jackwerth B (1995) Fettalkoholpolyglycoside – eine neue Tensidgeneration mit besonderer Hautverträglichkeit. Skin Care Forum 12:4
32. Schrader, K, Rohr M (1996) Methods for measuring the skin-cleansing effect of surfactans in comparison with skin roughness and compatibility. Clin Dermatol 14:57-65

CHAPTER 8

Methods for Antiperspirant and Deodorant Efficacy Evaluations

J.E. Wild, J.P. Bowman, L.P. Oddo

Introduction

Claims support documentation is a requirement for all types of products including cosmetic products. The globalization of products has made the documentation of a product's safety and efficacy parameters more important since these products may have to meet several various regulatory jurisdictions. In Europe, for example, the European Cosmetic Directive requires that products have documentation to support the claims made [1]. In the United States the requirement is essentially the same except that some products that are considered cosmetic in some regulatory jurisdictions are over-the-counter drug products in the United States.

Antiperspirant products are in this category and in the United States only certain active ingredients previously approved by the Antiperspirant Monograph may be used in products labeled as antiperspirants. An active ingredient not on this list must go through the new drug approval process before it can be used in this capacity.

Our primary focus in this chapter will be to describe methods for determining the efficacy of products that will be labeled as antiperspirants.

Product Definition

There are some misunderstandings in the minds of consumers and cosmetic scientists about the product category known as antiperspirants. The confusion is centered around the three terms namely antiperspirant and deodorant and what has become a relatively new term primarily used in Europe "dry deodorant".

An antiperspirant product is designed to inhibit sweat production at the site of application and since it inhibits the sweat which acts as a culture medium for bacteria to potentially degrade and form malodor, antiperspirants can also be called deodorants. On the other hand a product formulated to only have deodorant activity may control malodor through absorption, masking (i.e., fragrance) and/or by antibacterial activity. Its main function is to reduce or prevent odor, not sweat production. The term dry deodorant describes a product that delivers some level of sweat reduction and also controls malodor.

For a product to be labeled as an antiperspirant in the United States it must demonstrate its capacity to reduce underarm sweat production to a level which is statistically significantly greater than 20% reduction and be formulated within the Category 1 guidelines of the Antiperspirant Drug Products for Over-the-Counter Human Use; Tentative Final Monograph [2]. Products not formulated within these guidelines will require submissions as new drugs.

Antiperspirants are considered cosmetic products in other parts of the world and are not subject to the efficacy requirements as established by the United States Food and Drug Administration.

Methods for Evaluating Antiperspirant Efficacy

There are three approaches for evaluating antiperspirant efficacy:
1. Visual
2. Instrumental
3. Gravimetric

Visualization Methods

There are various techniques that use starch-iodine or other suitable indicators which produce colored spots at the site of sweat droplets and several authors have published this type of method for determining antiperspirant activity. Kuno [3] has provided an overview of the early work done using colormetric techniques. These methods' and/or adaptations are used primarily as screening tools which indicate activity but do not quantify the level of antiperspirant reduction.

Instrumental Methods

Instrumental methods employ hygrometry, electrical conductance or impedance, and thermography to evaluate the efficacy of antiperspirant products. These methods are also considered screening tools and are not employed as typical standard antiperspirant efficacy evaluation techniques [4]. The most recently published method by Buelfeldt, Frase and Gassmueller [5] describes a test with 16 sites on the back used to compare eight test materials each with an adjacent control. The sweat collected on cellulous pads was eluted and the eluates were measured for electrical conductance. The authors reported results which were comparable to gravimetric axillary collections.

Gravimetric Methods

Gravimetric techniques were developed in order to quantify the actual amounts of sweat produced during specific time intervals and under specific conditions. After suitable times and conditions were established, antiperspirant applications were made and reduction in the quantity of sweat output was then determined. Gravimetric analysis became the method of choice for determining antiperspirant efficacy and continues to be the most used method today [4].

Three methods have been reported as techniques for induction of sweating: (1) Ambient temperature and humidity [6], (2) controlled hotroom environment [7], and (3) emotional sweating [8].

The most common method used for inducing sweat is the environmentally controlled hotroom maintained at approximately 100°F±2°F and 35%–40% relative humidity. Ambient conditions and emotional stimulations can also be used to induce perspiration but the hotroom is perhaps the easiest to control.

The gravimetric method, with minor modifications, published by Majors and Wild 1974 [7], has become the standard method for evaluating antiperspirant efficacy. The conclusions from their studies are still considered valid by many investigators today [9].

The following sections outline this gravimetric method for analyzing antiperspirant activity.

Objectives

An antiperspirant study is usually conducted for one of two objectives: (1) To evaluate the test article to determine if the percent reduction in axillary sweat at specified post-treatment intervals meets the OTC Monograph standard for antiperspirant labeling; (2) to compare the antiperspirant efficacy of two or more test articles at specific post-treatment intervals.

Experimental Design

There can be two experimental design objectives. (1) To evaluate the percent reduction in axillary sweat. The study is conducted following a paired comparison test design where one axilla is treated with a test article and the opposite axilla is either treated with a placebo or left untreated. (2) To compare the efficacy of two or more test articles. The study is conducted using a paired comparison design where one axilla is treated with one test article (A) and the contralateral axilla is treated with a different test article (B).

Test Material

The study sponsor should provide enough test articles that each subject can be assigned an individual sample or a pair of samples. The test materials are often coded to blind their identity.

Subject Selection

A critical aspect of all clinical evaluations is the selection of subjects to participate in the study. A sufficient number of subjects should be recruited to participate in a conditioning period to assure that the desired number of subjects participate in the test period.

The appropriate number of subjects will be an important consideration when designing an antiperspirant study. Typical studies employ 30–60 subjects per treatment cell which should produce results that are within 5%–10% of the true value [10].

Prior to participation in the test period all subjects must participate in a conditioning period lasting a minimum of 17 days. During this time they must abstain from using any axillary antiperspirant products. They may be allowed to use a deodorant product during this time if the deodorant has proven to have no antiperspirant efficacy. Subjects should also be given a non-antimicrobial soap to use during the conditioning period and during the test period. However, they will be restricted from washing the axillae during the test period except under supervised conditions at the test facility.

Other criteria to consider when selecting subjects include:
- Age 18–65
- Acceptable annual physical examination
- Brief medical screening just prior to study initiation
- Provide signed informed consent.

Criteria to consider when excluding subjects from participation include:
- Axillary irritation
- History of irritation or sensitivity to axillary antiperspirant, deodorant or soap products
- Recurring history of infections, boils, abscesses or lymph node enlargement in the axilla
- Active psoriasis, eczema, skin cancer, tinea versicolor or a dermatological condition that may interfere with the study conduct
- Used systemic antibiotics or topical antibiotic medications in the axillary area within 2 weeks prior to the study
- Uses medication which could suppress either an irritant reaction or result in a drug reaction or interaction; or deemed to present the subject as unhealthy for participation (e.g., antihistamines, immunosuppressive agents, anticholinergics or corticosteroids)
- Medical condition(s), such as heart disease, uncontrolled hypertension, kidney disease, significant respiratory disease, epilepsy, diabetes, heat intolerance, significant cosmetic allergies or very sensitive skin
- History of any significant immunologic or infectious disease, such as hepatitis, tuberculosis, positive HIV or AIDS and systemic lupus erythematous, which could place the subject at risk or interfere with the results of the study
- Pregnant, lactating, or planning a pregnancy.

Procedure

Axillary Examinations

Subjects should also be screened for axillary irritation just prior to being accepted on the study. The axillary examination is conducted by the investigator's personnel using a suitable light source to illuminate the axillary area. These examinations should be conducted daily during the study and the findings should be documented.

Baseline Sweat Collection

The investigator has the option of including a baseline sweat collection in the test design. Baseline sweat volumes can be used to compare differences between highest and lowest rates of sweating among the test subjects in order to meet the OTC Monograph criteria. Subjects with baseline levels below 150 mg of sweat/20 min/axilla should be eliminated from the treatment period.

After being accepted on the study following baseline, each subject participates in a supervised wash. These supervised washes will also be conducted prior to each test article application.

Supervised Washes

The subjects will be instructed to wash according to the following procedure:
1. Wash right axilla for 10 s using a disposable towel saturated with a 2% aqueous solution of a mild soap.
2. Wet a fresh disposable towel under running water and rinse the axilla until all soap is removed.
3. Gently pat dry the axilla using a dry disposable towel.
4. Repeat for left axilla.

Treatment Assignment/Application

For each subject the determination of which axilla will receive which test article will be randomly assigned prior to the study start. Treatment assignments to the right and left axillae of a specific subject will remain the same throughout the study.

Each subject will receive four [4] treatment applications to the axillary areas (the number of treatment applications is dependent upon the study design). Test articles will be applied to uniformly cover approximately a 4×6 IN. area centered in the axillary vault. All applications will be made by a qualified technician. Treatment applications are made according to the sponsor's directions. Except for the test articles, no axillary antiperspirant is to be used by any subject during the treatment period.

The subjects should wait at the test facility for approximately 30 min–1 h following each test article application to allow time for drying and absorption of test articles.

The effect of the test article treatments on axillary sweating will be determined by sweat collections conducted at a specified interval following specified applications.

Evaluations

Sweat Collection Evaluation Intervals

Sweat collection evaluation interval time points should be chosen according to the objectives of the sponsor. Baseline and more than one evaluation timepoint are optional. Evaluation time points may be at 1, 2, 4, 8, 12, 24, and 48 h following any number of treatments. For a typical design, evaluations are done at baseline, 1 h after application No. 3, and 24 h after application No. 4.

Sweat Stimulation

Sweating is induced by having the subjects sit in a room maintained at 100°F±2°F and a relative humidity of about 35%. The temperature and humidity conditions in the hotroom should be continually monitored and recorded.

Sweat Collections

During the first 40 min of the sweat stimulation period, the subjects hold unweighed pads of Webril (non-woven cotton padding fabric) in the axillae. These pads are discarded following the 40-min period. This preliminary warm up period is followed by two successive 20-min collection periods, during which the subjects hold weighed Webril pads in the axillae. These pads are weighed in tightly capped polystyrene vials before and after use. The vials are labeled with the subject's number, axilla (right or left) and collection designation. To insure the correct assembly of the bottle, cap and pad after use, all three components of the right collection unit are distinctively marked. The first collection made with weighed pads is designated Collection B and the second Collection C.

Posture during the collection period is an important factor effecting the variability of sweat output. Therefore, during the collections with weighed pads, the subjects must sit in an erect position with both feet flat on the floor and with their arms resting against their sides in a symmetrical manner.

Insertion and removal of the weighed pads are made by laboratory technicians. The subjects are allowed to drink water as desired during the warm up period and between Collections B and C.

Test Schedule

A typical test schedule is shown in Table 1. Test schedules are modified to meet the objective(s) of the study.

Table 1. Typical test schedule

Day	Procedure
Days 1–17	Conditioning period
Day 18	Medical screening, baseline sweat collection, test article application No. 1, followed by approximately 1-h wait
Day 19	Test article application No. 2, followed by approximately 1-h wait
Day 20	Test article application No. 3, followed by approximately 1-h wait, post-treatment sweat collection
Day 21	Test article application No. 4, followed by approximately 1-h wait
Day 22	24-h post-treatment sweat collection

Statistical Analysis

When the objective of the test is to meet OTC Monograph requirements, the following statistical analyses are recommended. When baseline sweat collections are performed: The data will be analyzed using the Wilcoxon Signed Rank Test, which is recommended in the Guidelines for Effectiveness Testing of OTC Antiperspirant Drug Products, August 1982 [11]. The source data for this analysis are treated to control ratios adjusted for the ratio of right-to-left axillary sweating rates. These ratios are calculated using the post-treatment average B and C collections for each individual at each time period. The adjusted treated to control ratios for this analysis will be calculated as follows:

$$Z = (PC \times T)/(PT \times C)$$

where Z is the adjusted ratio, PC is the pretreatment measure of moisture for the control axilla, PT is the pretreatment measure for the test axilla, T is the treated measure for the test axilla, and C is the corresponding quantity for the control axilla.

The study results are analyzed by comparing the adjusted ratio to 0.80, the ratio which corresponds to a 20% reduction in moisture due to treatment. The hypothesis that reduction in perspiration exceeds 20% is tested statistically by subtracting 0.80 from Z for all subjects and testing the resulting number with the Wilcoxon signed rank test.

The hypotheses tested in the signed rank test are stated below:
- Ho: Median $Z \geq 0.80$
- Ha: Median $Z < 0.80$.

Hypothesis testing will be performed at the $\alpha = 0.05$ level. Rejection of the null hypothesis will justify the conclusion that at least 50% of the target population will obtain a sweat reduction of at least 20%.

When baseline sweat collections are not performed: The data will be analyzed using the Wilcoxon Rank Sum Test, which is recommended in the Guidelines for Effectiveness Testing of OTC Antiperspirant Drug Products, August 1982 [11]. The source data for this analysis are right-to-left ratios adjusted for 20% reduction due to treatment. These ratios are calculated using the post-treatment average B and C collections for each individual at each time period.

The adjusted right-to-left ratios for this analysis will be calculated as follows:
- For subjects treated on the right axilla: $X = R/(0.8L)$
- For subjects treated on the left axilla: $Y = (0.8R)/L$.

The hypotheses tested in the rank sum test are stated below:
- Ho: Median $X \geq Y$
- Ha: Median $X < Y$.

Hypothesis testing will be performed at the $\alpha = 0.05$ level. Rejection of the null hypothesis will justify the conclusion that at least 50% of the target population will obtain a sweat reduction of at least 20%.

Estimates of percent reduction are calculated using a method described by Dietrich [12].

When the objective of the study is to compare the efficacy of two or more active test articles there are two statistical methods that are most frequently employed. For both methods, the averages of the post-treatment B and C collection milligram data are transformed to their natural logarithms.

When baseline sweat collections are conducted: An analysis of covariance method described by Murphy and Levine [13] is utilized.

When baseline sweat collections are not performed: The method described by Wooding and Finkelstein [14] is employed.

Analyses are conducted for each post-treatment evaluation interval. Hypothesis testing is usually performed at the $\alpha = 0.05$ level.

Deodorant Claims

Methods for Evaluating Deodorant Efficacy

There are three approaches for evaluating the potential for efficacy of deodorant products:
1. In vitro microbiological evaluation
2. Chemical analysis
3. Clinical sensory evaluation.

In Vitro Microbiological Evaluations

These techniques are designed to demonstrate the products ability to inhibit the bacterial populations which are contributing to the breakdown of the body secretions and causing the formation of malodor. However, these techniques do not quantify the potential of actual malodor reduction or control [15].

Chemical Analysis

The use of chromatographic analytical methods, can be carried out to detect the chemical constituents of the malodor but again these techniques are limited by the complex nature and variation in composition of axillary malodor between individual subjects [16]. The analysis does not yield a quantified malodor assessment.

Clinical Sensory Evaluation

The use of sensory evaluation techniques is the primary method by which deodorant efficacy is determined. The American Society for Testing and Materials (ASTM) has established guidelines for axillary deodorant evaluation [17].

The standard practice describes specific topics for special consideration, these include:
– Test design
– Subject selection
– Subject restriction (prior to and during test)
– Odor judge selection
– Odor judge training
– Scaling techniques.

The performance of deodorant efficacy evaluations is made more complex than some other test methodologies because it requires a commitment to select, train and maintain a panel of qualified odor judges.

Conclusion

All consumers expect the products they purchase to be safe and effective for their intended use. The requirement for manufacturers to have documentation available to support these parameters will insure that consumers will not be put at risk and will derive the expected benefit from their purchases.

References

1. Anon (1993) 6th amendment to the council directive of 27 July 1976 on the approximation of the laws of the member states relating to cosmetic products (76/768/EEC)
2. Department of Health and Human Services, Food and Drug Administration (1982) Antiperspirant drug products for over-the-counter human use; tentative final monograph. Federal Register, vol 47
3. Kuno Y (1956) Human perspiration. Charles C Thomas, Springfield, Illinois, pp 43, 223–250
4. Felger CB, Rogers JG (1988) Clinical evaluation of antiperspirants. In: Laden K, Felger C (eds) Antiperspirant and deodorants. Marcel Dekker, New York, pp 293–307
5. Bulfeldt S, Frase T, Gassmueller J (1997) New sensitive method for assessment of antiperspirants with intrindividual comparison of up to eight formulations. In: Proceedings of In-Cosmetics '97, Kongresszentrum SÜD, Düsseldorf, pp 163–169
6. Jungermann E (1974) Antiperspirants: new trends in formulation and testing technology. J Soc Cosmet Chem 25:621
7. Majors PA, Wild JE (1974) The evaluation of antiperspirant efficacy: influence of certain variables. J Soc Cosmet Chem 25:139
8. Quatrale RP, Stoner KL, Felger CB (1977) A method for the study of emotional sweating. J Soc Cosmet Chem 28:91–102
9. Parisse AJ (1990) Antiperspirants. In: Waggoner WC (ed) Clinical safety and efficacy testing of cosmetics. Marcel Dekker, New York, pp 163–223
10. Bowman JP, Dietrich FH, II, Wild JE (1998) A discussion of data variability in antiperspirant testing. Cosmetics and Toiletries Manufacturer Worldwide Aston Publishing Groups, Hertfordshire, UK, pp 227–236
11. Department of Health and Human Services, Food and Drug Administration (1982) Guidelines for effectiveness testing of OTC antiperspirant drug products
12. Dietrich FH, II, Bowman JP, Fath BM, Wild JE (1993) A comparison of antiperspirant data analysis methods. J Soc Cosmet Chem 44:13–21
13. Murphy TD, Levine MJ (1991) Analysis of antiperspirant efficacy test results. J Soc Cosmet Chem 42:167–197
14. Wooding WM, Finklestein P (1975) A critical comparison of two procedures for antiperspirant evaluation. J Soc Cosmet Chem 26:255–275
15. Wild JE (1988) Clinical testing of deodorants. In: Laden K, Felger CB (eds) Antiperspirant and deodorants. Marcel Dekker, New York, pp 391–411
16. Baxter PM, Reed JV (1983) The evaluation of underarm deodorants. Int J Cosmet Sci 5:85–95
17. American Society for Testing and Materials (1987) ASTM Designation E1207-87, ASTM Annual Book of ASTM Standards, vol 15.07. Sensory practice for the sensory evaluation of axillary deodorancy

CHAPTER 9

Sunscreens

B. Gabard

Introduction

Sunlight is a part of our everyday life and has been endowed since ancient times with health-beneficial and life-supporting properties. However, sunlight can also be harmful to human skin. Excessive exposure causes erythema and sunburn. Cumulative effects of prolonged exposure are now increasingly recognised to be the possible cause of degenerative changes in the skin such as premature ageing and some skin cancers [1].

The solar radiation reaching the surface of the earth has been subdivided into three main spectral bands: infrared radiations (IR; wavelengths >760 nm); visible radiations (400–760 nm); ultraviolet radiations (UVR; 290–400 nm). The UVR from both sunlight and artificial sources is further subdivided into three sections termed UVA, UVB and UVC from the longer to shorter wavelengths: UVA from 320–400 nm, UVB from 290–320 nm, UVC <290 nm. Although the boundaries of these regions originally defined in 1932 at the 2nd International Congress on Light were slightly different (UVC <280 nm, UVB 280–315 nm, UVA 315–400 nm), this classification is now widely accepted [2, 3].

The short-wavelength UVC is absorbed by ozone in the highest part of the earth's atmosphere. Thus, sunlight's UVR at the surface of the earth is constituted by variable proportions of UVB and UVA. This variability is due to different factors such as latitude, height of the sun above horizon (time of the day), altitude, weather and atmospheric conditions etc. As a rule, the amount of UVA may be considered to be 10–20 times greater than that of UVB.

The biological effects of UVB have been thoroughly investigated: UVB is the principal cause of sunburn (erythema, peak intensity 20–24 h after exposure) and tanning (melanogenesis). Long-term UVB-radiation is mutagenic and cancerogenic, but on the other side promotes the synthesis of vitamin D and a thickening of the epidermis. Thickening and tanning is a natural defence reaction of the skin.

The importance of the biological effects of UVA has been only recently recognised. UVA induces significant photobiological reactions, mostly of indirect nature and requiring the presence of oxygen, such as an immediate (diminishing soon after exposure) and a delayed (peaking 10–12 h after exposure) erythemal reaction. It also causes an immediate tanning reaction (or immediate pigment darkening, IPD) and new melanin formation (melanogenesis, persistent pigment darkening PPD). However, UVA is about 600–1000 times less effective than UVB in producing these effects. The UVA tan response is not associated with an increased epidermal thickness and provides much less a protective effect against sunburn (UVB-induced erythema) than the UVB-induced tan. More importantly, there is now considerable evidence that UVA definitively contributes to long-term degenerative changes of the skin. Prolonged irradiation with UVA can induce inflammation, significant connective tissue damage, cancer formation and may also contribute significantly to UVB-induced carcinogenesis [2–5].

Therefore, there are two main concerns about the deleterious effects of sunlight exposure: acute effects (sunburn) and long-term risks (degenerative changes, carcinogenesis). Preventing or at least lessening these outcomes requires effective photoprotective measures and sunscreens.

Definitions

As pointed out by Pathak [6], there is no definition of „sunscreens" in the medical and leading English language dictionaries. The conventional approach defines sunscreens as "to screen the sun and to protect or shelter viable cells of the skin against potentially harmful effects of solar UVR". This has emerged with time and refers to the protective effect of different topical products called sunscreens, such as solutions, creams, lotions, oils, gels etc. against sunburn. However, in view of a growing photobiological knowledge about the mechanisms of UVR-effects in the skin, this definition must now be revised to include new concepts. Thus besides sunburn protection, modern sunscreens (or "photoprotectants" [6]) may not only contain chemicals that absorb, reflect or scatter UVR but also chemicals that interfere with secondary reactions such as generation of free radicals and reactive oxygen species in the skin, generation of inflammatory mediators, photoexcitation of different molecules etc. and ultimately exert long-term protective effects on degenerative skin damage. Consequently, non UVR-absorbing, -reflecting or -scattering molecules with a pharmacological action in the skin may also be incorporated in sunscreens, endowing the corresponding products with expanded properties [6].

Objectives

Different methods aiming at the support of the general claim "sun protection" will be reviewed shortly, as many recent publications on this subject exist. The extension of the "sunscreen" to the "photoprotectant" concept will be taken in account and new approaches investigated.

Prerequisites

It is not the purpose of this review to define the legal frame of the clinical studies required for claim support. The reader is referred to the corresponding monographs or publications covering extensively the general procedures concerning human studies, their legal frame and the pre-requisite information about the products to be tested [7–9] as well as the particular aspects of sunscreen testing [10–13].

Investigating the Claims

In Vivo Measurement of the Sun Protection Factor

Background

The photoprotective efficacy of a particular sunscreen is generally expressed as its sun protection factor (SPF). The SPF is a ratio of the time required for a given irradiation to produce minimal perceptible erythema (MED: minimum erythemal dose, the UVR-dose necessary to produce the minimal sunburn or minimal perceptible erythema 16–24 h after exposure) in sunscreen-protected skin to the time required for unprotected skin. Thus, the SPF is predominantly an indication of efficacy against UVB-light. The relative contribution of UVA-radiation to sunburn is considered to be 15–24% [6].

Methodology

Recent, methodologically most detailed guidelines about the in vivo measurement of the SPF of a sunscreen have been published in different countries and are briefly summarised in Table 1 for USA, Australia/New Zealand and Europe. The reader is referred to the detailed presentation and discussion of these guidelines in the corresponding monographs [10–13].

SPF measurement methods may be now considered world-wide as close to harmonisation [14]. Although subtle differences remain, the SPF value of a given sunscreen should now be the same within acceptable limits regardless of the measurement method used. The still legal but methodologically obsolete DIN method dated 1984 [15] has been omitted. It was mainly responsible for the differences between European and American SPF values of a sunscreen, that now should no more exist.

Comments

Light Source, Spectral Output, Exposure Dose
The spectral power distribution of a light source is determined by spectroradiometry [16]. A solar simulator is a lamp that emits a spectrum of radiations similar to that of terrestrial sunlight (within limits defined in the guidelines). For radiometric calculations, the exposure dose is expressed in joules per square meter and the spectral irradiance of the simulator in watts per square meter:

$$\text{Dose (J/m}^2) = \text{Irradiance (W/m}^2) \times \text{time (s)}$$

The exposure dose used for the determination of SPFs is the MED. The MED has the advantage of being related to the biological consequences of the exposure. To obtain the MED, the lamp irradiance has to be weighted by the effectiveness of the radiations at particular wavelengths to cause an erythemal reaction:

$$\text{Biologically effective irradiance (W/m}^2) = \text{Sum}[E\lambda \times e\lambda \times D\lambda]$$

where $E\lambda$ is the spectral irradiance ($W/m^2/nm$), $e\lambda$ a measure of the effectiveness of the radiation of wavelength λ in producing erythema relative to a reference wavelength (a ratio, thus without unit) and $D\lambda$ the wavelength interval used in the summation. The

Table 1. Comparative summary of SPF measurement methods in USA, Australia/New Zealand and Europa (COLIPA recommendations)

Country	USA	Australia/New Zealand	Europe (COLIPA)
Reference	12, 13	11	10, 28
Light source	Xenon arc solar simulator	Xenon arc solar simulator	Solar simulator
Spectral output	UVC output: <1% VIS>400 nm: <5%	Global daylight (Albuquerque) ±4 nm	Standard sun defined by spectral distribution of erythemal efficacy (limits within±3 SPF)
Reference sunscreens	Homosalate reference SPF 4	1. Homosalate reference SPF 4–5 (±2) 2. P3 Reference (same as COLIPA high SPF Std.) SPF 12.5–18.5 (±2)	1. P1 low (DIN K17N) SPF 4.0–4.4 2. P2 high (CTFA/JCIA std.) SPF 11.5–13.9 3. P3 high (Bayer C202/ 101) SPF 14.0–17.0
Test subjects	Minimum 20	Minimum10 (if SEM not greater than 7% of the mean SPF) Skin types I, II or III	Minimum 10, maximum 20 (95% CI within 20% of the mean SPF) Skin types I, II or III or colour typing ITA°>28°
Product application: area, location	2 mg/cm² 50 cm² On the back	2±0.1 mg/cm² 30 cm² On the back Product delivery method should be validated	2±0.04 mg/cm² 35 cm² On the back
Test sites	1 cm² recommended	Approximately 1 cm² separated by at least 1 cm	Minimum 0.4 cm², recommended 1cm² separated by at least 1 cm
Waiting time before irradiation	15 min	At least 15 min or according to product instructions	Irradiate as soon as possible after 15 min waiting time
Exposure	Constant flux variable time, 5 sites 1.25× incremental dose increase between sites	Constant flux variable time, at least 5 sites, 1.25× incremental dose increase between sites	Constant flux variable time, minimum 5 sites 1.25× incremental dose increase between sites
MED reading	Sequential determination unprotected/protected allowed Read after 16–20 h	Simultaneous determination unprotected/protected Read after 20±4 h	Simultaneous determination unprotected/protected Read after 16–24 h Colorimetric reading optional
SPF	Arithmetic mean of individual SPF values	Arithmetic mean of individual SPF values	Arithmetic mean of individual SPF values

guidelines require Eλ to be as close as possible to the spectral irradiance of midday, clear sky, summer sunlight (i.e. "standard sun" [10, 11, 16]). eλ is the CIE standard skin reference erythemal action spectrum [17]. The COLIPA guidelines consider the biologically effective irradiance, the American and Australian guidelines consider the spectral power of the lamp emission. Compliance of the spectral irradiance of the solar simulator with the "standard sun" spectrum is important. Sources too high in UVB will overestimate the SPFs, sources too high in UVA will lead to too low SPFs [18].

It must be kept in mind that the SPF is, per definition, at constant irradiation flux rate, a ratio of time (see section: "Background" above). The biologically effective exposure of the subjects during the measurements remains the same in protected and unprotected skin (i.e. the MED). Because the sunscreen action is to diminish the biologically effective irradiance the exposure time is increased to reach the endpoint, the MED. This follows a fundamental law of photochemistry, named reciprocity, stating that the magnitude of the response depends only on the absorbed dose of energy, and not on the intensity of the radiation or its duration [19]. This also explains why, theoretically, reapplication of the sunscreen just before reaching the sunburn threshold does not afford supplementary protection. In everyday practice, however, given the many factors that may influence sunscreen use, reapplication is recommended [20].

Test Subjects, Test Area

Skin type is defined from the individual sensitivity of unprotected skin to 30 to 40 min of sun exposure in early summer without previous sun exposure that season [3, 10]. In addition, the COLIPA guideline defines the individual typology angle ITA° expressing the coloration of the skin measured by reflectance colorimetry in the CIE (1976) L*a*b* colour space [10]. The ITA° appears particularly helpful to select the study participants. There is a considerable overlapping of the MED values of different skin types [21] and within individual subjects [22, 23]. On the other side, ITA° values seem to be closely related to MED values [24].

Substantial variability in the MED as a function of the anatomical location of the test area has been repeatedly shown. Recent results provide evidence that despite these significant differences between anatomical sites, the SPF might remain unaffected. However, it is important to stick to the guidelines recommendations in this respect and to make the measurements on the back, as these results remain controversial [22, 23, 25].

Product Application, Application Technique

The quantity of sunscreen used for SPF determination has been settled at 2 mg/cm² [10–13]. The obvious dependency of SPF on appropriate application of the sunscreen has been known for a long time [26, 27]. Matching the guidelines requirements as close as possible is fundamental. For this reason, a most detailed description of a suitable application technique has been published [28]. The importance of this factor is underlined by the requirements of the Australian/New Zealand guideline to validate the product delivery method [11]. Validation is: "establishing documented evidence that the procedure used does what it purports to do based on a pre-planned validation protocol" (FDA/PIC-citation). A very recent technique for quantitative assessment of sunscreen application may be used for this purpose [29].

Sunscreen amount on the skin deserves a further comment: In everyday practice, the amount used by the consumers is lower than 2 mg/cm² and has been estimated on average between 0.5 [30] and 1.5 mg/cm^2 [27, 29, 31]. Therefore, a decreased real SPF is likely, and has been measured at least for a high-protection sunscreen [27].

Colorimetric MED Evaluation

Non-invasive bioengineering methods are increasingly used in dermatology [32]. This has been recognised by the COLIPA. In addition to the colorimetric skin typology ITA°, the guideline proposes an optional colorimetric determination of the MED [10, 28]. The usefulness of different non-invasive measurement methods in UVR-induced erythema has been recently investigated by several research groups [22, 33–35]. In particular, chromametry seems to be very helpful to investigate the effects of sunscreens on non-Caucasian, e.g. black skin [22, 33].

SPF Labelling

The newest proposition from the FDA limits the maximum allowable SPF at 30 [12, 13]. It has been concluded that the additional benefits from SPFs>30 (at this level, already 96.7% of UVR are absorbed) are outweighed by the increased exposure of the consumer to the sunscreen ingredients. Similarly, the Australian/New Zealand Standard lifted the maximum SPF that may be claimed from 15+ to 30+ [11], stating that "15+, correctly applied, is expected to provide adequate protection for most people who avoid overexposure to the sun". Both guidelines give an optional category description (Table 2) which in our eyes represents a simple, straightforward and useful information for the consumer. The Australian/New Zealand Standard joins water resistance claims and the category description (see section "Water and sweat resistance", below).

In Vitro Measurement of the SPF

Background

The in vivo measurement of sunscreen efficacy is a complicated and time-consuming procedure not really suitable for broad screening during product development. Many publications deal with the problem of the in vitro determination of SPFs. The problem's

Table 2. Comparative summary of category descriptions

Country	USA [12, 13]		Australia/New Zealand [11] Maximum water resistance time t claim (SPF measured after t water contact)	Europe (COLIPA)
Category description				
Minimal	SPF 2 to <4	SPF 2 to <4	SPF: no claim	SPF 2 to 5
Moderate	SPF 4 to <8	SPF 4 to <8	SPF: t=40 min	SPF 6 to 11
High	SPF 8 to <12	SPF 8 to <15	SPF: t=80 min	SPF 12 to 19
Very high	SPF 12 to <20	SPF > 15 (broad spectrum protection should be fulfilled)	15 to 20, t=2 h 20 to 25, t=3 h ≥25, t=4 h	SPF ≥20
Ultrahigh	SPF 20 to 30			

solution is not simple. The in vitro SPFs must correlate with the results of in vivo phototesting, the costs must remain low and the materials needed must be readily available. As quoted by Kelley et al. [36], many substrates have been tested for sunscreen application, including wool, synthetic skin casts, pig skin, mouse or human epidermis. Satisfactory results were obtained only with skin casts or isolated epidermis, but these substrates are difficult to obtain. The surgical adhesive tape method developed by Diffey and Robson [37] thus appears attractive.

Methodology

Diffey and Robson have published a detailed description of their in vitro method using a piece of surgical Transpore tape as substrate [37]. In our laboratories, this method is routinely used in the following way [38]: The Transpore tape is stuck onto a light-diffusing double-ground quartz plate. The sunscreens are spotted onto the tape from a pre-weighted syringe at a rate of 2 mg/cm^2 and spread evenly with a gloved finger. The light source is a 150 W Xe arc lamp equipped with a UG11 filter absorbing visible and IR light. The light passing through the sample (Quartz plate+tape) is collected by a 4-inch integrating sphere and enter a spectrometer. Spectroradiometric measurements are performed in 5 nm steps between 290 and 400 nm before and after sunscreen application. The calculation of the SPF is performed as described by Diffey and Robson [37], using here, too, the spectral irradiance of midday, clear sky, summer sunlight and the CIE standard skin reference erythemal action spectrum for weighting the data. To our knowledge, two equipments are commercially available for performing in vitro SPFs measurements [39].

Comments

The SPF obtained with this method need a critical examination and do not ultimately replace the in vivo determination. In our hands, correlation of the in vitro SPF with the in vivo SPF is satisfactory (with some exceptions) for sunscreens containing chemical UV-filters, but poorer for sunscreens containing mineral pigments such as TiO$_2$ or ZnO [38]. A poor correlation is also observed for high protection sunscreens with in vivo SPF$\geq$20. Some difficulties have been pointed out [36]. Using human stratum corneum (skin surface biopsy) as substrate may be a possibility of improving the reliability of the method [40]. Recently, use of human epidermis has been shown to overcome the difficulties associated with the in vitro measurements of high SPF sunscreens, but this again raises the question of substrate availability [41].

Despite undeniable limitations, this in vitro technique has the advantage of allowing the comparison of an unlimited number of products during development, provided the results are critically evaluated. It further provides more and very valuable information about a particular product, particularly in view of the rising concern about UVA protection (see section: "UVA Protection" below and [42]).

UVA Protection

Background

As already stated, there is increasing awareness that exposure of the skin to UVA-radiation can induce deleterious changes in the skin, including tumour development

[4, 5, 43]. The appearance of high-SPF sunscreens has led consumers to remain longer in the sun and consequently to be exposed to increased UVA-doses. More and more sunscreens now claim UVA-protection. There is a considerable debate on the suitable ways of measuring a biologically relevant UVA-protection [4, 5, 44]. Numerous publications describe in vivo as well as in vitro techniques, but at the present moment no index of UVA-protection (in the sense of the SPF) has been generally accepted.

Methodology

The measuring techniques have been recently summarised and critically reviewed [44]. They include in vivo and in vitro techniques:
In vivo:
 Immediate pigment darkening (IPD) [45]
 Persistent (or delayed) pigment darkening (PPD) [45]
 UVA-erythema
 Phototoxic protection factor

In vitro:
 Diffey method [42, 46]: The broad-spectrum rating is based on the wavelength λc for which the area under the absorption spectrum from 290 nm to λc amounts to 90% of the integral of the absorption spectrum from 290 to 400 nm.
 Australian/New Zealand Standard [11]: Three measurement possibilities are offered, using spectral transmission analysis (1) of a solution in a particular solvent (after centrifugation if necessary), (2) of a thin film (thickness 8μ) and (3) of a thick film (thickness 20 μm) of the sunscreen under investigation. In cases 1 and 2, light transmission between 320 and 360 nm shall be only 10% from blank transmission, in case 3 1%. Sunscreens fulfilling these requirements may be labelled "broad-spectrum protection" if otherwise their SPF amounts to at least 4.

Comments

Protection factors measured with the IPD and/or PPD methods may be useful but their determination is difficult [44]. The indication of one or two additional numbers on the packaging may be confusing for consumers, as these numbers cannot be interpreted in the way of the SPF (SPF 10: 10 times prolongation of my personal time to sunburn for my unprotected skin, but what about a PPD factor of 10 for example?). Furthermore, in common with other determination methods for UVA-protection, the significance of these factors in relation to the long-term biological effects of UVA is unknown.

 For practical reasons, we favour an in vitro measurement, that presents the advantage of expressing the UVA-protection in relation to UVB-protection. Two possibilities exist, exemplified by the Australian/New Zealand approach [11] or the Diffey approach [42, 46]: The Australian/New Zealand Standard [11] gives a detailed description of an in vitro method for evaluation of UVA-protection (see section "Methodology" above). This is the only method published in an official guideline. The answer is of the yes/no type. This simple approach assumes that decreasing the UVA light transmission by the required amount will also diminish the biological effects. This affirmation is of course questionable, but at the present moment it has been neither denied nor approved.

The Diffey index of broad spectrum protection takes into account that "...why should volunteers be exposed to sources of radiations with spectra that will never be encountered (i.e. lamp filtered to emit only UVA), why should as an endpoint a bio-logical effect be used which nobody wants to protect against (pigment darkening)...". It has the advantage of being based on solar light emission spectrum, of being easily measured in vitro and of giving a simple classification of sunscreens in categories such as "no", "low", "moderate" or "high UVA-protection".

Together with the SPF, which is considered to primarily represent protection in the spectrum range 290 to 340 nm [44], the Australian yes/no answer or the better Diffey classification gives a very valuable and understandable information for the consumer about the product he is going to buy and for the dermatologist who may read from the broad-spectrum reading which wavelength represents the limit where 90% UVR is ab-sorbed. This may be of importance for some patients. However, here too, no assumpti-ons are made about the relevance to immediate or long-term photobiological damages and degenerative skin changes.

IR Protection

Background

In addition to the SPF or UVA-protection, some sunscreens are now labelled as IR-pro-tecting. Most of the products bearing this indication are sunscreens containing mine-ral pigments such as TiO_2 and ZnO. These materials are optimised for UVR-protection by eliminating a significant light absorption in the wavelength domain ≥400 nm, thus removing by the way the problematic cosmetic appearance of preparations containing pigmentary (particle size » 200 nm) and not micronized or ultrafine material (particle size »10–50 nm; [47, 48]). Therefore, careful measurements and product optimisation are needed before claiming a significant IR-protection.

Few studies investigated the effects of IR on the skin. IR, inseparably linked to sun-light and perceived as heat, is implicated in erythema "ab igne" and elastotic degene-ration. Studies investigating the interactions of IR and UVR have shown controversial results [49–52]. It is generally accepted that IR enhances the effects of UVR [49, 50, 52], but on the other side recent developments point to a possible protective effect of short-term hyperthermia against UVB-induced changes [53].

Methodology

IR protection of a sunscreen was investigated using the immediate erythema induced by IR in a similar way to the determination of the SPF [49]. The doses were increased by a factor of $\sqrt{2}$. Protection factors of 1.4 on average were measured using this techni-que. A more recent study used colorimetry and only one IR-dose on protected and un-protected skin, and in addition measured the infrared reflection coefficient of the sun-screens. The sunscreens were classified in three groups: (I) products with anti-erythe-mic properties simultaneously reflecting IR. (II) products with no anti-erythemic pro-perties but still reflecting IR and (III) products showing anti-erythemic properties but no IR-reflection [52].

Comments

Clearly much more studies are presently needed about this controversial issue, which is not explicitly addressed in the most recent monographs on sunscreens nor in the Standard Australia/New Zealand [10–13].

Water and Sweat Resistance

Background

Substantivity characterises the property of a sunscreen to maintain its degree of protection under adverse conditions, such as repeated water immersion or sweating. Due to the outdoor use of sunscreens in conditions where water immersion is usual and abundant sweating may be encountered, water- and sweat-resistance is very important [54, 55]. Several in vitro and in vivo methods have been published for evaluating the substantivity of a given sunscreen. In vitro methods have not gained widespread use, but may be used during product development for a rough estimate of the product substantivity. However, human testing is considered to be the most acceptable and definitive method [55].

Methodology

Different methods have been published for estimating in humans the substantivity of a sunscreen. They were recently summarised (Table 3; [56]). However, only two of these methods are actually agreed and published in corresponding guidelines [11–13]. Briefly:
FDA guideline: A product is claimed to be "water-resistant" if it retains the same category description (Table 2) after 40 min water immersion (2×20 min time periods separated by a 20 min rest period without towelling). It may be claimed "very water-resistant" if this is the case after 4 immersion periods of 20 min each. The claim "water-proof" is no longer allowed [12]. Products carrying the claims "water resistant" or "very water resistant" may also claim to be "sweat resistant" because the FDA concluded that the immersion test is a more severe test than a sweating test [12, 13, 55].
Australian/New Zealand guideline: The SPF of the sunscreen is determined after immersion of the test subjects for not less than 40 min (2×20 min time periods separated by a 5 min rest period without towelling) in either a swimming pool or a spa. Where water resistance of greater than 40 min is to be tested, the schedule of alternating 20 min immersion/5 min rest is continued. The SPF measured after immersion determines the category classification of the sunscreen. Any claim of water resistance is to be qualified by a statement of the time for which the water resistance has been tested, up to the maximum claimable time (Table 2). No statement is made about sweat resistance.

Comments

An important point which favours the FDA or Australian approach for the determination of sunscreen substantivity is the fact that the MED of unprotected skin is mea-

Table 3. Comparative summary of measurement methods for the determination of water resistance

Method	USA[a]	Australia/New Zealand[b]	Greiter[c]	Schrader[d]
Water contact	2×20 min or 4×20 each separated by 20 min without towelling	2×20-min periods as needed each separated by 5 min without towelling	2 min 21 s[e]	2 min 21 s
Equipment/ Immersion	Swimming pool or whirlpool jacuzzi	Swimming pool or spa pool (indoors)	Shower	Laminar water flow, Aperture 83×2 mm
Water		Swimming pool: 23–28°C, pH 6.8–7.2 Spa pool: fresh water, 33±2°C, pH 6.8–7.2, water circulation 16 min, air circulation 4 min	Output: 210 l/h Temp.: 23°C	Quantity: 7 l Temp.: 23°C
Other conditions		Swimming pool protected from direct sunlight Spa pool: Approx. 1.8×1.8 m, subjects sitting, test sites completely immersed but not impinged on directly by air or water jets	Distance from the back: 40 cm Angle of the jet direction to skin surface: 45°	
Claim	SPF within the same category description after: 2×20 min: Water resistant 4×20 min: Very water resistant	SPF after immersion, immersion time (see Table 2) Maximum claim: 4 h water resistance for SPF≥25	% Water resistance	SPF after water contact >50% before: water resistant

[a] [12, 13], [b] [11], [c] From [85], [d] [56]
[e] Statement on p. 263 in [85]: "A shower time of 2 min 21 s with a water flow of 210 l/h, a water temperature of 23°C and a room temperature of 22°C is equivalent to 40 min swimming in chlorated pool
water at 24.5°C (air temp. 37°C)."

sured on wet, previously immersed areas. This is not the case in some of the methods
outlined in Table 3, and in our eyes constitutes a major drawback, as it is well-known
that skin sensitivity to UVR is altered by exposure to water [57]. Actually, these recent
results confirm former statements and give background to the use of fresh water for
substantivity testing [55, 57].

The different approaches of the substantivity problem by the FDA and the Australian guidelines deserve a further comment. For Standard Australia, the impression
should not be given that the sunscreen is effective for a longer period than the SPF
value would allow. Nowadays, it is technically possible to achieve long water resistance
times through particular formulation, but it is not correct to claim 4 or 8 h water resistance for a product with a SPF of 4 for example. Therefore, a clear restriction on the
claim "water resistant" has been incorporated in the Australian guidelines.

Last, this discussion underlines the usefulness of a category description of the product. Rather than the SPF (which of course should still be indicated), the classification
of the sunscreen in a category (Table 2) joins together information about the level of
protection (minimum to very high), the UVA-protection (very high protection

products must display broad protection) and the level of substantivity and/or water resistance time.

Photostability

Background

The availability of high-SPF sunscreens claiming UVA-protection has given concern about a possible light-induced alteration of their chemical components, because consumers may stay in the sun for longer periods of time. Although photochemistry, photostability and/or light-induced chemical reactions are a general problem in the context of cosmetic products, this is of particular importance for sunscreens [58–60]. Chemical UV-filters are, of course, in first line, because of their deliberate selection as UVR-absorbing molecules. Although one may argue that photostability is taken in account during the in vivo measurement of SPF, because photodegradation of the UV-filters would lead to a reduced protection, longer exposure times and the variable proportion of UVA that may be encountered in daily practice are not considered during the regular, well-standardised SPF measurement procedure.

Methodology

A COLIPA working group has recently published a detailed proposal for investigating the photostability of UVB-filters and a modified protocol for UVA-filters [61]: A liquid film from a suitable solvent containing the UV-filter at a relevant concentration is irradiated on a glass surface with 5 or 10 standard MEDs from a Xe arc light source filtered with a WG 320/2 mm filter. After irradiation, the UV-filters are analysed by spectrophotometry or HPLC. In the case of UVA-filters, the protocol remains almost similar with the exception of a 15% increased exposure time and the introduction of a polymeric film (Myla D50) between the light source and the sample to simulate the presence of UVB-filters.

Another proposal from Diffey et al. [62] uses a slight modification of its in vitro model already described (see section: "Methodology" under "In Vitro Measurement of the SPF" above). The sunscreens are dispensed at the rate of 1 mg/cm^2 onto two quartz plates with roughened surfaces. The light source is a Xe arc lamp optically filtered to simulate summer sunlight. One of the plates is exposed to the light, the other remains in the dark. The SPF is measured 3 times consecutively on the exposed and on the non-exposed plate after energy doses of 18, 36 and 54 J/cm^2. A chemical analysis of the UV-filters incorporated in the sunscreens may be added.

Comments

It has been already known for some time that some UV-filters, particularly of the cinnamate series, are less photostable than others [60] On the other side, benzophenones for example are known to be very photostable [58, 60]. The problem of photostability is now becoming more important due to the high SPFs and the concomitant increased UVA-exposure. High SPFs may be obtained by rising the concentrations of the UV-filters in the sunscreen formulations up to the allowed maximum and/or by increasing the numbers of filters associated in the preparation. Therefore, not only the photostability of a single filter is important, but also interactions of filters with each other must be investigated: Certain filters may show a stabilising effect on others [63]. It is also known that the photostability of some molecules depends on the solvent used and/or on the vehicle in which they are formulated [58, 60]. For these reasons, preference is to be given to methods investigating the filters in their environment, that means in the sunscreen formulation, such as the Diffey method [62].

Photochemical reactions due to UVR are inextricably coupled with the chemistry of free radicals. The photostability of UV-filters should be considered within a more general frame, such as the extension of the "sunscreen" concept to the "photoprotectant" concept, as pointed out in the section "Definitions" above. The role of free radicals and of reactive oxygen species (ROS) is now been examined as a possible cause of chronic skin damage. Thus, incorporation of molecules being able to control free radical formation and/or ROS not only should improve the photostability of a given sunscreen, but in addition should be beneficial in terms of the so-called photo- or actinic ageing of the UV-exposed skin.

Antioxidants and Free Radical Scavengers

Background

The generation of free radicals and ROS by sunlight, and particularly by UVR, was considered until recently as at most an academic curiosity. It is now accepted that exposure of the skin to UVR leads to the generation of a multitude of free radical species. These, and the derived ROS cause injury by reacting with molecules such as lipids, proteins, nucleic acids and by depleting the skin of its natural endogenous antioxidant defences [64, 65]. This is a paradoxical situation particular to the skin, since a normal reaction to the oxidative stress imparted by UVR would lead to an up-regulation of the defence systems [64].

The cutaneous antioxidant defence system is complex, multilayered, and far from being completely understood. Briefly, it contains enzymic, non-enzymic and inducible elements [66]. This classification, however, remains academic if action mechanisms are considered, because all parts together form a well-organised, interlinked network working against oxidative stress by scavenging ROS and other free radicals, and by removing, repairing or regenerating used biomolecules. The different action mechanisms have been recently reviewed [64–67].

Consequently, it is not surprising that, although an overwhelming evidence suggests that antioxidants will be effective at inhibiting UV damage to the skin, investigations of the possible protective effects of different molecules have till now shown only modest benefit. Besides problems of formulation, costs, or local bioavailability (for example, the stratum corneum is the most susceptible skin layer for UVR-induced depletion of vitamin E), there often has been investigated only one molecule at a time. The multifactorial and interlinked nature of the system requires combinations of different molecules for proper protection. This has been recently confirmed by showing a dramatic improvement in photoprotection after the topical application of vitamin C, vitamin E and melatonin in combination compared to the single substances alone [68].

Future, improved sunscreen formulations will be based on combinations of UV-filters and of antioxydant molecules of different types. These formulations will present the great advantage of working on several lines of attack. By combining a diminution of the biologically effective irradiance and an improved antioxidant defence, they will be better adapted to oppose the myriad of events triggered in the skin by UVR insult and culminating in the actinic erythema as an end-point [69, 70].

Methodology

There are many recent publications describing different models for the investigation of an antioxidant effect. Animal and human studies have been performed, and a thorough review of these experiment is given in [65]. Both short-term (e.g. UVR-induced erythema) and long-term (e.g. skin wrinkling or tumour incidence) effects have been investigated.

Comments

Numerous chemicals potentially active as antioxidants with different mechanisms of action are presently under study. Therefore, several methodological approaches are and will remain necessary. The subject extends far beyond the cosmetic area, medicinal applications are being investigated [71]. Furthermore, recent studies have shown that topical antioxidants as sunscreens must be applied before UVR-exposition to properly work [65, 72]. This rises the question of combining topical sunscreens with systemic dosing of antioxidants in particular situations [73].

Photoageing

Background

Skin undergoing long-term sun exposure experiences a number of morphologic and functional alterations termed dermatoheliosis and presents a sallow yellow discoloration, pigmentation changes, wrinkles, loss of elasticity, dryness and small tumours. These alterations are distinct from those following chronological ageing [51, 54, 74, 75]. Besides loss of connective tissue, accumulation of material in the dermis with histological staining characteristics of elastin is observed. For this reason, these changes are generally termed solar elastosis. Further analysis has revealed that the poorly structured material accumulating in the dermis is composed of normal constituents of elastic fibres, among them glycosaminoglycans, elastin and fibrillin. Experimental studies with animal models have shown that UVB is responsible for the dermal connective tissue destruction, and that UVA significantly contributes to the solar elastosis. Therefore, sunlight as such is of concern in photoageing or dermatoheliosis of human skin [51, 75].

Methodology

Several studies have underlined the value of non-invasive bioengineering techniques in the study of aged skin [76–78]. Most recent results have shown that even differences between chronological (intrinsic) ageing and photoageing can be detected and quantified by these techniques [78]. The value of sunscreens in the protection against dermatoheliosis has been repeatedly demonstrated in several models [51, 79–81].

Comments

There is no doubt that sunscreens can protect the exposed skin against dermatohelio-sis. This has been demonstrated in animals models and in human studies [51, 54, 75]. Particularly, high SPF sunscreens were demonstrated of value in persons at risk for skin cancer because they reduced the number of new precancerous lesions and increased the rate of remission of existing ones [75, 82]. In this respect, Kligman and Kligman have shown that the dermatoheliosis is not irreversible, and that what appears as the degenerative changes outlined above ("Background") is the result of the balance between destruction and repair under challenge by solar irradiation. When the irra-diation stress is relieved, either by sunlight avoidance or by the use of broad-spectrum sunscreens, the balance is shifted toward repair [51].

Conclusion

The increasing awareness about the damaging effects of sunlight has led not only to a significant demand for more protection from sunscreens, but also to a widening of the concept of photoprotection and a to a change in current concepts about sunscreen mo-de of action.

The demand for more protection is clearly reflected by the steady increase in the primary index of photoprotection, the SPF. The SPF-values of the majority of the products found on the market, at least in Europe, are now comprised between 10 and 20, compared to 2–8 at the end of the 1980s [83]. Sunscreens with SPF >30 are now available. These facts are reflected by the adaptation of the official guidelines, as dis-cussed in the section "Comments" under "In Vivo Measurement of the SPF", but simultaneously concern about the increased exposure of the consumers in relation to the benefit of such high protection factors has been expressed. It must be also kept in mind that modern daily use skin care cosmetics often contain incorporated UV-filters, thus providing additional exposure to these substances. There is now a general agree-ment that occasional use of sunscreens with SPFs between 15 and 20 are expected to provide an adequate protection to the great majority of the population unless special situations are encountered [84].

The traditional "sunscreen" concept has been now enlarged to "photoprotection", including UVA-radiation and its consequences, skin photoageing i.e. dermatoheliosis, solar elastosis and precancerous lesions. This is due to the increased knowledge about the action mechanisms of UVR in the skin. Photoprotection may thus be achieved with molecules different from the classical UV-filters acting through absorption and/or scattering of UVR. Antioxidants or related molecules are the prototypes of such active substances fitting in this widened concept. Combinations of different active molecules with classical UV-filters are most promising. The SPF could be in the future accompa-nied by a "mutation protection factor" reflecting the protection against interactions of UVR with the cellular genes. However, much research is to be done regarding proper experimental models because long-term effects are investigated.

Up to now, mandatory labelling of the products is the SPF. This acknowledges the fact that consumers now are aware of the SPF system. Category descriptions are optio-nal. In our opinion, category descriptions should be considered in first line in place of the SPF as the best way to provide complete information, because they are able to take in account the widening of the "sunscreen" into the "photoprotection" concept. A category description could include UVB- and UVA-protection (broad-range rating), possibly indications about protection against long-term effects and about other claims such as water resistance, thus providing the consumer with broad and understandable information about the product.

Finally however, these progresses should not be understood as an encouragement to use high-SPFs sunscreens and to stay longer in the sun. On the contrary, most benefits are awaited when consumers are encouraged to avoid excessive sun exposure and to prudently and frequently use good sunscreens.

References

1. Müller I (1997) Sun and man: An ambivalent relationship in the history of medicine. In: Altmeyer P, Hoffmann K, Stücker M (eds) Skin cancer and UV radiation. Springer, Berlin Heidelberg New York pp 3–12
2. Epstein JH (1997) The biological effects of sunlight. In: Lowe NJ, Shaath NA, Pathak MA (eds) Suncreens: Development, evaluation, and regulatory aspects, 2nd edition Marcel Dekker New York Basel Hong Kong, pp 83–100
3. Pathak MA (1991) Sunscreens: Principles of photoprotection. In: Mukhtar H (ed) Pharmacology of the skin. CRC Press Boca Raton Ann Arbor London pp 229–248
4. Schaefer H, Rougier A (eds) (1996) UVA and the skin (I). Eur J Dermatol 6:219–238
5. Schaefer H, Rougier A (eds) (1997) UVA and the skin (II). Eur J Dermatol 7:203–228
6. Pathak MA (1997) Photoprotection against harmful effects of solar UVB and UVA radiation: An update. In: Lowe NJ, Shaath NA, Pathak MA (eds) Suncreens: Development, evaluation, and regulatory aspects, 2nd edn. Marcel Dekker New York Basel Hong Kong pp 59–79
7. Seidenschnur EK (1995) FDA and EEC regulations related to skin: Documentation and measuring devices. In: Serup J, Jemec GBE (eds) Handbook of non-invasive methods and the skin. CRC Press Boca Raton Ann Arbor London pp 653–665
8. COLIPA-The European cosmetic, toiletry and perfumery association (1997) Guidelines for the evaluation of the efficacy of cosmetic products.
9. Davis JB, McNamara SH (1998) Regulatory aspects of cosmetic claims substantiation. In: Aust LB (ed) Cosmetic claims substantiation. Marcel Dekker New York Basel Hong Kong pp 1–20
10. COLIPA – The European cosmetic, toiletry and perfumery association (1994) Sun protection factor test method.
11. Australian/New Zealand Standard (1997) Sunscreen products-Evaluation and classification.
12. Murphy EG (1997) Regulatory aspects of sunscreens in the United States. In: Lowe NJ, Shaath NA, Pathak MA (eds) Suncreens: Development, evaluation, and regulatory aspects, 2nd edn. Marcel Dekker New York Basel Hong Kong pp 201–213
13. Griffin ME, Bourget TD, Lowe NJ (1997). Sun protection factor determination in the United States. In: Lowe NJ, Shaath NA, Pathak MA (eds) Suncreens: Development, evaluation, and regulatory aspects, 2nd edn. Marcel Dekker, New York Basel Hong Kong, pp 499–512
14. Evison J (1997) Broad spectrum sun protection: the issues and status. Cosmetics & Toiletries 112(6):35–41
15. Deutsches Institut für Normung eV (1985) Experimentelle dermatologische Bewertung des Erythemschutzes von externen Sonnenschutzmitteln für die menschliche Haut. DIN 67501
16. Diffey BL (1997) Dosimetry of ultraviolet radiation. In: Lowe NJ, Shaath NA, Pathak MA (eds) Suncreens: development, evaluation, and regulatory aspects, 2nd edn. Marcel Dekker, New York Basel Hong Kong, pp 175–188
17. McKinlay AF, Diffey BL (1987) A reference action spectrum for ultraviolet induced erythema in human skin. Chem Ind Eng 6:17–22
18. Uhlmann B, Mann T, Gers-Barlag H, Alert D, Sauermann G (1996) Consequences for sun protection factors when solar simulator spectra deviate from the spectrum of the sun. Int J Cosmet Sci 18:13–24
19. Sayre RM, Kaidbey KH (1990) Reciprocity for solar simulators used in sunscreen testing. Photodermatol Photoimmunol Photomed 7:198–201
20. Odio MR Veres DA, Goodman JJ, Irvin C, Robinson LR, Martinez J, Kraus AL (1994) Comparative efficacy of sunscreen reapplication regimens in children exposed to ambient sunlight. Photodermatol Photoimmunol Photomed 10:118–125

21. Snellman E, Jansén CT, Leszczynski K, Visuri R, Milan T, Jokela K (1995) Ultraviolet erythema sensitivity in anamnestic (I-IV) and phototested (1–4) caucasian skin phototypes: the need for a new classification system. Photochem Photobiol 62:769–772
22. Cordier M, Adhoute H, Benveniste JM, Marchand JP, Privat Y (1991) Comparison of the minimum erythematous dose on two distinct anatomical sites. Nouv Dermatol 10:134–136
23. Soon Park B, Il Youn J (1998) Topographic measurement of skin color by narrow-band reflectance spectrophotometer and minimal erythema dose (MED) in Koreans. Skin Res Technol 4:14–17
24. Ferguson J, et al (1996) Collaborative development of a sun protection factor test method: A proposed European standard. Int J Cosmet Sci 18:203–218
25. Iveson RD, Guthrie DM, Veres DA, Doughty D (1995) A study of the effect of anatomical site on sun protection factor efficiency using a novel UV delivery device. J Soc Cosmet Chem 46:271–280
26. Brown S, Diffey BL (1986) The effect of applied thickness on sunscreen protection: in vivo and in vitro studies. Photochem Photobiol 44:509–513
27. Gottlieb A, Bourget TD, Lowe NJ (1997) Sunscreens: Effects of amounts of application on sun protection factors. In: Lowe NJ, Shaath NA, Pathak MA (eds) Suncreens: Development, evaluation, and regulatory aspects, 2nd edn. Marcel Dekker, New York Basel Hong Kong, pp 583–588
28. Ferguson J (1997) European guidelines (COLIPA) for evaluation of sun protection factors. In: Lowe NJ, Shaath NA, Pathak MA (eds) Suncreens: Development, evaluation, and regulatory aspects, 2nd edn. Marcel Dekker, New York Basel Hong Kong, pp 513–525
29. Rhodes LE, Diffey BL (1996) Quantitative assessment of sunscreen application technique by in vivo fluorescence spectroscopy. J Soc Cosmet Chem 47:109–115
30. Bech-Thomsen N, Wulf HC (1992/1993) Sunbather's application of sunscreen is probably inadequate to obtain the sun protection factor assigned to the preparation. Photodermatol Photoimmunol Photomed 9:242–244
31. Diffey BL, Grice J (1997) The influence of sunscreen type on photoprotection. Br J Dermatol 137:103–105
32. Serup J, Jemec GBE (eds) Handbook of non-invasive methods and the skin. CRC Press Boca Raton Ann Arbor London, 1995
33. Jonker DL, Summers RS, Summers B (1994) Constitutive skin tone and sunscreen effects-UV-induced skin darkening in negroid skin. Cosmetics & Toiletries 109(2):51–58
34. Procaccini EM et al. (1997) Thirty hour's evaluation of UVB-induced erythema by chromometry and microflowmetry. Dermatology 195:317–320
35. Lock-Andersen J Gniadecka M, deFine Olivarius F, Dahlstrøm K, Wulf HC (1998) Skin temperature of UV-induced erythema correlated to laser Doppler flowmetry. Skin Res Technol 4:41–48
36. Kelley KA, Laskar PA, Ewing GD, Dromgoole SH, Lichtin JL, Sakr AA (1993) In vitro sun protection factor evaluation of sunscreen products. J Soc Cosmet Chem 44:139–151
37. Diffey BL, Robson J (1989) A new substrate to measure sunscreen protection factors throughout the ultraviolet spectrum. J Soc Cosmet Chem 40:127–133
38. Gabard B, Treffel P, Bieli E, Schwab S (1996) In vitro Messung des Sonnenschutzfaktors. Akt Dermatol 22 [Suppl 1]:25–30
39. Equipment 1: SPF Measurement System, Glen Spectra Ltd., 2–4 Wigton Gardens, Stanmore, Middlesex HA7 1BG UK (Tel. +44 181 204 9517; Fax +44 181 204 5189; E-mail: gs@isa-gs.demon.co.uk) Equipment 2: SPF-290S Sunscreen Protection Analyser System, Optometrics USA, Inc., Nemco Way, Stony Brook Industrial Park, Ayer, MA 01432 USA (Tel. +01 978 772 1700; Fax +01 978 772 0017; E-mail: opto@optometrics.com)
40. Pearse A, Edwards C (1993) Human stratum corneum as a substrate for in vitro sunscreen testing. Int J Cosmet Sci 15:234–244
41. Stokes RP, Diffey BL (1997) In vitro assay of high-SPF sunscreens. J Soc Cosmet Chem 48:289–295
42. Diffey BL (1997) Indices of protection from in vitro assay of sunscreens. In: Lowe NJ, Shaath NA, Pathak MA (eds) Suncreens: Development, evaluation, and regulatory aspects, 2nd edn. Marcel Dekker, New York Basel Hong Kong, pp 589–600
43. Lavker RM, Kaidbey KH (1997) A rationale for the development and use of sunscreens that protect from ultraviolet B as well as total ultraviolet A radiation. Hospitalis 67:190–193
44. Lowe NJ (1997) Ultraviolet A claims and testing procedures for OTC sunscreens: A summary and review. In: Lowe NJ, Shaath NA, Pathak MA (eds) Suncreens: Development, evaluation, and regulatory aspects, 2nd edition Marcel Dekker New York Basel Hong Kong pp 527–535
45. Chardon A, Moyal D, Hourseau C (1997) Persistent pigment darkening response as a method for evaluation of ultraviolet A protection assays. In: Lowe NJ, Shaath NA, Pathak MA (eds) Suncreens: development, evaluation, and regulatory aspects, 2nd edn. Marcel Dekker, New York Basel Hong Kong, pp 559–582
46. Diffey BL (1994) A method for broad spectrum classification of sunscreens. Int J Cosmet Sci 16:47–52

47. Stamatakis P, Palmer BR, Salzman GC, Allen TB (1990) Optimum particle size of titanium dioxide and zinc oxide for attenuation of ultraviolet radiation. J Coatings Technol 62(789):95–98
48. Anderson MW, Hewitt JP, Spruce SR (1997) Broad-spectrum physical sunscreens: Titanium dioxide and zinc oxide. In: Lowe NJ, Shaath NA, Pathak MA (eds) Suncreens: Development, evaluation, and regulatory aspects, 2nd edn. Marcel Dekker, New York Basel Hong Kong, pp 353–397
49. Pujol JA, Lecha M (1992/1993) Photoprotection in the infrared radiation range. Photodermatol Photoimmunol Photomed 9:275–278
50. Moyal D, Chardon A, Hourseau C (1993) Infra-red erythema and the part it plays in actinic erythema. Eur J Dermatol 3:64–67
51. Kligman LH, Kligman AM (1997) Ultraviolet radiation induced skin aging. In: Lowe NJ, Shaath NA, Pathak MA (eds) Suncreens: Development, evaluation, and regulatory aspects, 2nd edn. Marcel Dekker, New York Basel Hong Kong, pp 117–137
52. Violin L Girard F, Girard P, Meille JP, Petit-Ramel M (1994) Infrared photoprotection properties of cosmetic products: correlation between measurement of the anti-erythemic effect in vivo in man and the infrared reflection power in vitro. Int J Cosmet Sci 16:113–120
53. Kane KS, Martin EV (1995) Ultraviolet B-induced aptoposis of keratinocytes in murine skin is reduced by mild local hyperthermia. J Invest Dermatol 104:62–67
54. Lowe NJ, Friedlander J (1997) Sunscreens: Rationale for use to reduce photodamage and phototoxicity. In: Lowe NJ, Shaath NA, Pathak MA (eds) Suncreens: Development, evaluation, and regulatory aspects, 2nd edition Marcel Dekker New York Basel Hong Kong pp 35–58
55. Kaidbey K (1990) Substantivity and water resistance to sunscreens. In: Lowe NJ, Shaath NA (eds) Suncreens: development, evaluation, and regulatory aspects, 1st edn. Marcel Dekker, New York Basel Hong Kong, pp 405–410
56. Schrader K, Schrader A (1994) Die Sonnenschutzfaktorbestimmung: Prüfung der Wasserresistenz. Akt Dermatol 20:130–134
57. Schempp CM, Blümke C, Schöpf E, Simon JC (1997) Skin sensitivity to UVB-radiation is differentially increased by exposure to water and different salt solutions. Arch Dermatol 133:1610
58. Rieger MM (1997) Photostability of cosmetic ingredients on the skin. Cosmetics Toiletries 112(6):65–72
59. Brand-Garnys EE, Brand HM (1998) Photochemistry on the skin: More than sun care only! SÖFW 124:155–159
60. Shaath NA, Fares HM, Klein K (1990) Photodegradation of sunscreen chemicals: Solvent considerations. Cosmetics Toiletries 105(12):41–44
61. Berset G et al. (1996) Proposed protocol for determination of photostability. I: Cosmetic UV filters. Int J Cosmet Sci 18:167–177
62. Diffey BL et al (1997) Suncare product photostability: a key parameter for a more realistic in vitro efficacy evaluation. Eur J Dermatol 7:226–228
63. Forestier S, Lang G (1997) Photostable suncare products: Major progress in sun protection. In: Altmeyer P, Hoffmann K, Stücker M (eds) Skin cancer and UV radiation. Springer, Berlin Heidelberg New York, pp 314–319
64. Darr D, Pinnell SR (1997) Reactive oxygen species and antioxydant protection in photodermatology. In: Lowe NJ, Shaath NA, Pathak MA (eds) Suncreens: Development, evaluation, and regulatory aspects, 2nd edn. Marcel Dekker, New York Basel Hong Kong, pp 155–173
65. Thiele JJ, Dreher F, Packer L (1998) Antioxydant defense systems in skin. In: Elsner P, Maibach HI (eds) Drug vs cosmetics: cosmeceuticals? Marcel Dekker New York pp (in press)
66. Applegate LA, Frenk E (1995) Cellular defense mechanisms of the skin against oxidant stress and in particular UVA radiation. Eur J Dermatol 5:97–103
67. Black HS, Rajan B (1997) Antioxydants and carotenoids as potential photoprotectants. In: Lowe NJ, Shaath NA, Pathak MA (eds) Suncreens: Development, evaluation, and regulatory aspects, 2nd edn. Marcel Dekke,r New York Basel Hong Kong, pp 139–153
68. Dreher F, Gabard B, Schwindt D, Maibach HI (1998) Topical melatonin in combination with vitamins E and C protects skin from UV-induced erythema: a human in vivo study. Br J Dermatol 139:332–339.
69. Darr D, Dunston S, Faust H, Pinnell S (1996) Effectiveness of antioxydants (Vitamin C and E) with and without sunscreens as topical photoprotectants. Acta Derm Venereol (Stockh) 76:264–268
70. Bissett DL, McBride JF (1996) Synergistic topical photoprotection by a combination of the iron chelator 2-furildioxime and sunscreen. J Am Acad Dermatol 35:546–549
71. Hadshiew I, Stäb F, Untied S, Bohnsack K, Rippke F, Hölzle E (1997) Effects of topically applied antioxidants in experimentally provoked polymorphous light eruption. Dermatology 195:362–368
72. Dreher F, Denig N, Gabard B, Schwindt D, Maibach HI (1999) Effect of topical antioxidants on UV-induced erythema formation when administered after exposure. Dermatology 198:52–55

73. Gollnick HPM Hopfenmüller W, Hemmes C, Chun SC, Schmid C, Sundermeier K, Biesalski HK (1996) Systemic beta carotene plus topical UV-sunscreen are an optimal protection against harmful effects of natural UV-sunlight: results of the Berlin-Eilath study. Eur J Dermatol 6:200–205
74. Fisher GJ, Wang ZQ, Datta SC, Varani J, Kang S, Vorhees JJ (1997) Pathophysiology of premature skin aging induced by ultraviolet light. N Engl J Med 337:1419–1428
75. Gilchrest BA (1996) A review of skin ageing and its medical therapy. Br J Dermatol 135:867–875
76. Levêque JL Porte G, deRigal J, Corcuff P, Francois AM, Saint-Leger D (1988) Influence of chronic sun exposure on some biophysical parameters of the human skin: an in vivo study. J Cutan Aging Cosmet Dermatol 1:123–127
77. Richard S, deRigal J, deLacharriere O, Berardesca E, Levêque JL (1994) Noninvasive measurement of the effect of lifetime exposure to the sun on the aged skin. Photodermatol Photoimmunol Photomed 10:164–169
78. Quan MB, Edwards C, Marks R (1997) Non-invasive in vivo techniques to differentiate photodamage and ageing in human skin. Acta Derm Venereol (Stockh) 77:416–419
79. Harrison JA, Walker SL, Plastow SR, Batt MD, Young AR (1991) Sunscreens with low sun protection factor inhibit ultraviolet B and A photoaging in the skin of the hairless albino mouse. Photodermatol Photoimmunol Photomed 8:12–20
80. Boyd AS Naylor M, Cameron GS, Pearse AD, Gaskell SA, Neldner KH (1995) The effects of chronic sunscreen use on the histologic changes of dermatoheliosis. J Am Acad Dermatol 33:941–946
81. Bernstein EF, Brown DB, Takeuchi T, Kong SK, Uitto J (1997) Evaluation of sunscreens with various sun protection factors in a new transgenic mouse model of cutaneous photoaging that measures elastin promoter activation. J Am Acad Dermatol 37:725–729
82. Marks R (1997) Reduction of actinic keratoses by sunscreens. In: Lowe NJ, Shaath NA, Pathak MA (eds) Suncreens: development, evaluation, and regulatory aspects, 2nd edn. Marcel Dekker, New York Basel Hong Kong, pp 189–198
83. Diffey BL (1998) Sun protection: have we gone too far? Br J Dermatol 138:562–563
84. Schauder S (1997) Sunscreens in Europe: recent developments. In: Altmeyer P, Hoffmann K, Stücker M (eds) Skin cancer and UV radiation. Springer, Berlin Heidelberg New York, pp 276–295
85. Greiter F (1987) Aktuelle Technologien in der Kosmetik. Hüthig, Heidelberg, pp 262–263

CHAPTER 10

Self- or Sunless Tanning Lotions

S. B. Levy

Introduction

With increasing awareness of the hazards of ultraviolet light exposure, self-tanning or sunless tanning preparations have steadily become more popular as a safer means of achieving a tanned appearance. Better product aesthetics, ease of use and experience with using these preparations have also contributed to wider use. As available products have proliferated in the marketplace, claims regarding performance and efficacy of self-tanning lotions have been refined and broadened for promotion to an enlarging consumer base.

A brief review of the chemistry, mechanism of action and performance of the active ingredient in self tanners, dihydroxyacetone, will allow a critical examination of claims regarding their use. A more detailed review of the chemistry and application of dihydroxyacetone containing sunless or self-tanning lotions is available elsewhere [5].

Definition

Dihydroxyacetone (DHA) is the active ingredient in self tanners responsible for darkening the skin by staining. DHA is classified in the International Cosmetic Ingredient Dictionary and Handbook [12] as a colorant or a colorless dye. Products containing DHA should not be confused with bronzers intended to produce a darker color on the skin by the use of water soluble colorants. So-called tan accelerators containing tyrosine and other ingredients and tanning promoters containing psoralens require UV exposure to effect skin coloration. They will not be discussed here.

Chemistry

DHA ($C_3H_6O_3$) is a white, crystalline hygroscopic powder. This three-carbon sugar forms a dimer in freshly prepared aqueous solution. With heating to effect a solution in alcohol, ether, or acetone, it reverts to the monomer. DHA is stable between pH 4 to 6, but above pH 7 efficacy is lost with the formation of brown colored compounds. A buffered mixture at pH 5 is most stable. Heating above 38°C will also effect stability. DHA can react with oxygen and nitrogen containing compounds, collagen, urea derivatives, amino acids, and proteins which should be avoided in the formulation of the vehicle. Most cosmetic preparations contain 3.0–6.0% DHA.

Mechanism of Action

The site of action of DHA is the stratum corneum. Tape stripping of the skin quickly removes the color [6], as does mechanical rubbing. Microscopic studies of stripped stratum corneum and hair reveal irregular pigment masses in the keratin layers [3]. DHA reacts with free amino groups available as amino acids, peptides and proteins supplied by the keratin to form brown products or chromophores referred to as melanoidins [13]. Melanoidins have some physicochemical properties similar to naturally occurring melanin [7].

Application

Following application of a typical DHA containing self tanning lotion, color change can be observed within an hour. This color change can be seen under a Wood's light within 20 minutes. Maximal darkening may take 8 to 24 hours to develop. Individuals often make several successive applications every few hours to obtain their desired color. Depending on anatomical location, this color can be maintained with repeat applications every one to four days. The face requires fewer applications to achieve desired appearance but more frequent reapplication than the extremities.

Depth of color correlates with the thickness and compactness of the stratum corneum. Palms and soles stain deepest necessitating washing hands after application. Hair and nails color but not mucous membranes without a keratin layer. Rougher hyperkeratotic areas over the knees, elbows and ankles will take up the color more unevenly as will older photoaged skin with keratoses and mottled pigmentation. Color will be retained for longer periods in these areas.

Usage directions generally provided with self tanning products follow from these observations. The skin may be prepared with a mild form of exfoliation. Careful even application is directed, not skipping areas, with lighter application around elbows, knees, and ankles to avoid excessive darkening in these latter areas. Care needs to be taken around the hairline where lighter hair may darken. Hands need to be washed immediately after use to avoid darkening of the palms, fingers and nails. Clearly care, skill and experience are necessary to achieve the desired results with these formulations.

Claims

Based on our preceding discussion, more than with most cosmetic products, individual application technique dictates if performance claims are met. Additionally, the user's skin type and age will in large part determine satisfaction with these products. This needs to be borne in mind as we consider performance claims for this category of products. However, the formulator can have a significant impact on product performance by selection of the DHA containing vehicle.

Cosmetic Efficacy

The emphasis with self tanners is on readily visible performance claims. Such claims will rely on actual controlled supervised use testing as opposed to indirect in vitro or instrumental methods.

Duration with Onset of Action

The time of onset of perceptible color may be specified, generally within one to several hours. Depending on frequency of application and concentration of DHA, the duration of effect can be stated, up to 3 or 4 days. Frequency of cleansing and bathing may also impact on duration in a given individual. Claims such as fast acting or longer lasting may require comparative testing with other available products in the marketplace. Water resistance may be claimed, particularly relative to other cosmetic products such as bronzers.

Color

The color achieved with these products is the most significant product claim for users. Older DHA formulas were associated with an orange color, frequently objectionable to consumers, limiting their success in the marketplace. Newer products claim to provide a "natural" or "golden" tan with "natural looking color". By formulating with a lower concentration of DHA, supplied as a pure material, at appropriate pH and in a stable vehicle allowing for better penetration, superior color is obtained.

The color achieved remains, however, very much dependent on skin type. Medium complected individuals with skin photoypes II or III, as opposed to those who are lighter or darker will obtain a more pleasing color. Individuals with underlying golden skin tones will achieve better results than rosy, sallow or olive complected persons. Older individuals with rough hyperkeratotic skin and mottled pigmentation or with freckles may be displeased by irregular color emphasizing these attributes.

Products indicating a shade for specific skin types such as light, medium or dark may be particularly helpful to the consumer. These skin types may be listed with Fitzpatrick phototypes [1]. By varying the concentration of DHA in these products, individuals with lighter complexions will achieve better results. Less experienced users will also benefit from starting with a lower DHA concentration product more forgiving of application technique. Claims relating to evenness of color, "streak-less", "non-streaking" or "self-adjusting" are very application technique dependent.

Aesthetics

As with all cosmetic products aesthetic claims are vehicle dependent. They may be formulated as appropriate for oily, normal or combination skin types. The total formulation and use testing will determine if a product "spreads easily", "absorbs quickly", or is "fast drying". The latter claim may allow a user to "dress more quickly" following product application. DHA incorporated into some vehicles may be associated with a noticeable odor. An odor-free claim is sometimes made.

Moisturization

The vehicle also determines a self-tanning product's qualities as a moisturizer. Individual emollient and humectant ingredients are components of many vehicles desirable for incorporation of DHA in emulsion systems. The resulting product's effect on the feel, comfort, conditioning, resiliency, moisture content and barrier function of the skin may be assessed instrumentally as described in other sections of this book. Likewise, changes in fine lines and wrinkles may be assessed separately.

Additives

With interest in "active treatment" ingredients in skin care products, some have been incorporated in DHA-containing formulations. Vitamins, botanical extracts, antioxidants, anti-irritants and even alpha hydroxy acids have been added. Any benefits to the final product are obviously concentration, pH and vehicle dependent. Ideally, additional benefits are claimed on the basis of actual product testing and not simply the addition of an ingredient.

Sunscreen Efficacy

Sunscreen incorporated in a self-tanning product has a profound effect on product claims and it warrants a separate, more detailed discussion. Sun Protection Factor (SPF) claims may be made based on the addition of chemical sunscreen ingredients and appropriate testing. Claims, product labeling and ingredient disclosure are subject to regulation by the country in which the product is sold.

In the United States the Tentative Final Over-the-Counter Drug Products Monograph on Sunscreens [11] lists DHA as an approved sunscreen ingredient when used sequentially with lawsone (2-hydroxy-1,4-napthoquinone). The European Economic Community Directive does not list DHA as a permitted UV filter. DHA itself has at most a modest effect on SPF [10]. The brown color obtained with its use does absorbs in the low end of the visible spectrum with overlap into long UVA and may provide some UVA protection[4].

Consumers using DHA-containing tanning products need to be cautioned that despite a perceived darkening of their skin, these products provide minimal sun protection. Products labeled with SPF provide the stated level of protection for a few hours after application; but not for days a visible color change is still perceptible. After-sun products containing DHA which claim to prolong the duration of a tanned appearance may be particularly confusing to consumers.

Safety

The visible color change associated with the use of self tanners might suggest to users that these products are hazardous. Based on the chemistry of DHA and its toxicological profile, it can be considered relatively non-toxic. Contact dermatitis to DHA has only rarely been reported [9]. As with other topical products with active ingredients, such as sunscreens, much of the reported sensitivity is secondary to other ingredients in the vehicle [2]. All ingredients in the formulation need to be reviewed for safety. Ultimately, testing the final product dictates the stated claims.

The basis for the specific claims which follow have all been reviewed more thoroughly in other sections of this book for a broader range of products. Other than consideration for self tanners containing sunscreen, substantiating safety in these products should be done by similar protocols.

Allergy testing may be performed via modified Draize repeat insult patch test. Testing for subjective and objective irritancy is done via extended supervised use testing. In stating the product is suitable for those with "sensitive skin", panels of individuals appropriately identified as having sensitive skin need to undergo such testing. Rigorous product formulation and testing performed with a sufficient number of subjects may allow a hypoallergenic claim. A truly fragrance-free product also supports the latter claim. Testing for comedogenicity and acnegenicity is also done with the appropriate panelists by standard protocols[8]. The exact definition of a product claimed to be "dermatologist-tested" is most problematic.

Conclusion

Considering the well documented hazards associated with ultraviolet light exposure, self or sunless tanning products can be considered a safe way to tan. This claim is further supported by the benign toxicologic profile of dihydroxyacetone. Claims related to the tanned appearance achieved may be documented by supervised use testing. The results obtained with these products are dependent on final formulation, individual application technique and the consumer's complexion type. Consumers need to be clearly informed that these products do not offer significant protection against UVB. If formulated with standard sunscreens, the duration of UV protection is more short lived than the skin color change.

References

1. Fitzpatrick TB (1988) The validity and practicality of sunreactive skin types I through IV. Arch Dermatol 124:869–871
2. Foley P, Nixon R, Marks R, Frowen K, Thompson S (1993) The frequency of reactions to sunscreens: results of a longitudinal population–based study on the regular use of sunscreens in Australia. Br J Dermatol 128:512–518
3. Goldman L, Barkoff J, Blaney D, et al (1960) Investigative studies with the skin coloring agents dihydroxyacetone and glyoxal. J Invest Dermatol 35:161–164
4. Johnson JA, Fusaro RM (1987) Protection against long ultraviolet radiation: topical browning agents and a new outlook. Dermatologica 175:53–57
5. Levy SB (1992) Dihydroxyacetone–containing sunless or self-tanning lotions. J Am Acad Dermatol 27:989–993
6. Maibach HI, Kligman AM (1960) Dihydroxyacetone: a suntan-simulating agent. Arch Dermatol 82:505–507
7. Meybeck A (1977) A spectroscopic study of the reaction products of dihydroxyacetone with amino acids. J Soc Cosmet Chem 16:777–782
8. Mills OH, Berger RS (1991) Defining the susceptibility of acne-prone and sensitive skin populations to extrinsic factors. Dermatol Clin 9:93–98
9. Morren M, Dooms-Goossens A, Heidbuchel M, et al (1991) Contact allergy to dihydroxyacetone. Contact Dermatitis 25:326–327
10. Muizzuddin N, Marenus KD, Maes DH (1997) UV-A and UV-B protective effect of melanoids formed with dihydroxyacetone and skin. Poster 360 presented at the 55th Annual Meeting of the American Academy of Dermatology, San Francisco
11. Tentative Final Over-The-Counter Drug Products Monograph on Sunscreens (1993). Federal Register 58:28194–28302
12. Wenninger JA, McEwen GN ur, eds. (1997) International Cosmetic Ingredient Dictionary and Handbook⁷ᵗʰed. The Cosmetic, Toiletry and Fragrance Association
11. Wittgenstein E, Berry HK (1961) Reaction of dihydroxyacetone (DHA) with human skin callus and amino compounds. J Invest Dermatol 36:283–286

CHAPTER 11

Antidandruff

U.-F. Haustein, P. Nenoff

Clinical Picture of Dandruff

Dandruff or pityriasis capitis is defined as the noninflammatory excessive production of small flakes of dead skin on the scalp. To a certain degree this is a normal or physiological process, because the dead epidermal cells of the scalp skin are replaced constantly and flake off after about 1 month. This condition first becomes a cosmetic problem with increasing severity of scaling and itching. Patients do not go to the doctor until the detached scales drift unaesthetically among the hair shafts or fall on the collar and shoulders where they become visible.

Dandruff is characterized by white, often dry, sometime greasy, loose scaling together with a mild pruritus of the scalp (Fig. 1). These symptoms may occur in isolation or together. Pityriasis amiantacea with accumulation of "asbestos-like" scales occurs as an extreme form.

Seborrhoeic dermatitis (SD) is defined as a chronic inflammatory disorder that principally affects sebaceous areas. These are mainly the scalp, face with nasolabial

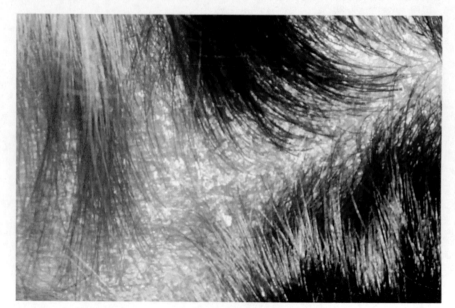

Fig. 1. Dandruff or pityriasis capitis: mild form of seborrhoeic dermatitis

folds, retroauricular region, auditory canals, forehead and eyebrows, and the upper trunk. This dermatosis is characterized by redness, itching and scaling of the skin. This may or may not be fortuitously associated with seborrhoea or with baldness. SD has a higher prevalence in persons with acquired immunodeficiency syndrome (AIDS) than in other persons.

Some dermatologists consider these to be different diseases. However, more and more the opinion is accepted that dandruff represents a mild form or an early stage of SD.

Dandruff is relative rare in childhood but becomes a cosmetic affliction in adolescent and adult people. At an age of 20 years nearly about 50% of caucasians are affected in some degree. Beyond the age of 50 years pityriasis capitis appears only seldom and then in a less intense form.

Aetiology and Pathogenesis

Role of Lipids and Hormones

Despite the fact that today it is well accepted that seborrhoea is not an important factor for SD this disorder is frequently associated with seborrhoea [38]. In addition, the age incidence suggests that SD may be related to the hormones, in particular to androgens. Androgenic hormones are responsible for stimulation of sebaceous glands. At least, incidence of SD decreases in pregnancy. Against that, an increased incidence is found in periods of emotional stress, in alcoholics and AIDS patients [40].

Previously, there were some investigations favouring the role of lipids as cause of SD. Konrad and Cernikova [24] found an increase of cholesterol and triglycerides and a decrease of squalenes and free fatty acids in SD. Gloor et al. [16] demonstrated identical whole lipids but different lipid composition. Patients with SD showed significantly higher concentrations of cholesterol and triglycerides but lower concentrations of free fatty acids, wax esters and squalenes in SD. This speaks for an increase of epidermal skin surface lipids in comparison to sebaceous gland lipids. The relative high concentration of free fatty acids which is a result of bacterial lipolysis in sebaceous glands or at the skin surface could possibly be due to a change of microbial micro flora of the skin. By way of contrast, Kligman and Leyden [23] found in SD an unchanged lipid composition and sebaceous gland secretion whereas an enhanced production of cells of the horny layer and keratinization occurs.

It has also been postulated that SD may reflect a nutritional deficiency of certain vitamins resulting in SD-like eruptions. A recent study of the serum essential fatty acid pattern from 30 subjects with infantile SD suggested a transiently impaired function of the enzyme delta 6–desaturase [43].

Dandruff and *Malassezia furfur*

Both SD and dandruff are strongly associated with the presence of the lipophilic yeast *Malassezia furfur* (formerly called *Pityrosporum ovale*). Although the exact mechanism remains to be proved, the pathogenic role of *M. furfur* in these skin disorders is more and more accepted now. *M. furfur* is a very common resident of the lipid-rich surfaces of the human skin [27]. There is no doubt that *M. furfur* is the aetiologic agent of pityriasis versicolor, *Malassezia* folliculitis, and *Malassezia* intertrigo. *M. furfur* is rarely capable of causing even systemic infections preferably in immunocompromised patients receiving fat emulsions infused through central venous lines.

The successful use of antimycotics, especially ketoconazole, in the treatment of SD and dandruff confirmed the hypothesis that *M. furfur* infection is aetiologically important.

An aetiological role for the *Malassezia* yeasts in SD was proposed already in the nineteenth century [36]. Thereafter, Malassez [26] described a *Pityrosporum*-like microorganism which was thought to be responsible for pathogenesis of pityriasis capitis. Subsequently, Unna [44] and Sabouraud [36] confirmed these observations and the aetiological agent was called *Pityrosporum ovale*. However, in the 1960ies and 70ies of our century the hypothesis failed to gain acceptance and the increased number of these micro-organisms found in SD of the scalp was regarded to be a secondary colonization of the rash [23]. The pathogenesis of pityriasis capitis or dandruff was separated from that of SD. The former was thought to be due to epidermal hyperproliferation, and the latter more to an inflammatory process [22]. The hyperproliferation hypothesis was thrown into doubt by Shuster et al. [41]. He concluded that the terms of Koch's postulates were fulfilled by *M. furfur* as the primary aetiological agent for the clinical pictures both of dandruff and SD.

M. furfur occurs in both hyphal and yeast form in skin lesions and in culture, but it has been observed only in yeast phase in normal human skin (Figs. 2, 3). The colonization starts during puberty when the sebaceous glands become active. Bandhaya [2]

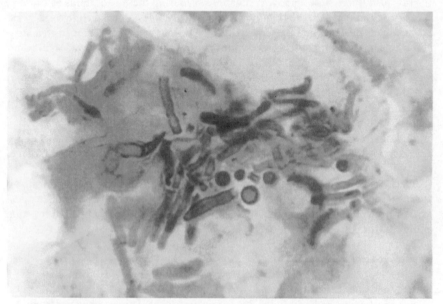

Fig. 2. *Malassezia furfur* in pityriasis versicolor. Microscopically, round yeast-like fungal cells together with short hyphal elements are visible in horny scales from skin lesion. Potassium hydroxide preparation with cresyl true red staining

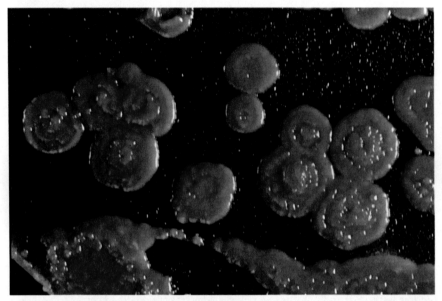

Fig. 3. *Malassezia furfur.* Typically, colonies are smooth, sometimes glistening, and creamy to yellowish brown with an intact margin. Growth at 37° C on Sabouraud 4%–glucose agar supplemented with 2% olive oil and 0.2% Tween 80

investigated the normal skin of 200 volunteers in an age range 20–30 years. All of the subjects studied harboured *M. furfur* at every site tested, and had high counts on the head and upper trunk regions of high sebum excretion rate. Moreover, the number of *M. furfur* yeast cells is significantly higher in dandruff-affected area of the scalp than in controls [21].

In the last 2 or 3 years the genus *Malassezia* has been revised using morphology, physiology, ultrastructure, and molecular biology. As a result the genus has been enlarged to include seven species comprising the three former taxa *M. furfur*, *M. pachydermatis*, and *M. sympodalis*, and four new taxa, *M. globosa*, *M. obtusa*, *M. restricta*, and *M. slooffiae* [18]. With the exception of *M. pachydermatis*, the species have an absolute requirement in vitro for a supplementation of long-chain fatty acids in the medium, hence the term lipophilic yeast, applied to the members of this genus. *M. pachydermatis* is mainly isolated from animals, but of the others, no one species is associated with SD in either AIDS or non-AIDS patients or the other above mentioned *Malassezia*-associated skin disorders. This suggests that the development of lesions is not caused by specific infections with a single organism. On the other hand, there is also no evidence that the phenotypic feature varies among different *Malassezia* strains isolated from SD, such as for example their ability to adhere to keratinocytes [19].

Early attempts to quantitate *M. furfur* on normal human skin were limited by inefficient recovery media [21]. Leeming and Notman [25] carried out the most reliable quantitative study of the carriage and distribution of *M. furfur* on normal human adult skin. They found that the population density was highest on the upper trunk (1.1×10^4 colony forming units [CFU] cm^{-2} on the chest; 8.9×10^3 CFU cm^{-2} on the back; 10^3 CFU cm^{-2} on the cheek, 3×10^4 CFU per swab from the ear). McGinley et al. [27]

carried out quantitative microbiological investigations of the scalp, showing that *M. furfur* accounts for 46% of the total microflora in normal individuals, 74% in the presence of dandruff and even 83% in SD. The finding that the population density of *M. furfur* in dandruff is twice as high as on a nonaffected scalp is still unclear. Is it a true increase of the yeast cell population density in dandruff, or is it only due to an enlargement of the skin surface as a result of scaling?

In addition, several other authors reported on the significantly higher density of *M. furfur* yeast cells in scalp regions with dandruff than in unaffected control individuals [21]. Recently, Piérard-Franchimont et al. [35] demonstrated immunohistochemically the amount of yeasts in SD and dandruff, which was in agreement to most previous published microscopic studies. In contrast to that, they stressed that the culture methods for assessment of *M. furfur* cell count yield exceedingly low numbers of colonies per surface area compared with the number of *M. furfur* present in squamae. This means that yeasts are present inside and not at the surface of most of the clumps of corneocytes in SD. They concluded that if this is responsible for the huge discrepancy in numbers, SD should be considered the "disease of the dead *M. furfur*".

A further hypothesis for the involvement of *M. furfur* in the pathogenesis of SD is a direct effect of the yeast cells on stimulatory response. *Malassezia* produces a lot of potential irritants, including lipase activity. They are capable of producing unsaturated free fatty acids and unsaturated triglycerides by peroxidation [19].

Immune Response to M. furfur

The immune status of the host rather than the characteristics of the organism per se is thought to play a major aetiological part in *Malassezia*-associated disease [2, 42]. However, findings concerning the immune reactivity to *M. furfur*, which is thought to be of primary importance, are contradictory. Serum IgG antibodies against *M. furfur* have been reported to be elevated in SD [28]. However, because other authors could not confirm these results, the serum IgG antibody titre seems to be of minor importance in SD [3, 4]. The evidence that SD is more common in AIDS patients suggests that immunological mechanisms may be involved. In earlier studies Bergbrant et al. [5] found T cell abnormalities in patients with SD and an inverse correlation between the levels of IgG antibodies against a protein antigen from *M. furfur* and the severity of SD. Because this immune reaction is T-lymphocyte dependent these results could suggest an immunoweakness in the patients as an explanation of the abnormal reaction in the skin against the saprophyte *M. furfur*. Patch testing with *Malassezia* antigen of patients with SD did not show contact sensitization to the yeast [33]. On the other hand, previously it was demonstrated that application of killed organisms to skin both of humans and also of rabbits can indeed lead to clinical changes similar to those observed in SD [19]. High numbers of HLA–DR4-positive lymphocytes in the blood of patients with SD lead to the suggestion that an intermittent activation of the immune system may be occurring. The predominance of CD4 phenotypic lymphocytes was also proven in tissue samples from skin sites affected with SD, whereas the number of CD1a-positive epidermal cells is similar in both normal and lesional skin [19]. In addition, elevated circulating Leu 7- and Leu 11-positive lymphocytes are found, suggesting an increased number of natural killer cells [19].

Piérard-Franchimont et al. [35] were able to demonstrate that *M. furfur* was always covered with the antibody to factor XIIIa, suggesting the presence of a transglutaminase in the yeast cell wall. This factor XIIIa-related transglutaminase present in fungal cell walls could act as an adhesion molecule to biological substrates. Deposits of IgG and C3 were present underneath and in close apposition to collections of *M. furfur* in SD, and absent in control materials. Therefore, these findings indicate a host response located specifically at the site of *M. furfur* suggesting an unique inflammatory reaction to this yeast in SD and dandruff.

Neuber et al. [32] have clearly demonstrated that peripheral blood mononuclear cells from patients with SD show a diminished cellular immune response to *M. furfur* antigens. An increased lymphocyte proliferation response to *M. furfur* antigen was observed in the controls but not in patients with SD. In addition, they found that IL-10 secretion was significantly increased after stimulation with *M. furfur* extract. IL-10 is known to inhibit monocyte/macrophage-dependent T-cell proliferation and cytokine synthesis. Therefore, increased IL-10 secretion in SD may explain low proliferation as well as reduced IL-2 and IFNγ secretion and the disturbed cellular immunity to *M. furfur*. The results of Neuber et al. [32] support the assumption that strong skin colonization with *M. furfur* in SD is due to an altered cellular immunity, which may be induced by increased IL-10 secretion.

In Vitro Activity of Azoles Against *M. furfur*

Based on the suggested role of the yeast *M. furfur* in the pathogenesis of SD and dandruff, the different antidandruff agents that are suitable for topical treatment of these disorders have to be tested in vitro in order to determine their efficacy to inhibit the growth of *M. furfur*. A useful method of in vitro susceptibility testing of *M. furfur* strains isolated from patients with *Malassezia*-associated skin alterations is the agar dilution method. Media for both cultivation and maintenance of this lipophilic microorganism have to contain olive oil and the detergent Tween 80 to enable growth of the yeast. We perform both cultivation and susceptibility testing at a temperature of 37°C, but the use of lower temperatures down to 26°C has also been described by others.

Agar dilution tests to determine the minimum inhibitory concentrations (MIC) of true antifungals but also other substances were performed on D.S.T. agar (D.S.T.=Diagnostic Sensitivity Test Agar, Unipath, Oxoid, Basingstoke, Hampshire, England), pH adjusted to 5.7. Most antifungals were suspended in dimethyl sulfoxide and further diluted in sterile distilled water. The final concentration of dimethyl sulfoxide in the medium was 4% or lower. Controls were done with agar containing dimethyl sulfoxide without antifungal to rule out any inhibitory effect of the solvent. Serial two-fold dilutions of the agents ranging from 0.006 to 100 µg ml^{-1} were prepared in D.S.T. agar containing additionally 2% olive oil and 0.2% Tween 80, which were added later to allow growth of the lipophilic yeast. For susceptibility testing 6-day-old cultures of *M. furfur* on Sabouraud 4% dextrose agar with olive oil were used. *M. furfur* cell aliquots were prepared as suspensions in olive oil, sterile distilled water and Tween 80 (3:5:2). These suspensions were vortexed twice for 20 s. Plates were inoculated with a multipoint inoculator. The yeast cell suspension (approximately 10^8 CFU ml^{-1}) was inoculated onto antifungal-containing media using a multipoint inoculator that delivered 3–4 µl per spot, resulting in a final amount of 3–4×10^5 CFU. Results were recorded after incubation at 37°C for 96 h. The lowest drug concentration at which a strain showed no

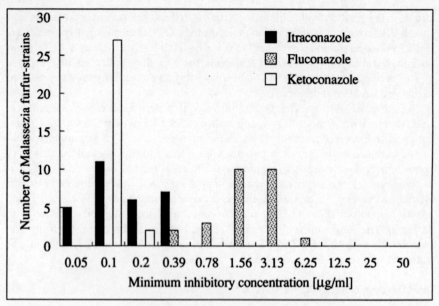

Fig. 4. MIC values of the azole antifungals ketoconazole, itraconazole and fluconazole against *Malassezia furfur*

growth was considered to be the MIC. Growth controls were carried out on the medium without the active antifungal agent.

A new method for microdilution susceptibility testing was recently published by Schmidt and Rühl-Hörster [39]. Preincubation of the *M. furfur* strains and also the susceptibility testing were carried out in medium A according to Leeming and Notman [25]. Because of the underlying turbidity of the medium, growth or growth inhibition of the fungi has to be determined by a nonturbidimetric method using Alamar Blue, an oxidation–reduction indicator, based on the colorimetric detection of metabolic activity. The original colour of the solution is blue. The MIC was determined as the lowest drug concentration that maintained a blue or a blue-pink hue. Wells with growth were pink-red in colour.

The in vitro antifungal activity of ketoconazole, several other azole and polyene antimycotics but also of antiseborrhoeic and antipsoriatic agents against M. furfur was demonstrated in recent studies. Van Cutsem et al. [45] showed that ketoconazole had a greater in vitro activity against *M. furfur* than zinc pyrithione or selenium disulfide.

Recently, we demonstrated the inhibitory effect of ketoconazole but also of different other azole antimycotics against *M. furfur* in vitro [29]. In accordance with Faergemann [12,13], ketoconazole was more effective in vitro against *M. furfur* than the other azole derivatives – itraconazole, fluconazole, tioconazole, clotrimazole – and the polyene natamycin (Figs. 4, 5).

Experimental *Malassezia* Dermatitis in Animals

Van Cutsem et al. [45] assessed in an animal model the efficacy of four shampoos – 2% ketoconazole, 1% and 2% zinc pyrithione and 2.5% selenium disulfide – in experi-

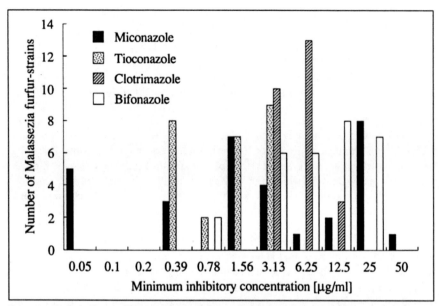

Fig. 5. MIC values of topically applied azole antimycotics against *Malassezia furfur*

mental pityrosporosis. The guinea pigs were inoculated on each of 7 consecutive days on intact skin. The lesions were scored for erythema, folliculitis, and hyperkeratosis 24 h after the last inoculation and after treatment. Final evaluations were performed 13 days after infection (10 days after last shampoo application). Treatment with undiluted and diluted (1:10) shampoos showed consistently superior clinical and mycological results for ketoconazole shampoo. Van Gerven and Odds [46] obtained comparable results in experimental *M. furfur*-induced dermatitis, also in guinea pigs. Among the imidazole antifungal agents tested, ketoconazole cream and shampoo showed the most potent efficacy when compared to bifonazole 1%, clotrimazole 1%, flutrimazole 1% and miconazole 2%. It has to be mentioned, however, that the relatively newly developed azole derivative, sertaconazole, as 2% gel and cream, showed no reduction in lesion severity to below control.

Clinical Trials in Dandruff

A randomized, double-blind, placebo-controlled trial of ketoconazole 2% shampoo versus selenium disulfide 2.5% shampoo in the treatment of moderate to severe dandruff over a period of 4 weeks was carried out by Danby et al. [9]. They showed that the mean total adherent dandruff score declined throughout the treatment period, with both ketoconazole 2% and selenium disulfide 2.5% shampoos significantly better than placebo at all visits. Ketoconazole was statistically superior to selenium disulfide at day 8 only. Both medicated shampoos were significantly better than placebo for reducing irritation and itching.

Recently, Peter and Richarz-Barthauer [34] reported on the results of a multicentre, double-blind, placebo-controlled trial on the treatment and prophylaxis of scalp SD and dandruff with 2% ketoconazole shampoo. In 575 patients presenting with moderate to severe SD and dandruff of the scalp, 2% ketoconazole shampoo was used twice weekly for 2–4 weeks, producing an excellent response in 88%. SD and dandruff have a strong tendency for chronicity and relapse of the skin alterations. In nearly all cases, a long-lasting prophylactic treatment is necessary. Interestingly, of those patients who responded in this study, 312 were included in a prophylactic phase lasting 6 months. These patients were treated with the active preparation (shampoo with ketoconazole) once weekly, once every other week, alternating with placebo (shampoo without ketoconazole), or with placebo only once weekly. Relapse of SD occurred in 47% of patients in the placebo group, compared with 19% in the active treatment group and 31% of patients in the active/placebo group. The rate of absorption of the ketoconazole 2% shampoo was shown to be <1%, which emphasizes the safety of this preparation.

Although in all studies performed a significant difference from placebo was found, it was noticed that about one-third of the placebo-treated patients presented with a noticeable improvement of their scalp conditions. One could therefore argue that more frequent shampooing could passively remove dandruff and unmask the effect of ketoconazole. This is why Arrese et al. [1] performed a double-blind, placebo-controlled study to evaluate the efficacy of ketoconazole 0.5% and 1% shampoos when used once daily over a period of 2 weeks. This trial revealed the clearly superior effect of ketoconazole 0.5% and 1% shampoo over placebo in the treatment of dandruff. Moreover, a dose-dependent activity of ketoconazole was demonstrated. In the past it was shown that a relapse of dandruff occurs more quickly when the frequency of shampooing with a nonmedicated shampoo is lower than the frequency of use of an antifungal agent, which can be explained by a faster recolonization of the scalp by *M. furfur*.

Modern shampoos designed for treating dandruff and SD were developed on the basis of the proven antifungal effect of their active ingredients against *M. furfur*. The antidandruff shampoos should remove the scales, alter corneocyte binding and diminish yeast cell reproduction of *M. furfur*. Removal of the squames is important both for the direct cosmetic effect and also for the indirect effect of interrupting the cyclic process of yeast cell accumulation followed by blocking the release of proinflammatory mediators. Goffin et al. [17] conducted a study to quantify the effect of eight proprietary antidandruff shampoos on the human stratum corneum using a squamometric in vivo bioassay and a corneosurfametric ex vivo bioassay. Besides the shampoos containing active antifungal agents one additional shampoo, which contained only a mild surfactant, was assessed. Surfactants present in shampoos are interfacially active substances which interact with the stratum corneum. The authors were able to demonstrate differences among antidandruff shampoos in their interaction with stratum corneum, in particular the activity against corneocyte clumping. Significant differences in mildness were disclosed between some test shampoos and the selected mild reference surfactant. It is concluded that the formulation of shampoos for treatment of dandruff should not be overlooked.

Systemic Treatment with Ketoconazole

Although the response of SD and dandruff to systemic ketoconazole has helped to consolidate understanding of their fungal aetiology, the safety and cost of systemic ketoconazole limit its use for these conditions. As long ago as in 1984, Ford et al. [15]

conducted a randomized, double-blind, placebo-controlled cross-over study of the systemic application of 200 mg ketoconazole daily in 19 patients with SD of the scalp and other body sites. The body and scalp lesions and the itching regressed considerably and significantly with ketoconazole in all but 5 patients, 3 of whom subsequently responded to a higher dose.

It is reported that oral ketoconazole 200 mg daily decreases sebum excretion in patients suffering from acne vulgaris and seborrhoea. This is explained by its antiandrogen action. However, topically applied ketoconazole is not percutaneously absorbed and cannot influence the glandular synthesis of androgens and thus the sebum excretion. Surprisingly, Dobrev and Zissova [10] observed an increase of scalp lipid level in half the patients suffering from SD of the scalp treated with 2% ketoconazole

Table 1. Treatment options for dandruff

Generic name	Trade name	Concentration (%)	Usage
Ketoconazole[a]	Terzolin solution	2	Once to twice/week
Clotrimazole[a]	SD Hermal cream	2	Once to twice/week
Ciclopirox olamine	Stieprox solution	1	Once to twice/week
Selenium disulfide[a] [2]	Selsun suspension Selukos suspension Ellsurex paste	2.5	Once to twice/week
Zinc pyrithione[a]	De-squaman N hermal cream	1	Once/week, in severe cases up to three times/week
Coal tar[a] [3]	Bernifer scalp gel	0.5	Once to twice/week
	Polytar solution	0.3 Juniper tar 0.3 Wood tar 0.07 Coal tar	Once to twice/week
Benzoyl peroxide[a]	Benzoyl peroxide liquidum medical shampoo	2.5	Once to twice/week
Salicylic acid[b] [1]	Psorimed solution	10	Twice to three times/week
	Squamasol solution and gel	10	Twice to three times/week
Corticosteroids[c] [7]	Alpicort solution [1]	0.2 prednisolone 0.4 salicylic acid	Once/day, overnight for 2(–4) weeks
	Ultralan crinale solution [1]	0.5 fluocortolone-21 pivalate 1 salicylic acid	Once to twice/day, overnight, for 2(–4) weeks
	Ecural solution	0.1 mometasone furoate	Once/day, overnight, for 2(–4) weeks
	Lygal scalp tincture [2]	0.2 prednisolone 1 salicylic acid 0.3 dexpanthenol	Once to twice/day, for 2(–) weeks
Lithium succinate [1]	Efadermin ointment [1]	8 lithium succinate 0.5 zinc sulfate	Twice/day for about 4 weeks

[a] The listed agents for treatment of seborrhoeic dermatitis of the scalp are used as shampoos. These shampoos can be used two or three times a week. After application shampoos should be left on the hair and scalp for at least 5–10 min. After that the preparation can be removed by rinsing with warm water
[b] Application of the solution by massaging into the scalp. It should be left for 10–30 min. After that it can be removed by rinsing with warm water
[c] Application of the solutions as indicated without rinsing out

shampoo for 4 weeks. It is assumed that the ketoconazole shampoo does not influence the sebum production but improves its delivery onto the skin surface. This is probably due to the removal of the follicular occlusion. The possible underlying pathogenetic mechanism may be that the yeasts colonizing the pilosebaceous duct were destroyed, which contributes to the elimination of the follicular inflammation and occlusion. The more efficient flow of sebum leads to the reduction of *Malassezia* yeasts and bacteria colonizing the pilosebaceous ducts. In addition, ketoconazole shampoo could reduce the follicular occlusion regardless of the incidence of *M. furfur*.

Role of Antiseborrhoeic Agents

Therapy of SD with antiseborrhoeic agents such as selenium disulfide and zinc pyrithione was already in use before the introduction of antimycotics – especially ketoconazole – for SD treatment. The therapeutic effect of antiseborrhoeic agents in SD was thought to be a function of their anti-inflammatory action. Previously, we demonstrated the good in vitro efficacy both of selenium disulfide and zinc pyrithione against all tested *M. furfur* strains from patients with SD. Zinc pyrithione in particular was very effective against *M. furfur* in vitro. MICs of zinc pyrithione were comparable to those of the true antimycotic agents being investigated. These results support the assumption that SD is fungal in origin (Fig. 6).

Additionally we could demonstrate the in vitro susceptibility of *M. furfur* to the antipsoriatic drugs liquor carbonis detergens and dithranol, but in accordance with findings of Bunse and Mahrle [7] it was found a less effective growth inhibition than was obtained with the in vitro efficacy of antimycotic and also antiseborrhoeic drugs.

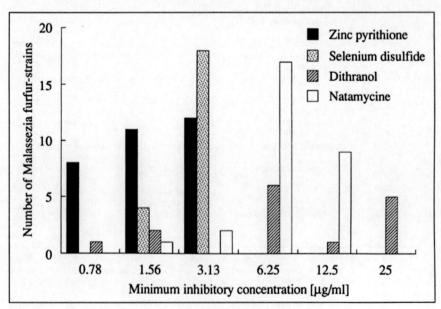

Fig. 6. MIC values of antiseborrhoeic and antipsoriatic agents as well as the polyene natamycin against *Malassezia furfur*

It is concluded that the test agents commonly used against SD exert their efficacy, at least in part, by way of inhibition of *M. furfur*.

Coal Tar

Coal tar gels have been shown to be efficacious in the treatment of SD of the scalp. It has been suggested that an antifungal mode of action of the coal tar gel may be responsible, at least in part, for this therapeutic efficacy.

The antimicrobial effect of a coal tar gel on the growth of 54 *M. furfur* strains isolated from patients suffering from SD, dandruff, and pityriasis versicolor was demonstrated in an in vitro assay [31]. At MIC values from 625–10,000 µg ml⁻¹ – corresponding to 3–50 µg ml⁻¹ coal tar – complete growth suppression of the *M. furfur* isolates tested was found. The only exceptions were two *M. furfur* strains isolated from dandruff, whose growth could not be inhibited with concentrations of less than 10,000 µg ml⁻¹. This may be explained by the observation that different *M. furfur* strains developed varying growth behaviour under in vitro conditions. Especially the two yeast isolates just mentioned showed a very strong and fast growth compared with other *M. furfur* strains, possibly indicating an increased virulence of certain strains.

The results of this study concerning the in vitro activity of coal tar gel are in accordance with a recent report of Wright et al. [47]. For one *M. furfur* strain investigated (ATCC 12078) they could demonstrate that the coal tar gel exhibits fungistatic effects in vitro at MIC values in the range of a 1:640–1:768 dilution, corresponding approximately to 7 µg ml⁻¹ coal tar. The broader range of MIC values achieved in the study is due to the number of 54 different yeast strains tested. Although slightly higher inoculum densities were used ($3-4\times10^5$ CFU vs. $2-4\times10^4$ ml⁻¹ in [47]), comparable inhibitory concentrations were obtained. In previous investigations MIC values of 0.1 µg ml⁻¹ for ketoconazole were found. Other azoles such as tioconazole and clotrimazole inhibited growth of *M. furfur* at MIC from 0.39 to 3.13 and 3.13 to 6.25 (12.5) µg ml⁻¹, respectively. For antiseborrhoeic agents such as selenium disulfide and zinc pyrithione, which were used for the treatment of SD even before the introduction of antimycotics, MIC values ranging from 1.56 to 3.13 and 0.78 to 3.13 µg ml⁻¹ were demonstrated. The calculated MIC values of 3–50 µg ml⁻¹ for coal tar do not exceed very much the antifungal activity of classical antimycotics and other investigated antiseborrhoeic agents.

In addition, the in vitro activity of the gel formulation without coal tar on 22 *M. furfur* strains was investigated. Also the base of the coal tar gel itself was able to inhibit growth of *M. furfur* in vitro, but higher concentrations of 5,000–10,000 µg ml⁻¹ were necessary for growth suppression. The gel base appears to be a less potent inhibitor of in vitro growth of *M. furfur*.

The in vitro susceptibility of the *M. furfur* strains to coal tar – the active substance of the gel – was also investigated. It could be demonstrated that coal tar alone has an antifungal potential on *M. furfur* in vitro. In accordance with previous results, MIC values of 250–5000 µg ml⁻¹ for coal tar were found. These data are also in agreement with those of Bunse and Mahrle [7], who demonstrated a half-maximal growth inhibition of *M. furfur* by liquor carbonis detergens at 1850 µg ml⁻¹. Nevertheless, the usual therapeutic concentrations of the agent, i. e. approximately 5–10% for coal tar, may also be able to inhibit growth of *M. furfur* in vivo. The experimentally determined MICs for coal tar markedly exceed the theoretically calculated coal tar gel MIC values provided by a 0.5% coal tar gel. Presumably both coal tar as the active agent and the gel base contribute to the in vitro activity of the coal tar gel against *M. furfur* like a summation effect. It is concluded that the tested coal tar gel but also the antiseborrhoeic and antipsoriatic agent coal tar itself, which are commonly used for dandruff and SD therapy, exert their efficacy, at least in part, through inhibition of *M. furfur*.

Lithium Succinate in Seborrhoeic Dermatitis

Lithium succinate ointment has been shown to be effective in the treatment of SD. Thus, Boyle et al. [6] reported that there was no growth inhibition of *M. furfur* in vitro until a concentration of 150 mg lithium succinate/l. Regarding the fact that the usual ointment contains 8% lithium succinate and 0.05% zinc sulfate we tested in vitro susceptibility of *M. furfur* strains to lithium succinate at markedly increased concentrations of the agent.

The effectiveness of topical lithium succinate ointment of SD was shown in preliminary studies. A significantly higher number of patients treated with lithium succinate ointment than of those treated with placebo showed remission or marked improvement. Because the growth of *M. furfur* was not significantly inhibited by lithium succinate in former studies it was suggested that lithium succinate probably acts as an anti-inflammatory agent [8]. Previously, it was shown that lithium is able to block the release of arachidonic acid, resulting in an inhibition of the release of different pro-inflammatory mediators produced by metabolism of this fatty acid, i. e. prostaglandin E_2, 6 keto-prostaglandin F, prostaglandin E_1, and thromboxane B_2 [20].

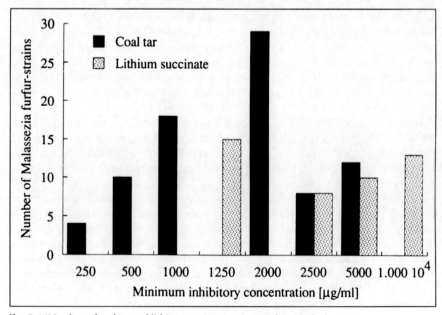

Fig. 7. MIC values of coal tar and lithium succinate against *Malassezia furfur*

Our own results show that lithium succinate is able to inhibit growth of all tested *M. furfur* strains in vitro, but at much higher concentrations (Fig. 7). MIC values between 1,250 and 10,000 µg per ml agar gave the most pronounced anti-*Malassezia* activity [30].

An antifungal activity has been explained on the basis that the blocking of the fatty acid release might deprive the yeast of essential nutrients. More recently, it has been suggested that lithium could also have some direct antifungal effect [11].

However, when calculated as percentage lithium succinate of the agar, the above-mentioned concentrations correspond to 0.125–1% lithium succinate content, presumably far below the 8% content of the lithium succinate ointment, confirming the assumption that the effectiveness of lithium succinate on SD is at least partly due to inhibition of the growth of *M. furfur*.

The Allylamine Terbinafine

Recently, Faergemann et al. [14] demonstrated a new topical treatment option in a study of 20 patients with SD of the scalp. They used the allylamine antifungal agent terbinafine in a 1% solution once daily over a period of 1 month and achieved a cure in 61% of patients, who were still free of lesions 2 weeks after stopping treatment.

Salicylic Acid

Use of salicylic acid in the treatment of squamous skin disorders has a very long history. Even in quite low concentrations, salicylic acid is known to exhibit bactericidal activity, which is pH-dependent. The bactericidal efficacy is probably due to an enzyme inhibition. In addition, it is also effective against *Candida* spp. and other fungi. We can only speculate on whether the growth of *M. furfur* can be inhibited by salicylic acid. Beyond it, at a concentration of ≥5%, salicylic acid shows keratolytic features. The cohesion between stratum corneum cells is diminished and disintegrated, followed by loosening of connecting intercellular substance. Increased proliferation leads to impairment of the keratinization process, with the resulting detachment of great cell complexes. Preparations for topical therapy of dandruff contain up to 10% salicylic acid.

Corticosteroids

Corticosteroid are also known to be effective in the treatment of SD. In a previous study it was demonstrated that hydrocortisone 1% solution alone when compared with miconazole and the combination of miconazole plus hydrocortisone, exhibited a good efficacy in therapy for dandruff. Moreover, the combination of miconazole and hydrocortisone was significantly more active than hydrocorticone alone when used twice monthly as prophylactic treatment for 3 months.

Conclusion

In conclusion, dandruff or pityriasis capitis is a very common skin disorder of the scalp which is now considered as a mild or early form of SD. For the persons affected by dandruff, the permanent scaling first of all represents a great cosmetic affliction. Today, it is accepted that the lipophilic yeast *M. furfur* is at least partly responsible for maintenance of the typical skin alterations, scaling and itching. For this reason, the treatment of dandruff is based on the use of shampoos and topical preparations containing antifungal agents, e. g. ketoconazole. Besides this, the efficacy of antiseborrhoeic substances for the treatment of dandruff, e.g. coal tar, selenium disulfide, and zinc pyrithione, is possibly also due to their antimycotic activity against *M. furfur*. Thus, it should also be taken into account that they exert additional antiseborrhoeic, anti-inflammatory and antiproliferative effects on the skin.

References

1. Arrese JE, Piérard-Franchimont C, De Doncker P, Heremans A, Cauwenberg G, Piérard GE (1996) Effect of ketoconazole-medicated shampoos on squamometry and *Malassezia ovalis* load in Pityriasis capitis. Cutis 58: 235–237
2. Bandhaya M (1993) The distribution of *Malassezia furfur* and *Malassezia pachydermatis* on normal human skin. Southeast Asian J Trop Med Public Health 24: 343–346
3. Bergbrant I-M, Faergemann J (1990) The role of *Pityrosporum ovale* in seborrheic dermatitis. Semin Dermatol 9: 262–268
4. Bergbrant IM (1991) Seborrhoeic dermatitis and *Pityrosporum ovale*: cultural, immunological and clinical studies. Acta Derm Venereol Suppl (Stockh) 167:1–36
5. Bergbrant IM, Johansson S, Robbins D, Bengtsson K, Faergemann J, Scheynius A, Soderstrom T (1991) The evaluation of various methods and antigens for the detection of antibodies against *Pityrosporum ovale* in patients with seborrhoeic dermatitis. Clin Exp Dermatol 16: 339–343
6. Boyle J, Burton JL, Faergemann J (1986) Use of topical lithium succinate for seborrheic dermatitis. Br Med J 292: 28.
7. Bunse T, Mahrle G (1992) Anthralin is a potent inhibitor of *Pityrosporum orbiculare/ovale in vitro*. Acta Derm Venereol (Stockh) 72: 72–73
8. Cuelenaere C, De Bersaques J, Kint A (1992) Use of topical lithium succinate in the treatment of seborrheic dermatitis. Dermatology 184: 194–197
9. Danby FW, Maddin WS, Mergesson LJ, Rosenthal D (1993) A randomized, double–blind placebo–controlled trial of ketoconazole 2% shampoo versus selenium sulfide 2.5% shampoo in the treatment of moderate to severe dandruff. J Am Acad Dermatol 29: 1008–1012
10. Dobrev H, Zissova L (1997) Effect of ketoconazole on scalp sebum level in patients with seborrhoeic dermatitis. Acta Derm Venereol (Stockh) 77: 132–134.
11. Efalith Multicenter Trial Group (1992) A double-blind, placebo-controlled, multicenter trial of lithium succinate ointment in the treatment of seborrheic dermatitis. J Am Acad Dermatol 26: 452–457
12. Faergemann J (1988) Activity of triazole derivatives against *Pityrosporum orbiculare in vitro and in vivo*. Ann NY Acad Sci 544: 348–353
13. Faergemann J (1992) *Pityrosporum* infections. In: Flewski BE (ed.) Cutaneous fungal infections. Igaku–Shoin New York, pp. 69–83
14. Faergemann J, Jones TC, Hettler O, Loria Y (1996) *Pityrosporum ovale* (*Malassezia furfur*) as the causative agent of seborrhoeic dermatitis: new treatment options. Br J Dermatol 134 [Suppl 46]:12–15
15. Ford GP, Farr PM, Ive FA, Shuster S (1984) The response of seborrhoeic dermatitis to ketoconazole. Br J Dermatol 111:603–607
16. Gloor M, Wiegand I, Friederich HC (1972) Über Menge und Zusammensetzung der Hautoberflächenlipide beim sogenannten seborrhoischen Ekzem. Dermatol Monatsschr 158: 759–764
17. Goffin V, Piérard-Franchimont C, Piérard GE (1996) Antidandruff shampoos and the stratum corneum. J Dermatol Treat 7:215–218
18. Guého E, Midgley G, Guillot J (1996) The genus *Malassezia* with description of four new species. Antonie van Leeuwenhoek 69:337–355
19. Hay RJ, Graham-Brown RAC (1997) Dandruff and seborrhoeic dermatitis: causes and management. Clin Exp Dermatol 22:3–6
20. Horrobin DF (1990) Effect of lithium on essential fatty acid and prostaglandin metabolism. In: Bach RO, Gallichio VS (eds) Lithium and cell physiology. Springer, Berlin Heidelberg New York, pp 137–149

21. Ingham E, Cunningham AC (1993) *Malassezia furfur.* J Med Vet Mycol 31:265–288
22. Ive FA (1991) An overview of experience with ketoconazole shampoo. Br J Clin Pract 45:279–284
23. Kligman AM, Leyden JJ (1983) Seborrhoeic dermatitis. Semin Dermatol 2:57–59
24. Konrad B, Cernikova M (1963) Biochemische Untersuchung bei Dermatitis seborrhoica. Dermatol Wochenschr 147:383–385
25. Leeming JP, Notman FH (1987) Improved methods for isolation and enumeration of *Malassezia furfur* from human skin. J Clin Microbiol 25:2017–2019
26. Malassez L (1874) Notes sur le champignon de la pilade. Arch Physiol Norm Pathol [Ser 2] 1:203–212
27. McGinley KJ, Leyden JJ, Marples RR (1975) Quantitative microbiology of the scalp in non-dandruff, dandruff, and seborrheic dermatitis. J Invest Dermatol 64:401–405
28. Midgley G, Hay RJ (1988) Serological responses to *Pityrosporum* (*Malassezia*) in seborrhoeic dermatitis demonstrated by ELISA and Western blotting. Bull Soc Mycol Med 17:267–276
29. Nenoff P, Haustein U-F (1994) In vitro susceptibility testing of *Pityrosporum ovale* against antifungal, antiseborrheic and antipsoriatic agents. J Eur Acad Dermatol Venereol 3:331–333
30. Nenoff P, Haustein U-F, Münzberger C (1995) *In vitro* activity of lithium succinate against *Malassezia furfur.* Dermatology 190:48—50
31. Nenoff P, Haustein U-F, Fiedler A (1995) The antifungal activity of a coal tar gel on *Malassezia furfur in vitro.* Dermatology 190:311–314
32. Neuber K, Kröger S, Gruseck E, Abeck D, Ring J (1996) Effects of *Pityrosporum ovale* on proliferation, immunoglobulin (IgA, G, M) synthesis and cytokine (IL-2, IL-10, IFNγ) production of peripheral blood mononuclear cells from patients with seborrhoeic dermatitis. Arch Dermatol Res 288:532–536
33. Nicholls D, Midgley GM, Hay RJ (1990) Patch testing against *Pityrosporum* antigens. Clin Exp Dermatol 15:75
34. Peter RU, Richarz-Barthauer U (1995) Successful treatment and prophylaxis of scalp seborrhoeic dermatitis and dandruff with 2% ketoconazole shampoo: results of a multicentre, double-blind, placebo-controlled trial. Br J Dermatol 132:441–445
35. Piérard-Franchimont C, Arrese JE, Piérard GE (1995) Immunohistochemical aspects of the link between *Malassezia ovalis* and seborrheic dermatitis. J Eur Acad Dermatol Venereol 4:14–19
36. Rivolta S (1873) Parassin Vegetali, 1st edn. Giulio Speirani, Turin, pp 469–471
37. Sabouraud R (1904) Maladies du cuir chavelu. II. Les maladies desquamatives. Pityriasis et alopécies peliculaire. Masson, Paris, pp 295
38. Schaich B, Korting GHC, Hollmann J (1993) Hautlipide bei mit Seborrhoe- und Sebostase-assoziierten Hauterkrankungen. Hautarzt 44:75–80
39. Schmidt A, Rühl-Hörster B (1996) In vitro susceptibility of *Malassezia furfur.* Arzneimittelforschung 46:442–444
40. Schürer NY (1993) Die fette Haut. Zeitschr H + G 68: 636–640
41. Shuster S (1984) The aetiology of dundruff and the mode of action of therapeutic agents. Br J Dermatol 3:235–242
42. Sohnle PG (1988) *Pityrosporum* immunology – a review. In: Torres-Rodriguez JM (ed) Proceedings of the X. Meeting of the International Society for Human and Animal Mycology. JR Prous Science, Barcelona
43. Tollesson A, Fritz A, Berg A, Karlman G (1993) Essential fatty acids in infantile seborrheic dermatitis. J Am Acad Dermatol 28:957–961
44. Unna PG (1887) Seborrhoeic eczema. J Cutan Dis 5:449–453
45. Van Cutsem J, Van Gerven F, Fransen J, Schrooten P, Janssen PAJ (1990) The *in vitro* antifungal activity of ketoconazole, zinc-pyrithione, and selenium sulphide against *Pityrosporum* and their efficacy as a shampoo in the treatment of experimental pityrosporum in guinea pigs. J Am Acad Dermatol 22:993–998
46. Van Gerven F, Odds FC (1995) The anti-*Malassezia furfur* activity *in vitro* and in experimental dermatitis of six imidazole antifungal agents: bifonazole, clotrimazole, flutrimazole, ketoconazole, miconazole and sertaconazole. Mycoses 38:389–393
47. Wright MC, Hevert F, Rozman T (1993) *In vitro* comparison of antifungal effects of a coal tar gel and a ketoconazole gel on *Malassezia furfur.* Mycoses 36:207–210

CHAPTER 12

Efficacy of Barrier Creams (Skin Protective Creams)

H. Zhai, H.I. Maibach

Introduction

The concept of barrier creams (BC) has been around since the early 20th century. In practice, their utilization remains the subject of a lively debate; some suggest that inappropriate BC application may induce additional irritation rather than benefit [1–5].

To evaluate BC efficacy, in vivo and in vitro methods have been developed. In particular, recent bioengineering techniques provide more accurate quantitative data than supplied by traditional clinical studies dependent on visual scoring.

We review the investigative details of pertinent scientific literature, and summarize methodology and efficacy of BC.

Barrier Creams (BC)

BC are designed to prevent or reduce the penetration and absorption of various hazardous materials into skin, preventing skin lesions and/or other toxic effects from dermal exposure [1, 2, 4–7]. The term BC is also called "skin protective creams (SPCs)" or "protective creams (PCs)", as well as "protective ointments", "invisible glove", "barrier", "protective" or "pre-work" creams and/or gels (lotions), "after-work" emollient, etc. [7–9]. Frosch et al. [4] suggest the term "skin protective creams" which seems more appropriate since most products do not provide a barrier comparable to stratum corneum.

Methodology and Efficacy Of BC

In 1940, Schwartz et al. [10] introduced an in vivo method to evaluate the efficacy of a vanishing cream against poison ivy extract utilizing visual erythema on human skin. The test cream was an effective prophylaxis against poison ivy dermatitis where compared to unprotected skin.

Sadler et al. [11] performed qualitative tests to evaluate the efficiency of barrier creams. One method used the fluorescence of a dyestuff and eosin as an indicator to measure penetration and the rates of penetration of water through barrier creams; this is rapid and simple, but provides only a qualitative estimate. They introduced an apparatus for measuring the permeability of films of barrier creams.

Wahlberg [12, 13] employed an isotope disappearance measurement technique for documenting the inhibiting effect of barrier creams on chromate (^{51}Cr) percutaneous absorption in guinea pigs (Table 1; Fig. 1) [13]. In this series 2,4 [Indulona (Slova-

Table 1. Influence of Indulona and Ivosin on the percutaneous absorption of 0.017 M chromate solution $K \times 10^5$ min^{-1}. (Modified from [13])

Series No.	Barrier cream	Volume applied ml/cm2	Interval[a] (min)	<3.4 (n)	3.4–6.6 (n)	6.7–10.1 (n)	10.2–13.5 (n)	13.6– (n)	Mean relative absorption $K \times 10^5$ min^{-1} 10 exp.	χ^2(c), analysis of variance (v) compared with series 1
1	No barrier cream			–	4	4	–	2	8.8±1.4b	–
2	Indulona	0.05	1	3	2	4	–	1	(5.7–6.7)c	0.05< p<0.10 (c)
3	Indulona	0.10	1	–	3	4	1	2	9.0±1.2b	p>0.2 (v)
4	Indulona	0.10	15	4	1	3	2	–	(5.5–6.8)c	0.02< p<0.05 (c)
5	Indulona	0.15	1	–	5	–	5	–	8.2±0.1b	p>0.2 (v)
6	Ivosin	0.025	1	2	2	3	3	–	(6.7–7.3)c	0.10< p<0.20 (c)
7	Ivosin	0.05	1	7	1	2	–	–	(2.1–4.5)c	0.001< p<0.01 (c)
8	Ivosin	0.10	1	8	–	2	–	–	(1.8–4.5)c	p<0.001 (c)
9	Ivosin	0.10	15	5	5	–	–	–	(2.5–4.2)c	0.001< p<0.01 (c)
10	Ivosin	0.15	1	5	3	2	–	–	(3.2–4.7)c	0.001< p<0.01 (c)

[a] Interval between application of barrier cream and test substance.
[b] Standard error.
[c] See text.

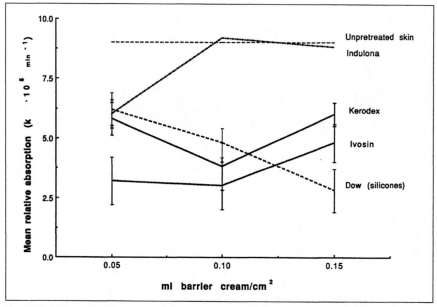

Fig. 1. The effect of barrier creams on the percutaneous absorption of a 0.017 M aqueous solution of chromate. Three different volumes per unit area (ml/cm²) were studied. (Modified from [13])

kofarma, Hlonovec, CSSR) contains Na_2H_2 ethylenediaminetetraacetate (EDTA), $CaNa_2$EDTA and acidum ascorbicum as active ingredients] and 6–10 [Ivosin (Hermal-Chemie Kurt Herrmann, Hamburg) contains the hydrochloride of a copolymerizate of p-divinyl benzol and p-m-dimethylaminomethylstyrol] absorption decreased as a result of pretreatment. In some cases the disappearance technique was not sufficiently sensitive to permit quantitative determination. The disappearance measurements differentiated between different barrier creams, volumes per unit area and intervals between application of cream and chromate [13].

Langford [14] introduced in vitro studies conducted to determine the efficacy of the formulated FC-resin complex included solvent penetration through treated filter paper, solvent repellency on treated pigskin, and penetration of radio-tagged sodium lauryl sulfate through treated hairless mouse skin. The penetration rate of radio-tagged SLS/ethanol through hairless mouse skin is shown in Figure 2.

Reiner et al. [15] examined the protective effect of ointments both on guinea pig skin in vitro and on guinea pigs in vivo. The permeation of "toxic agent 4" through unprotected and protected skin within 10 h is plotted in Figure 3 as a function of time. The permeation values were determined radiologically and enzymatically. Permeation of "toxic agent 4" was markedly reduced by polyethylene glycol ointment base and ointments containing active substance. In in vivo experiments on guinea pigs mortality was greater after applying the toxic agent to unprotected skin. All formulations with nucleophilic substances markedly reduced the mortality rate.

Lachapelle et al. [16–19] utilized a guinea pig model to evaluate the protective value of barrier creams and/or gels by laser Doppler flowmetry and histological assessment.

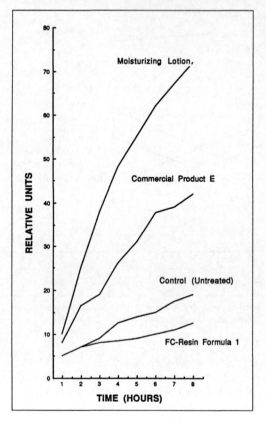

Fig. 2. Penetration rate of radio-tagged sodium lauryl sulfate/ETOH through hairless mouse skin. (Modified from [14])

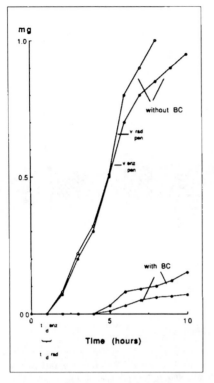

Fig. 4 shows a bar chart with y-axis labeled μg/ml, ranging from 0.00 to 0.25. Two bars labeled A (n=4) and B (n=4).

Fig. 3. Permeation of the "toxic agent 4" through unprotected and protected skin as a function of time. *Clear dots*, radiological data; *filled dots*, enzyme data; *BC*, reactive PEG ointment such as S4-S8. (Modified from [15])

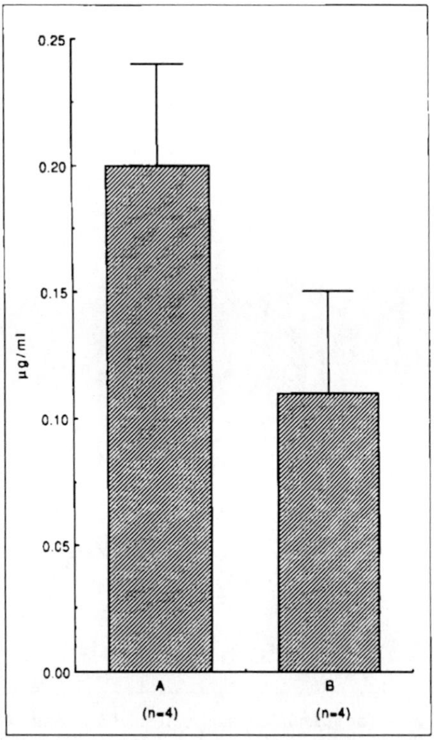

Fig. 4. Mean ± SD (μg/ml) of blood levels of n-hexane in two groups of guinea pigs exposed for 30 min. A, control group; B, gel-pretreated group ($p<0.05$). (Modified from [18])

In addition, the blood concentration of n-hexane of the control group and the gel-pretreated group was determined. Figure 4 shows partial results [19]. They correlated invasive (blood levels) and noninvasive techniques.

Loden [7] evaluated the effect of barrier creams on the absorption of (^{3}H)-water (^{14}C)-benzene and (^{14}C)-formaldehyde into excised human skin. The control and the barrier-cream-treated skins were exposed to the test substance for 0.5 h, whereupon absorption was determined. The experimental cream "water barrier" reduced the absorption of water and benzene but not formaldehyde. Kerodex 71 cream slightly reduced benzene and formaldehyde absorption. Petrogard and "Solvent barrier" did not affect the absorption of any of the substances studied (Fig. 5). One advantage of the method is the use of human skin. The effects of the barrier cream on the skin and the test substance mimic the in vivo situation. Another advantage is that the method is quantitative.

Frosch et al. [2–4, 20, 21] developed the repetitive irritation test (RIT) in the guinea pig and in humans to evaluate the efficacy of BC using a series of bioengineering tech-

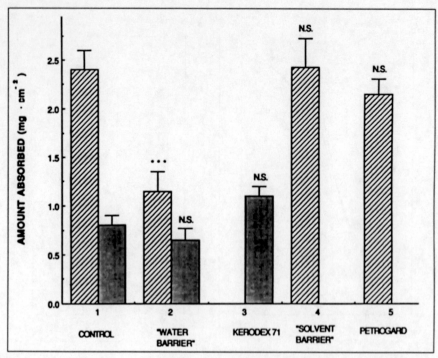

Fig. 5. The amount of water absorbed into control skin and skin treated with barrier creams during 0.5 h of exposure. Skin from two donors was used (*hatched and dotted columns*). Values are means ± SE of the number of experiments within parenthesis. ***$p<0.001$; N.S., not significantly different from control. (Modified from [7])

niques. The cream pretreated and untreated test skin (guinea pig or humans) were exposed daily to the irritants for 2 weeks. The resulting irritation was scored on a clinical scale and assessed by biophysical techniques' parameters. Some test creams suppressed irritation with all test parameters; some failed to show such an effect, and even exacerbated (Fig. 6) [4].

Treffel et al. [22] measured in vitro on human skin the effectiveness of barrier creams against three dyes (eosin, methylviolet and oil red O) with varying n-octanol/water partition coefficients (0.19, 29.8 and 165, respectively). BC efficacy was assayed by measurements of the dyes in the epidermis of protected skin samples after 30 min application. Penetration depths of the dyes into the stratum corneum are shown in Figure 7. The total color change (ΔTCC) (%) related to the number of the cellophane tape strips made from the skin sample controls. The dyes were present in high amounts in the superficial layers of the stratum corneum; ΔTCC due to eosin in the first strip was lower than that obtained with both the other dyes (not statistically significant). Oil red O penetrated in greater amounts into the deeper stratum corneum. The amount of the three dyes at the bottom of the stratum corneum remains, however, low. The efficacy of barrier creams against the three dyes showed in several cases data contrary to manufacturer's information. There was no correlation between the galenic parameters of the

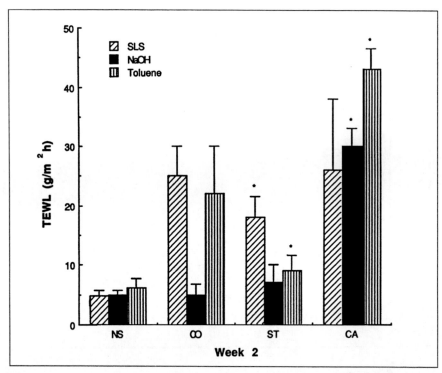

Fig. 6. The effect of barrier creams: Stokoderm Salbe (ST) and Contra Alkali Creme (CA) in the guinea pig model after 2 weeks of treatment with three irritants (SLS, sodium lauryl sulfate; NaOH, sodium hydroxide; toluene). CO, control animals; NS, normal skin (untreated). Shown are the data of the transepidermal water loss (TEWL). Significant differences from control animals and barrier cream-treated animals are indicated by $^*p<0.05$. (Modified from [4])

assayed products and the protection level, indicating that neither the water content nor the consistency of the formulations influenced the protection effectiveness.

Fullerton and Menne [23] evaluated that the protective effect of EDTA barrier gels against nickel contact allergy using in vitro and in vivo methods. The amount of 30 mg of barrier gel was applied on the epidermal side of the skin in vitro and a nickel disc was applied above the gel. After 24 h application, the nickel disc was removed and the epidermis separated from the dermis. Nickel content in epidermis and dermis was quantified by adsorption differential pulse voltammetry (ADPV). The distributions of nickel in epidermis and dermis after 24 h of occluded application of the two nickel discs made from alloy A and alloy B is in Figure 8. The amount of nickel in the epidermal skin layer after application of the barrier gels was significantly reduced compared to the untreated control.

In vivo patch testing of nickel-sensitive patients was performed using nickel discs made of metal alloy A and Carbopol barrier gel systems with and without added EDTA (gel type A and B). Test preparations and nickel discs were removed 1 day post application and the sites evaluated. Reduction in positive test reactions was highly significant.

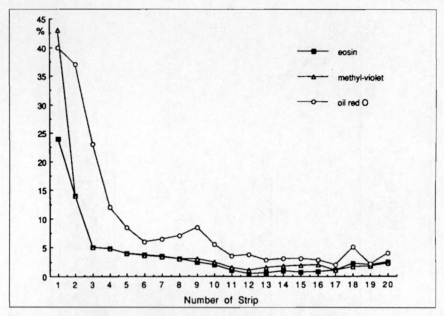

Fig. 7. Δ total color change measurement in the stratum corneum expressed in percentages. (Modified from [22])

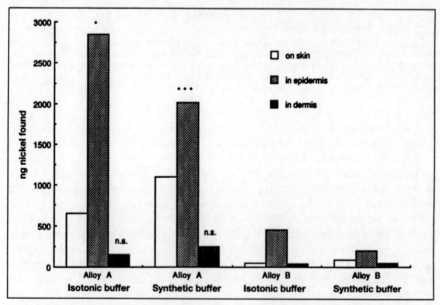

Fig. 8. Distribution of nickel in epidermis and dermis after 24 h occluded application of two nickel discs made from alloy A and alloy B. Recipient mediums were isotonic phosphate buffer and synthetic sweat (skin from donor A). Statistics: two-sample t-test comparing mean skin compartment distribution of nickel after application of alloy B and alloy A. Comparison for isotonic phosphate buffer and synthetic sweat as recipient medium, respectively. *n.s.*, No significance; *$p<0.05$; ***$p<0.001$. (Modified from [23])

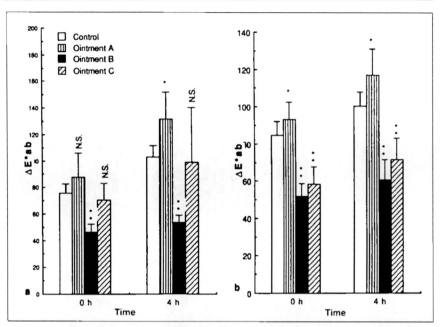

Fig. 9a,b. The amount of methylene blue (a) and oil red O (b) absorbed into control skin and skin treated with barrier creams. Results expressed as the means±SD of ΔE^*ab. Statistical differences in comparison to the control indicated by $*p<0.05$ to $**p<0.01$; N.S., not significant. (Modified from [5])

Zhai [5] developed an in vivo method in human skin to measure the effectiveness of skin protective creams against dye indicator solutions: methylene blue in water and oil red O in ethanol, representative of model hydrophilic and lipophilic compounds. Solutions of 5% methylene blue and 5% oil red O were applied to untreated and protective cream pretreated skin with the aid of aluminum occlusive chambers, for 0 h and 4 h. At the end of the application time, the materials were removed, and consecutive skin surface biopsies (SSB) obtained. The amount of dye penetrating into each strip was determined by colorimetry. Two creams exhibited effectiveness, but one cream enhanced the cumulative amount of dye (Fig. 9).

Zhai et al. [24] introduced a facile approach to screening protectants in vivo in human subjects. Two acute irritants and one allergen were selected: sodium lauryl sulfate (SLS) representative of irritant household and occupational contact dermatitis, the combination of ammonium hydroxide (NH4OH) and urea to simulate diaper dermatitis, and Rhus to evaluate the protective effect of model materials on allergic contact dermatitis. Test materials were spread over onto test areas, massaged, allowed to dry for 30 min, and reapplied with another 30-min drying period. The model irritants and allergen were applied with an occlusive patch for 24 h. Inflammation was scored with an expanded ten point scale at 72 h post-application. Most test materials statistically suppressed the SLS irritation and Rhus allergic reaction rather than NH4OH and urea induced irritation (Fig. 10).

Zhai et al. [25] utilized an in vitro diffusion system to measure the protective effective of Quaternium-18 bentonite (Q18B) gels to prevent the penetration of 1% [35S]-SLS

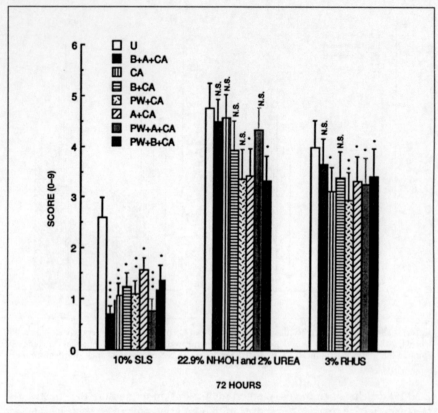

Fig. 10. Efficacy of protective materials against skin irritation following treatment by two acute irritants [10% sodium lauryl sulfate (SLS), 22.9% NH⁴OH, and 2% urea] and one allergen (3% Rhus). Results expressed as the means±SE. Statistical differences in comparison with untreated skin site. *p<0.05; **p<0.01; ***p<0.001. N.S., not significant. (Modified from [24])

Table 2. Cumulation amount of [35S]-SLS and protection effect percent. Values are means ± standard deviation of percent dose of applied dose. (Modified from [25])

	Control	A	B	C
Receptor fluid	0.43±0.4	0.05±0.05**	0.08±0.05**	0.15±0.2*
Skin content	14.19±11.1	5.3±7.3	3.95±4.1	4.7±3.5
Skin wash	78.6±12.7	83.81±12.0	83.19±14.9	83.76±10.6
Protection effect (%)		88	81	65

Statistical differences in comparison with the control. *p<0.05; **p>0.01

through human cadaver skin. The accumulated amount of [35S]-SLS in receptor cell fluid was counted to evaluate the efficacy of the Q-18B gels over a 24 h period. These test gels significantly decreased SLS absorption when compared to the unprotected skin control samples (Table 2). The percent protection effect of three test gels against SLS percutaneous absorption was from 88%, 81%, and 65%, respectively (Fig. 11).

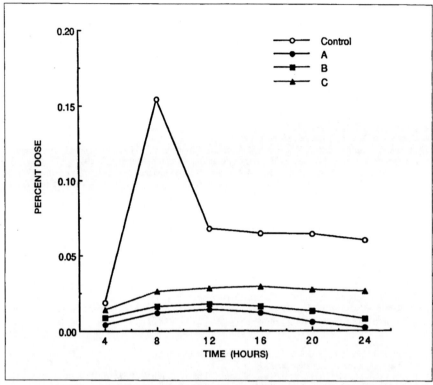

Fig. 11. The cumulative amount absorbed into control skin and skin treated with three gels during 24 h of exposure. Values are means of percent dose of applied dose. (Modified from [25])

Conclusions

1. Some BC reduce the local damage due to various irritants and allergens.
2. Using inappropriate BC may enhance irritation rather than benefit.
3. In vitro methods are recommended in screening procedure for barrier cream candidates because of their simplicity, speed, and safety.
4. Animal skin may be used to generate kinetic data. Percutaneous absorption in pigs and monkeys shows a closer similarity to that in humans. But no one animal, with its complex anatomy and biology, will simulate the penetration in humans for all compounds. Therefore, the best estimate of human percutaneous absorption is determined by in vivo studies in humans.
5. Noninvasive bioengineering techniques are valuable in quantifying the inflammation response to various irritants and allergens when BC are to be evaluated.
6. The accuracy of measurements of the efficacy of barrier creams depends on the use of proper methodology.
7. Above all, the clinical efficacy of BC should be assessed in real rather than in experimental circumstances.

In the end, in spite of the power of these models, well controlled field trials are required to define the relationship of the model to the occupational setting. Nevertheless, appropriate use of models should lead to formulation refinement and a greater mechanistic insight.

References

1. Lachapelle JM (1996) Efficacy of protective creams and/or gels, in prevention of contact dermatitis. In: Elsner P, Lachapelle JM, Wahlberg JM, Maibach HI (eds) Prevention of contact dermatitis. Curr Probl Dermatol. Karger, Basel, p 182
2. Frosch PJ, Schulze-Dirks A, Hoffmann M, Axthelm I, Kurte A (1993) Efficacy of skin barrier creams. I. The repetitive irritation test (RIT) in the guinea pig. Contact Dermatitis 28:94
3. Frosch PJ, Schulze-Dirks A, Hoffmann M, Axthelm I (1993) Efficacy of skin barrier creams. II. Ineffectiveness of a popular "skin protector" against various irritants in the repetitive irritation test in the guinea pig. Contact Dermatitis 29:74
4. Frosch PJ, Kurte A, Pilz B (1993) Biophysical techniques for the evaluation of skin protective creams. In: Frosch PJ, Kligman AM (eds) Noninvasive methods for the quantification of skin functions. Springer-Verlag, Berlin Heidelberg New York, pp 214
5. Zhai H, Maibach HI (1996) Effect of barrier creams: human skin in vivo. Contact Dermatitis 35:92
6. Zhai H, Maibach HI (1996) Percutaneous penetration (dermatopharmacokinetics) in evaluating barrier creams. In: Elsner P, Lachapelle JM, Wahlberg JM, Maibach HI (eds) Prevention of contact dermatitis. Curr Probl Dermatol. Karger, Basel, p 193
7. Loden M (1986) The effect of 4 barrier creams on the absorption of water, benzene, and formaldehyde into excised human skin. Contact Dermatitis 14:292
8. Guillemin M, Murset JC, Lob M, Riquez J (1974) Simple method to determine the efficiency of a cream used for skin protection against solvents. Br J Ind Med 31:310
9. Goh CL (1991) Cutting oil dermatitis on guinea pig skin. II. Emollient creams and cutting oil dermatitis. Contact Dermatitis 24:81
10. Schwartz L, Warren LH, Goldman FH (1940) Protective ointment for the prevention of poison ivy dermatitis. Public Health Rep 55:1327
11. Sadler CGA, Marriott RH (1946) The evaluation of barrier creams. Br Med J 23:769
12. Wahlberg JE (1971) Absorption-inhibiting effect of barrier creams. Dermatosen 19:197
13. Wahlberg JE (1972) Anti-chromium barrier cream. Dermatologica 145:175
14. Langford NP (1978) Fluorochemical resin complexes for use in solvent repellent hand creams. Am Ind Hyg Assoc J 39:33
15. Reiner R, Roßmann K, Hooidonk CV, Ceulen BI, Bock J (1982) Ointments for the protection against organophosphate poisoning. Arzneimed Forsch/Drug Res 32:630
16. Mahmoud G, Lachapelle JM, Neste DV (1984) Histological assessment of skin damage by irritants: its possible use in the evaluation of a "barrier cream". Contact Dermatitis 11:179
17. Mahmoud G, Lachapelle JM (1985) Evaluation of the protective value of an antisolvent gel by laser Doppler flowmetry and histology. Contact Dermatitis 13:14
18. Mahmoud G, Lachapelle JM (1987) Uses of a guinea pig model to evaluate the protective value of barrier creams and/or gels. In: Maibach HI, Lowe NJ (eds) Models in dermatology. Karger, Basel, p 112
19. Lachapelle JM, Nouaigui H, Marot L (1990) Experimental study of the effects of a new protective cream against skin irritation provoked by the organic solvents n-hexane, trichlorethylene and toluene. Dermatosen 38:19
20. Frosch PJ, Kurte A, Pilz B (1993) Efficacy of skin barrier creams. III. The repetitive irritation test (RIT) in humans. Contact Dermatitis 29:113
21. Frosch PJ, Kurte A (1994) Efficacy of skin barrier creams. IV. The repetitive irritation test (RIT) with a set of 4 standard irritants. Contact Dermatitis 31:161
22. Treffel P, Gabard B, Juch R (1994) Evaluation of barrier creams: an in vitro technique on human skin. Acta Dermatol Venereol 74:7
23. Fullerton A, Menne T (1995) In vitro and in vivo evaluation of the effect of barrier gels in nickel contact allergy. Contact Dermatitis 32:100
24. Zhai H, Willard P, Maibach HI (1998) Evaluating skin-protective materials against contact irritants and allergens. An in vivo screening human model. Contact Dermatitis 38:155
25. Zhai H, Buddrus DJ, Schulz AA, Wester RC, Hartway T, Serranzana S, Maibach HI (1998) In vitro percutaneous absorption of sodium lauryl sulfate (SLS) in human skin decreased by Quaternium-18 bentonite gels. Presented at the American Academy of Dermatology 56th Annual Meeting, Orlando, February 27, pp 113

CHAPTER 13

Anti-Cellulite

C. Rona, E. Berardesca

Introduction

Cellulite (local lipodystrophy) represents a very common cosmetic problem among women; the main clinical feature of this process is the appearance of "orange peel" skin in the areas affected [1–3].

The target of this disease is the subcutaneous tissue, which develops an altered blood and lymphatic microcirculation. As secondary events, accumulation of fat material and fibrotic changes occur.

Cellulite represents the most common lipodystrophic disease, which differs from diffuse adiposity, because it shows itself just in limited areas, such as abdomen, buttocks, trochanteric and perimalleolar area, anterior-, posterior-, medial and lateral thigh and knee [2]. Clinically it can be graded as follows [1,4]:
- 0=No cellulite
- 1=Slight dimpling of skin surface
- 2=Dimpling and skin depressions
- 3=Dimpling and depressed striations
- 4=Palpable nodules and depressed striations

Subjective symptoms more frequently reported by patients are:
- Heaviness and tension at lower limbs
- Cold feet
- Nightly cramps (rarely during the day)
- Paresthesias
- Pain, rarely spontaneous, generally induced by trauma, even slight.

Objective data more frequently reported by investigators are:
- Diffuse (orange peel) and local (mattress peel) uneveness
- Stretch marks
- Cutaneous colour changes (dischromic or hyperpigmented skin).

Clinical examination often reveals venous stasis and insufficiency at lower limbs on the basis of perimalleolar oedema, teleangectasiae and/or microvaricosity, varices and cutaneous trophic alterations.

Other peculiarities can be appreciated such as:
- Lack of elasticity
- Increase of skin plicability and doughiness
- Fine texture
- Micronodules, and, more easy to remark, macronodules, often painful at palpation.

Cellulite develops through progressive stages [4]:
- *Pre-cellulitic condition*: skin appears smooth and firm; ultrasound shows a thick dermis with minimal fluid retention; there is neither accumulation of linked collagen fibres nor elastin nodules. Adipocytes have regular diameter and are not engorged with lipids. No fatty deposits seem to protrude into the dermis. A thick blood and lymphatic vessels network supplies subcutaneous tissue of nourishment and oxygen, removing toxins and discarding elements.
- *Stage 1*: occurs at a deep cellular layer without cosmetic implications. Vessel walls become so permeable that they induce loss of fluids into the spaces between adipocytes (oedema), making the fatty layer to swell. Adipocytes become engorged with lipids, they are bigger and clump together. Furthermore, deranged lymphatic circulation makes it difficult to remove fluids that accumulate and promote oedema. At this stage, probably hormones play an important role. Many hypotheses have been proposed as regards to the causes of this metabolic alteration (involving changes of the levels of AMPc and Proteinkinase C), but no satisfactory explanation has been provided [5,6].
- *Stage 2*: dermal and subdermal involvement is much more marked. Adipocytes clumping together and collagen fibers linkage hamper blood circulation and cause homeostasis: all these events happen heterogeneously, so areas with a good microcirculation are near to severely damaged ones. Accumulation of fluids increases the heterogeneity of the subdermal region and the «orange peel» appearance becomes evident, because of the thinning of the epidermis and dermis.
- *Stage 3*: the vascular affection has more marked repercussions on dermis, giving rise to its metabolic alteration and thinning, due to the reduction in protein synthesis and the recovering processes. Adipocytes, cut off from supply and toxin removing processes, clump together, constituting micronodules surrounded by a thick and hard collagen layer and fatty masses. Skin palpation shows clearly orange peel phenomenon.
- *Stage 4*: micronodules clump together to form hard macronodules in dermal layer, whose dimensions range between 2 and 20 mm. Subjects often feel pain or trouble at this stage, because nerves can be compressed by nodules in involved areas [2].

Later stages are irreversible and refractory to any cosmetic treatment.

Pathogenesis

The pathogenesis of cellulite onset is still unknown. It results from blood and lymphatic microcirculation damage which gives rise to structural changes in fatty layer and surrounding collagen matrix. In particular, superficial microcirculation appears to be less efficient and this results in subcutaneous oedema due to alterated permeability of blood vessels; this condition can induce sclerosis and a reduced replacement of collagen fibers. An altered trophic reaction of adipocytes to endocrine and/or neuroendocrine stimuli, associated with oedema, vascular and fibrotic damage can also be present [7].

An increased accumulation of some unmetabolized compounds such as sugars, lipids and proteins can be transformed in triglycerides and stored in adipocytes. Therefore, there clearly seems to be a deranged lipolytic process in the onset of cellulite. Lipolysis is partially controlled by nerves: the β-adrenergic receptors activation or the α2-adrenergic receptors blockage promote lipolysis; in particular, β-adrenergic stimulation leads to an increase of AMPc levels due to an anti-phosphodiesterasic action; AMPc promotes the hydrolitic degradation of lipids, whereas α2-adrenergic receptors stimulation results in a reduction of AMPc intracellular levels with consequent inhibition of lipid release and therefore their degradation [3]. Cellulite is more marked in specific anatomical sites (thighs and buttocks in women) because of the presence of adrenergic receptors in these sites. Clinically, cellulite is more severe in women, because of the particular structure of the subcutaneous tissue (so called "mattress-like") at the interface between dermis and hypodermis, with small parallel collagen bands which link the dermis to the hypodermis giving rise to the "orange peel" appearance when deformed by lipid accumulation.

Noninvasive Techniques to Evaluate Cellulite

The purpose of cellulite treatment is to stimulate the inadequate blood and lymphatic circulation (massages, topical application of cosmetic products, electrolipolysis, mesotherapy and adequate diets). In particular, massage seems to play an important role in treating the cellulite condition in relation to the ability to smoothe the dermis-hypodermis junction even though the benefits of massage therapy are only temporary [8]. In general, the efficacy of cellulite treatments is often debated and objective studies are needed for claim support. Furthermore, cellulite is very difficult to investigate by bioengineering methods. The main noninvasive techniques helpful in monitoring some physical parameters related to the "cellulite" condition are discussed in the following sections.

Ultrasonography

Ultrasound is used to study the thickness and the quality of the connective tissue and the oedematous component of cellulite. When an ultrasound beam goes through differently structured portions of a tissue, it generates an echo according to the acoustic properties of the regions under examination; the echoes produce an electrical signal in the transducer, which is shown as an amplitude on an oscilloscope (A-mode). In B-mode scanning, the transducer is automatically moved tangentially over the skin surface and a number of A scans are depicted and processed electronically, resulting in a cross-sectional image of the skin in two dimensions. Frequencies between 10–15 MHz should be chosen for skin examination. With high frequencies it becomes more difficult to view in depth. To calculate total skin thickness, the time elapsed between the first echo (the interface between the sensor and the skin surface) and the second high amplitude echo (interface between dermis and hypodermis) is measured. Thickness of measured tissue equals transit time of the ultrasound through skin by normal speed of ultrasound in skin (1540 m/s) [9].

Laser Doppler Flowmetry

Laser Doppler flowmetry is an optical technique used to evaluate skin microcirculation which provides information on blood flow and erythema. The method consists of a

Ne-He laser source of 632 nm wavelenght applied to the skin via a small probe. The incident radiation enters the skin and is scattered and reflected by nonmoving tissue components and by mobile red blood cells encountered as the radiation penetrates to a depth of 1–1.5 mm. A portion of the scattered and reflected incident radiation exits the skin and is collected by a second optical fibre that carries the light back to a photodetector where it is converted to an electrical signal. Stationary skin tissue reflects and backscatters light at the same frequency as the incident source, while moving erythrocytes reflect the frequency shifted radiation. The shift increases with increasing velocity. The LDF extracts the frequency-shifted signal and derives an output proportional to the flux of erythrocytes of the blood flow. LDF is a reliable method to estimate cutaneous microcirculation [10].

Thermography

Anticellulite products are meant to increase local skin blood flow. By increasing the blood flow, they increase the local skin temperature. Thermography is an electro-optical method for imaging of temperature. The current technology used is based on the detection of infrared radiation emitted by the skin. A conventional colour thermogram uses a spectral colour range, where blue is cold and red-white is hot. Intermediary temperatures are shown in shades of green, yellow, orange, etc. [11].

Mechanical Properties

Bioengineering devices for the assessment of mechanical skin parameters differ greatly with regard to the physical principle behind the measurement. Devices based on tension, suction, torsion, vibration have been developed and used. Each particular approach has its own advantages and disadvantages, Anyhow, determination of skin distensibility, elasticity, hysteresis, has been quite standardised (at least in suction and torsion devices) and is currently used in quantification of cosmetic efficacy [12].

Plicometry

This technique implies the use of the Plicometer, a device which permits to evaluate the thickness of cutaneous plicae or folds, from which is possible to calculate the fat percentage in human body. The measurement is usually performed on the thigh, in a defined point, which can be determined measuring the half distance between the iliac crest and the centre of the knee as reference points. During measurements, the leg is relaxed. All measurements are performed in standard conditions which guarantee reliability and precision of data. In particular:
- Measurements are performed on dry skin
- The subject has to maintain the leg as relaxed as possible
- Measurements are performed always on the same site and each measurement is repeated twice for each data point
- The exact measuring point is set by using tape-measure
- Plicae are obtained by catching tissues between thumb and forefinger and gently pulling a little outside
- The plicometer has to be put on the precise point perpendicularly to the skin and 1 cm away from fingers keeping the plica.

Thigh Circumference Measurements

The evaluation of circumference provides a measure of the amount of the fatty layer under the area of examination. It is evaluated by tape-measure on hips, thighs, ankles as follows:

a) Hips: the tape-measure is positioned around the hips, putting it finally on the super-anterior iliac crest
b) Thigh: the-tape measure is placed around the thigh, marking the site of interest
c) Ankle: the tape-measure is placed around the ankle, exactly above the malleolar bone [4].

Study Procedure

An example of a study performed to assess the efficacy of anti-cellulite products is reported below.

Materials and Methods

A double-blind test was carried out on ten subjects, female volunteers. Two products (active and placebo) were applied on the left and right thighs respectively, twice a day, in a randomised and balanced manner, for 1 month. Environmental temperature and humidity were controlled during the study (18–20 C° and 40%–60% R.H.). Active product was based on escin, diosmin, acetylglucosamine and glucuronic acid in a liquid crystal emulsion (oleosomes); placebo was the base liquid crystal emulsion. Evaluation was performed by:

a) Clinical score, based on a grading scale (0–4) (see "Introduction")
b) Thigh circumference measurement
c) Noninvasive methods: skin thickness measured by pulsed ultrasound (A scan, Dermascan Cortex Technolgy, Denmark); biomechanical parameters (elasticity, distensibility, hysteresis) measured with a suction device (Dermaflex, Cortex Technology, Denmark) with a vacuum force set to 300 mbars
d) Cutaneous microcirculation measured by laser Doppler velocimetry (Periflux 2B, Perimed, Sweden).

Statistical analysis was made by Student's t-test for paired data (StatView, statistical package).

Results and Discussion

Results are shown in Table 1 and Figures 1–4. A general improvement in most parameters is generally recorded after treatment in both sites. However, tape-measurements of thigh circumference show a statistically significant decrease in the active treated site as compared to the placebo treated site ($p<0.007$) (Table 1; Fig. 1). Thickness of the subcutaneous fat, as measured by ultrasound, is decreased in both sites, even though significantly in the active-treated site ($p<0.0001$) (Table 1; Fig. 2). Comparison between the two sites after treatment shows significant differences ($p<0.03$) with lower fat thickness in the active treated-site. Skin microcirculation, as measured by laser

Table 1. Thigh circumference (cm), ultrasound (mm), laser Doppler velocimetry (perfusion units), and distensibility (mm) before and after treatment

	Baseline Active	Placebo	After treatment Active	Placebo
Thigh circumference	57.2±3.5[a]	57.15±4.8	56.35±3.1[a]	57.15±4.5
Ultrasound	0.86±0.1[a]	0.87±0.2	0.60±0.08[a,b]	0.80±0.19[b]
LDV	12.0±3.2	14.1±6.3	15.6±6.1	11.7±4.2
Distensibility	2.16±0.2	2.12±0.2	2.10±0.3	2.22±0.2

[a,b] Significant differences (see text for p values).

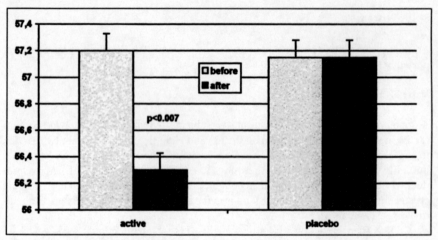

Fig. 1. Thigh circumference as measured by tape-measure. There is a significant reduction of diameter in the site treated with active product

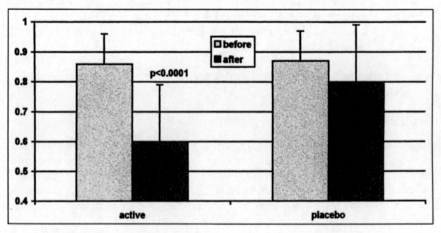

Fig. 2. Thickness of the subcutaneous fat layer as measured by ultrasound. A significant reduction on the site treated with active product is measured

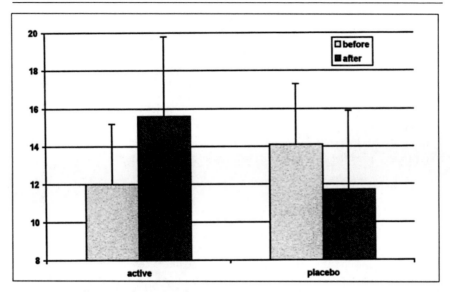

Fig. 3. Laser Doppler velocimetry (LDV). An improvement of blood flow (even though not statistically significant) is recorded on the active-treated site

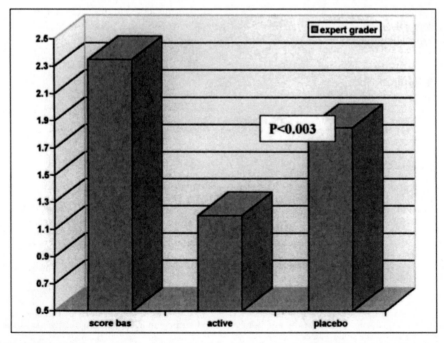

Fig. 4. Visual score expressed by an expert grader assessment. Active and placebo are significantly different ($p<0.003$)

Doppler velocimetry (Table 1; Fig. 3), shows an improvement of superficial skin blood flow in the active-treated site consistent with an improved microcirculation. The data is not statistically significant, probably due to the large standard deviation of the data induced by changes in the climatic conditions between basal and final recordings; however, on the contralateral site treated with placebo there is a decline in absolute values of microcirculation.

No significant differences were detected (Table 1) in mechanical parameters investigated and in particular in skin distensibility.

Clinical score, as expressed by an expert grader shows a significant reduction in the active treated site after therapy ($p<0.003$ vs placebo treated site).

Conclusion

In conclusion, the study shows that effective treatment of cellulite can be achieved and assessed. Ultrasound is the most reliable technique to assess the thickness of the subcutaneous fat and the amount of fat deposits at the interface between dermis and hypodermis. Laser Doppler velocimetry can give a good estimate of the improvement in skin microcirculation. The improvement in skin condition in the placebo treated sites is mainly due to massage subsequential to product application. It is known that massage can play an important role in modifying some physical properties of the skin resulting in a lower degree of cellulite [8]. Changes in other biophysical parameters, such as mechanical properties, have minor importance in this pathology and are less recommended. Furthermore, the study shows that improvement of skin microcirculation with topically applied diosmin in lesional skin associated with other compounds capable to reduce fluid retention can be helpful in controlling cellulite.

References

1. Curri SB, Ryan TJ (1989) Panniculopathy and fibrosclerosis of the female breast and thigh. In: Ryan TJ, Curri SB (eds) Cutaneous adipose tissue. Lippincott, Philadelphia, pp 107–119
2. Curri SB, Bombardelli E (1994) Local lipodystrophy and districtual microcirculation. Cosmet Toilet 109:51–65
3. Di Salvo RM (1995) Controlling the appearance of cellulite. Cosmet Toilet 110:50–59
4. Smith PW (1995) Cellulite treatments: snake oils or skin science. Cosmet Toilet 110:61–70
5. Gasparro V, Vettorello GF (1992) Treating cellulite. Cosmet Toilet 107:64–66
6. Vague J, Fenasse R (1965) Comparative anatomy of adipose tissue. In: Reynold AE, Cahill GF (eds) American handbook of physiology. Am Physiol Soc z25–34
7. Curri SB (1990) Inquadramento nosografico e classificazione delle panniculopatie da stasi. Flebologia 1:15–19
8. Lucassen GW, van der Sluys WLN, van Herk JJ, Nuijs AM, Wierenga PE, Barel AO, Lambrecht R (1997) The effectiveness of massage treatment on cellulite as monitored by ultrasound imaging. Skin Res Technol 3:154–160
9. Serup J (1995) Skin imaging techniques in bioengineering and the skin: methods and instrumentation. CRC Press, Boca Raton, pp 65–79
10. Bernardi L, Berardesca E (1995) Measurements of skin blood flow by laser doppler flowmetry in bioengineering and the skin: methods and instrumentation. CRC Press, Boca Raton, pp 13–28
11. Sherman-RA, Woerman-AL, Karstetter-KW (1996) Comparative effectiveness of videothermography, contact thermography, and infrared beam thermography for scanning relative skin temperature. J Rehabil Res Dev 33:377–386
12. Elsner P (1995) Skin elasticity in bioengineering and the skin: methods and instrumentation. CRC Press, Boca Raton, pp 53–64

CHAPTER 14

Methods for Claim Support in Cosmetology: Hair Cosmetics

L.J. Wolfram

Introduction

The history of claim substantiation has been an edifying example of an on-going interaction process between consumers, marketing and laboratory personnel in which various aspects of cosmetic attributes of a tissue have been characterized and then defined in terms of properties quantifiable by instrumental measurements. The ability to adapt some of the well established textile methodology has been of a great help in setting the claim support for hair on sound technical basis. One should be reminded, however, that the growing reliance on instrumental methods in no way diminishes the importance of sensory evaluation carried out on live heads in beauty salons or among the consumer panelists. Indeed, such tests have been and remain the cornerstone of the product development process for every hair care product. The discussion of the interplay between the sensory perception, psychophysics and instrumental measurement is, however, beyond the scope of this chapter and the reader is referred to an excellent reviews of this subject by Moskowitz [1] and Bush [2].

The great diversity of hair care products combined with the competitive market pressure to extol products performance in ever changing manner require a variety of tests and approaches to meet such a challenge. In this respect of considerable help have been recent advances in our understanding of the hair structure as well as an explosive growth of analytical techniques in the field of physics and chemistry. Yet, translating sensory perception and cosmetic attributes into a scientifically measured quantities remains demanding task. Occasionally the resolution is straightforward – claims for hair strengths or shine can be relatively simply derived from the tensile properties of hair and its surface reflectance, respectively. On the other hand, the attribute of hair conditioning is much more complex, encompassing hair softness, ease of combing, fly-away, etc. In this case an array of techniques involving both single fiber properties and those of fiber assemblies (hair tresses) are needed to obtain necessary support.

The purpose of this chapter is to provide a concise survey of physico-chemical techniques that are relevant to claim substantiation for hair care products. Much more detailed information on this subject can be found in recent publications by Ishi [3] and Stern et al. [4].

Single Fiber and/or Material Specific Techniques

Physical Properties

Tensile Properties

Ever since Speakman [5] provided the first comprehensive interpretation of the stress–strain behavior of keratin fibers, the measurements of tensile properties have been at the forefront of hair evaluation techniques. The simplicity of the measurement combined with the wealth of information it conveys, contributed greatly to its utilization and success. The load-extension curve (Fig. 1) displays three distinctly different regions; the initial, nearly linear, Hookean region (AB) is followed by the yield region (BC) where the fiber extends with relatively small increase in stress. As extension approaches 30% the fiber stiffens again signalling the onset of the post-yield region which continues until the fiber breaks.

Each of these regions reflects the different character of structural bonding within the fiber which can aid in monitoring the product-induced changes. The stiffness of the Hookean region is attributed to the elastic stability of hydrogen-bonded α-helices which, beyond the yield point, unfold reversibly into extended β configuration. The covalent disulfide cross-links appear, on the other hand, to be controlling factor in the bond network that opposes extension in the post-yield region.

Speakman's [5] observation that the keratin fibers which are extended no further than the yield region have the ability to recover fully their properties when relaxed in water proved of exceptional value in assessing simply and accurately the changes in fiber properties associated with chemical or physical treatment of hair. His technique involves determination of work required to stretch the hair 30% (calibration step) followed by overnight relaxation in water, subjecting the fiber to intended treatment and re-stretching. The change in work (RW30) expressed as the percentage of the calibrated value provides information of changes imparted by the treatment. As each hair is its own control, few tests suffice to generate reliable results and there is no need to account for variation in fiber diameter. This method has been extensively employed [6–9] as a test for hair damage in waving, bleaching, or coloring. By adjusting the pH of the testing solution, insight can be gained as to the coulombic (electrostatic) interaction in hair; testing in solvents other than water yields information on the accessibi-

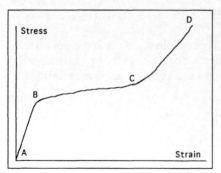

Fig. 1. The load–extension curve displays three distinctly different regions; the initial, nearly linear, Hookean region (*AB*) is followed by the yield region (*BC*) where the fiber extend with relatively small increase in stress. As extension approaches 30%, the fiber stiffens, again signalling the onset of the post-yield region which continues until the fiber breaks

lity of hair to various reagents. Over the years several modifications of the technique have been introduced, replacing the (RW) by the "index" value representing the ratio of work or force (treated/untreated) at 30%, 20%, or 15% extension [10]. Also, instead of single hair fibers, fiber bundles are used [11] and the hysteresis ratio (work of recovery/work of elongation) is employed in lieu of (RW) or the work index.

It is essential to point out that the mechanical properties of hair vary with the temperature, time and relative humidity at which the fibers are tested. Thus, strictly adhered-to testing procedures should be followed to assure the reproducibility of the results as well as their validity. In this regard, performing the tensile tests in water is often more convenient – the environment of 100% relative humidity is assured and the temperature control of the system is easy to maintain. Also, due to the plasticizing effects which water exerts on keratin, the interplay of structural bonding in the different regions of the stress–strain curve is easier to interpret.

While the techniques described above are very useful in portraying changes in hair resulting from product application, the intermittent stress relaxation measurements [12] permit insight into the process itself as it occurs in the fiber. This is of particular value for reactive treatments such as waving and straightening where the knowledge of the kinetics of the reaction process is essential in designing potential product improvements. The coincidental advantage of these measurements is that they are carried out at very low strain level which mimics the condition occurring in the practical use to of the product [13].

Bending and Torsional Properties

Inasmuch as the tensile properties are highly informative of the overall mechanical integrity of hair fibers, the most frequent deformations to which the latter are subjected in course of their resident life on the scalp are bending and torsion. Shampooing, setting or waving, combing and blow-drying all involve fiber displacement in which individual hairs are either bent or twisted. Clearly, the ability to evaluate such deformations is essential to successful modulation of these properties for enhancement of product performance.

Bending stiffness measurements, whether by static [14] or dynamic procedures [15] have shown that, in general, the bending behavior of keratin fibers, wet or dry, approximates to that expected from their tensile properties in the Hookean region. The methodology involved in measurement is difficult and cumbersome, and it is only recently that a much simpler technique was developed by Scott and Robbins [16]. A single hair fiber, weighed on both ends is draped over a wire and the distance (D) between the two vertical legs is determined. The value D is a measure of bending stiffness. Bogaty [17] was the first to point out the relevance and importance of torsional deformations both in impartation and maintenance of hair styles. By setting or waving of hair, helical coil configurations are formed and their performance can be viewed in the light of the engineering spring theory with respect to the effect of coil radius, its torsional stiffness and the hair diameter . Two general approaches have been used to measure torsional properties of hair fibers: the direct twist method of Morton and Permanyer [18] and the torsion pendulum method of Bogaty [17]. Both techniques yield reliable results, although the pendulum methods has an advantage in that a simple modification [19] of the technique permits examination of fibers both in air and in liquids.

Also, a "calibration" step similar to that used by Speakman [5] in tensile measurements is possible, and thus the torsion tests may be repeated several times on the same fiber.

Friction

Relative movement of two contacting surfaces is resisted by friction. Our tactile perception of hair softness, smoothness or springiness involves frictional contacts. Styling of hair or its combing entail continuous frictional displacement of adjacent hair fibers. It is thus not surprising that the measurement of friction is a requisite for characterization of surface properties of hair. A variety of methods has been used to measure the friction of fibers; highly popular has become the capstan method [20] in which a fiber with equal weights (one resting on a pan of a torsion balance) is draped over a cylinder. The latter can be made of glass, metal, horn, etc., or can have a layer of fibers. As the cylinder rotates the torsion balance indicates the developed frictional force. A recent improvement of this technique involves replacement of the torsion balance by an Instron tensile tester [21].

Optical Properties

Even though the term "optical properties" embraces wide range of attributes including refractive index, birefrigence, color, light scattering and spectroscopic properties, only the last three will be reviewed here. Of the three, the light scattering at the fiber surface appears to be the phenomenon of relevance to most of the consumers since it is the determining factor in the luster of hair.

Hair Luster

Most of the techniques of luster evaluation are based on the principle of measuring the intensity of light scattered from single fibers or hair tresses by means of a goniophotometer [22–24]. The data are then converted into the luster (shine) values by computing a ratio between specularly reflected and diffusively scattered light. Depending on the measurements protocol the luster values may vary somewhat. In order to verify the validity of a chosen formula it is customary to correlate the instrumental data with the subjective luster evaluations by trained observers.

A rapid technique for assessment of luster of hair has been recently developed (FJ Wortmann, personal communication, 1997). It is based on the measurement of the intensity of laser light scattered from single hair fibers by means of an Optical MultiChannel Analyser (OMA) that allows measurements at angular intervals of 1° in the range of 7°–173.5° in less than 1 s.

As an afterthought one should be reminded that while smooth surfaced fiber such as hair appears shiny, it is not the only factor involved as the luster can be effectively modulated by change of alignment of fibers, of their geometry (straight or curly) or color.

Hair Color

Irrespective of how many objective techniques might be available to define accurately the wavelength range and the intensity of the imparted color, it is the subjective evaluation of the dyed hair by experienced, professional hair colorists that makes the final call regarding the acceptance, or rejection of a new color formulation. Nevertheless, the objective measurements are used throughout the process of product development not only to assist the formulator in designing a color palette but to evaluate the stability of colored hair to shampoo, sweat, waving lotions, weathering, etc. (potential claim areas). This is done preferentially on hair tresses using commercially available spectrocolori meters [25]. The color values are expresses by lightness parameter "L" (for black L=0, for white L=100) and two chromaticity dimensions "a" and "b", where "a" is a measure of redness when the value is positive and greenness when negative, and "b" is a measure of yellowness when positive and blueness when negative. Additionally, spectral reflectance curves can be obtained over the entire visible spectrum range. Portable instruments – based on the same principle – have become now available and increasingly find their way into the beauty salons.

Spectroscopic Properties
Among the spectroscopic techniques the infra-red spectroscopy (IR) has been the most widely used in the structural investigations of keratin fibers [26, 27]. As the IR is based on absorption characteristics of specific molecular groups it can provide data on some aspects of the structure which are difficult to obtain otherwise. Thus, interaction of keratin with water or other sorbates can be followed by IR and assignments of binding sites made [28]. Incorporation of the Fourier Transform (FT) feature has significantly increased the sensitivity of the technique permitting virtually routine evaluation of fibers and assessment of changes brought about by treatments.

One of the applications was found in monitoring the oxidative cleavage of disulfide bonds of cystine that takes place during bleaching, coloring or weathering of hair [29]. In this case the cysteic acid content is used as an index of hair damage. With an ATR (attenuated total reflectance) it is possible to confine the IR absorption to the fiber periphery (up to thickness of 5 nm) and thus carry out the "optical sectioning" of the fiber. Such an approach has been exploited in following the interaction of keratin fibers with sodium sulfite and protein hydrolizates [30].

A recent report by Pande [31] draws attention to the potential of Raman spectroscopy as a highly sensitive tool for hair analysis. The technique is noninvasive and the measurements – in contrast to IR – are not affected by the presence of water. Also the spectra are significantly more detailed than those of IR over a broad range of wavelengths and this apparently permits the direct monitoring of disulfide bonds. Preliminary analysis of the amide I band in the Raman spectra suggests that the photo-induced damage of hair is more obvious in the cuticle and the amorphous matrix protein than in the α helical regions. It has been well known [32, 33] that keratin fibers fluoresce when excited with radiation in the 290–320 nm range, but it is only recently that this phenomenon has been skillfully put to use in evaluation of hair weathering [34]. The most significant single parameter in the weathering is solar radiation [35] and its absorption by hair is primarily mediated by the tryptophan residues and the melanin pigment. The changes in the latter – involving destructive photo oxidation process resulting in lightening of hair – are slow and thus not particularly well suited to serve as an index of light-induced damage. The assessment of cystine content appears to be more attractive in this regard but reliable determinations are either cumbersome or require fiber hydrolysis. On the other hand, the fluorescence measurements are rapid and non-invasive, and can be readily adapted to monitor the photo-decomposition of tryptophan residues in hair. A sensitive marker of hair photo-damage is thus available with a potential application for the evaluation of efficacy of sunscreens.

Physico-chemical Properties

Swelling

In spite of the fact that the surface of hair is highly hydrophobic, the keratinous substance of the fiber exhibits high affinity for water which at the saturation point (100% RH) represents almost one third of the fiber weight. The water absorption is accompanied by highly anisotropic swelling of hair – a 17% increase in hair diameter contrasts with 1% increase in fiber lengths. The equilibrium swelling is an accepted measure of the integrity of fiber structure. Any treatment that splits the covalent cross-links causes imbalance of Coulombic interactions or weakens the hydrogen bonds network, leading invariably to increased swelling. Conversely, the introduction of new cross-links or of bulky hydrophobic groups brings about decrease in swelling. The swelling of hair is thus clearly an useful indicator of product-induced changes. Two general approaches have been used to evaluate swelling of hair. In the first, swelling is monitored by microscopic examination of individual hair fibers [36], while the second relies on the measurement of the weight of sorbed liquid [37]. The microscopic technique is direct but tedious; the "liquid retention" method, on the other hand, is highly reproducible, easy to use and the results are more precise.

Supercontraction

The term was originally coined [38] to describe contraction of the stretched keratin fibers to a length less than its original. Unstretched hair fibers also contract when subjected to certain treatments and this phenomenon is now also referred to as supercontraction. It occurs on immersion of hair in boiling solutions of sodium bisulfite. The extent of supercontraction is a function of fiber cross-linking and thus particularly helpful in evaluation of properties of hair exposed to variety of treatments including weathering [35].

Chemical Properties

Amino-acid and Protein Analysis

Apart from lipids which amount to 3%–5% of the fiber weight, the hair is essentially pure protein and on hydrolysis yields 18 amino-acids. Until some years ago the amino-acid analysis (AA) was the only way to determine unequivocally the chemical changes resulting from various treatments of hair. The substantial cost of the AA equipment, combined with tedious and time consuming procedure prevented AA from becoming a routine method. The increased understanding of the reactivity of hair and of the reaction pathways of hair products generated a need for either a group – specific analysis or for noninvasive physical techniques. With regard to the latter a reference has already been made here of the determination of cysteic acid by IR and of tryptophan fluorescence measurements technique. Unfortunately no such simple method exists yet for determination of the combined cystine which as a major contributor to the stability of hair structure is of particular analytical interest. Some success has been obtained with ESCA (electron spectroscopy for chemical analysis) but the technique is primarily a surface probe [39]. A non-hydrolytic, polarographic analysis of cystine and cysteine in keratins was developed by Leach [40]. It is highly sensitive and was effectively employed with single fibers to determine the interfiber variation of cystine content [41]. A combination of radiotracer [42] and florescent [43] tagging, of the sulf-hydryl groups with subsequent microscopic analysis offers itself as a useful, though semiquantitative analytical tool for evaluation of distribution of cysteine residues in hair.

Occasionally an analysis of protein rather than of individual amino-acids is utilized for a specific purpose. Thus findings by Sandhu [44] that the damaged hair surface is highly vulnerable to abrasion led him to suggest that quantitative measurements of protein removed from hair by a standard abrasion test can serve as a sensitive method to assess the hair damage.

Alkali Solubility

Extraction of hair with aqueous alkali under standard conditions provides the basis of a solubility test for detection of both the disulfide and the peptide cleavage [45]. The test entails extraction with 0.1 M sodium hydroxide at 65°C for 1 h. The increase in alkali solubility caused by bleaching, coloring or weathering represents a useful index of fiber damage which may occur with these processes.

Properties of Fiber Assemblies

General Considerations

One can visualize the scalp hair as an assembly of fine, flexible fibers arranged in more or less orderly geometrical arrays. In most cases, the fiber arrangements will be generally parallel, although smaller, sub-assemblies (curls) might be at a variety of angles to each other. Individual fibers within the assembly are usually in a bent or slightly twisted configuration, and are in various states of contact with their neighbors. Such contacts represent sites of potential frictional restraint which is one of the important characteristics of fibrous assemblies. Although precise information regarding the mean density of contact points and the mean force per contact is difficult to obtain, in low density assemblies of almost parallel fibers, the number of contacts per unit length is proportional to β/d where β is packing density and d is the fiber diameter. For low density assemblies, the proportionality constant is close to unity and thus for a packing density of 0.02 the number of contacts per cm (with the average hair diameter of 80 µm) is 2.5. From five main types of deformation which a fiber in an assembly is subjected to, viz. transverse compression, longitudinal extension, longitudinal compression, torsion and bending, the latter two are probably the most relevant to the actual physical stimuli exerted onto the hair assemblies. High value of flexural rigidity of hair (10 dyne/cm^2) compared to other textile fibers implies that the bending and torsional (dry) deformation are less force-sensitive than frictional restraints, although a change in fiber geometry can either minimize (hair straightening) or intensify (waving, setting) the bending contributions. Overall, it is clear that substantial modulation of hair mass behavior is possible by manipulating interfiber friction.

Wetting of hair alters in a significant way the balance of interfiber interaction that exists in a dry assembly. One of the most important changes is the fall in bending modulus and a drastic decrease of torsional rigidity. Although this reduces the normal forces, the transverse swelling of hair can have the opposite effect. An usually strong force contribution is generated by the liquid trapped in the hair mass. While the minimal value of the force per contact is given by $2 \pi DT$ (~35 µN), the maximal attainable value of the interfiber force set up by the liquid meniscus in the case of parallel fibers is: $Fm=(8DET^2)1/3$ (~10 µN) where D is the diameter of the fiber, E is the transverse modulus of hair and T is the surface tension of the liquid. Deviation from parallel to perpendicular arrangement within an assembly (presence of curls for example) significantly lowers the contact force by over one order of magnitude as the $F_{II}/F\perp$~25.

Hair Combability

It takes usually no more than a touch or a gentle squeeze of hair strands and a single pass of a comb. In this brief moment the interplay of tactile sensation and the awareness of mechanical effort fuse together into a firm perception of hair "condition". Whether the coincidence that the tactile and combing attributes undergo directionally parallel changes, or the cumulative experience that easy combing does not go hand in hand with raspy feel, the hair combability, apart from being an important technique in its own right, has become an essential feature of support claims for hair conditioning.

Several instrumentation techniques for assessment of hair combability have been developed [46, 47], but the basic design is common to all and entails attaching a tress of hair to a strain gauge and measuring forces required to pull the comb through the tress under standard conditions. Both dry and wet combing can be evaluated this way as well as the detangling of hair. The combability tests have become a standard feature in evaluation methodology of virtually every hair care product but are of particular importance for assessment of efficacy of conditioners.

Hair Body

Hair body is doubtlessly one of the most desirable attributes of hair – it conveys bulk, liveliness, resilience. It is a complex property – a result of an interplay between the single fiber parameter such as friction, hair diameter, stiffness, geometry and the disposition of the individual fibers within the hair mass. The techniques which evolved to measure hair body address primarily three major structural properties of the hair mass: bulk volume, resistance to deformation and resilience [48, 49]. The Omega Loop test [49] measures the forces of compression and the recovery of a bent hair tress but the very configuration of the tress targets the bending stiffness as the major element in the deformation process. Such a focus on a single property of hair assembly is avoided in the Ring Technique [50] in which a freely hanging tress is pulled through a ring while continuous recording is made of the forces resisting the tress compression to which both the bending deformation and frictional restraints contribute. Successive passes of tress through the ring are used as a measure of resilience. Slightly different approach is employed in the Radial Compression technique [51] in which a freely hanging hair bundle is strangled as a recording is made of both the compression and recovery cycles.

The volume aspect of hair body is usually addressed by continuous recording of the contour of a tress rotated in front of a photocell and integrating the obtained data. Recently a volume measurement of hair tresses with the aid of an image analyzer was described [52].

Style Retention

Change in fiber configuration is an essential element of hair styling and the manipulative success of the latter relies primarily on the ability of hair to acquire and maintain permanent or temporary set. In the case of permanent setting the newly imparted set is stable to water and can only be attained by chemical processing of hair such as waving or straightening. The temporary set relies on water setting of hair as well as on its reinforcement by various setting aids such as gels, mousses and hairsprays. The techniques developed for the evaluation of set retention – and it is in the stability of the set configuration that the efficacy of the tested product reveals itself – while reflecting in procedural details, the differences of the setting process (permanent or temporary) adhere to similar test principles.

In a static hold test, the hair tresses (if single fibers are used then the hair–hair interaction aspect is missed) set in desired configuration are freely suspended in front of graduated panels and allowed to relax at a chosen humidity and temperature. Measurements are taken over time of the curl droop and the set retention efficacy calculated [54].

Static Charge

Unlike the combing where the comb material has little or no effect on the combing effort, the triboelectric charging of hair is almost entirely due to the comb-hair contact [55]. The resulting "fly-away" phenomenon is highly annoying as the hair becomes very unruly and difficult to comb. One of the main functions of a conditioning product is to either prevent or alleviate the static build-up. Most of the existing techniques for assessment of the static charge developed on hair during combing utilize the Faraday cage to collect the charge and an electrometer to measure it [56, 57]. The antistatic efficacy of shampoos and conditioners can be thus easily evaluated, but to assure optimal reproducibility, one ought to rely upon techniques in which the charge-generating step (hair combing) is automated and standardized.

Other Techniques

Microscopy

The very ability of a microscope to provide a magnified image of hair carries with it unique credibility and persuasiveness. It is thus not surprising that it has been widely used for claim support of product attributes which can capitalize on its features.

Light Microscopy

In spite of its limited resolving power, the light microscopy has been used in a highly reliable manner to provide evidence of internal hair damage [58], to follow the process of generation and repair of split ends [4], and, equipped with special attachment to detect the build-up of cationic polymers on hair or examine the penetration pathways of dyes [59, 60].

Scanning Electron Microscopy (SEM)

Owing to the unusual combination of high resolving power and great depth of focus, SEM has quickly gained a foothold among claim substantiation techniques. It is so far an unmatched tool for evaluation of hair surface providing highly accurate information on appearance of cuticle cells, on the nature of the surface damage or on the location and distribution of particulate materials on hair surface [61–63].

As only a small fraction of hair comes into view, caution should be exercised in evaluating the effects and a statistical approach to the analysis of SEM photographs is strongly recommended.

Atomic Force Microscopy (AFM)

AFM is a latecomer to this category but already shows some promise. Unlike SEM which requires coating of samples and high vacuum for their examination, AFM can operate in both air and water and is non-destructive to the samples. This extends vastly the scope of fiber testing, opening the way to in situ studies of the hair products [64].

Confocal Microscopy

This technique represents a new dimension in the light microscopy field and its application to hair has been reported recently [65]. Several aspects are worth noting: (a) confocal microscopy is particularly adapted to observations of rounded surfaces providing images with virtually no out-of-focus areas – this means greatly improved resolution over the conventional light microscope; (b) optical sectioning is possible thus opening the way to the nondestructive monitoring of penetration of materials through the whole thickness of hair.

Streaming Potential

Streaming potential measurements lie at the foundation of the newly developed Dynamic Electrokinetic and Permeability Analysis [66]. This elegant and highly sensitive technique is particularly effective in evaluating the interaction of hair with shampoos, conditioners and polymers providing information on binding such products to and removal from hair. This "fingerprinting" approach appears especially useful in studying the rinsability and build-up aspects of the products.

Dynamic Mechanical Analyser (DMA)

The importance of adequate and reliable characterization of properties of hair cannot be overstressed if one is to use them as a credible manner to support product claims. In most cases, however, the generation of such data is lengthy, requiring a variety of equipment. DMA [67] goes a long way to consolidate diverse measurements into a single instrument. Tensile, flexural and compression moduli can be readily measured over a wide range of temperatures along with the evaluation of the bending stiffness, creep recovery and storage modulus. In many instances a calibration step is possible thus allowing for repeat measurements or the fibers before and after treatment (Milczarek, Zielinski, personal communication, 1992).

Concluding Remarks

It is clear even from this brief survey that there is a plethora of techniques, methods, and approaches available to cosmetic scientists to develop sound, persuasive and often unique corroboration of product claims.

Hopefully, the process of claim substantiation can reach beyond the mere selection of meaningful techniques for verification of the desired attributes and also be of instructive value to the consumer in broadening their understanding of the scientific aspects of sensory perceptions.

References

1. Moskowitz HR (1980) The new psychophysics and cosmetics science. In: Breuer MM (ed) Cosmetic science, vol 2. Academic Press, London, pp 125–146
2. Bush P (1989) Arzt Kosmetol 19:270–315
3. Ishi MK (1997) Objective and instrumental methods for evaluation of hair care product efficacy and substantiation of claims. In: Johnson DH (ed) Hair and hair care. Marcel Dekker, New York, pp 261–302
4. Stern E, Gabbianelli A, Qualls A, Rahn J, Yang G, Meltzer N (1991) Views on claim support methods for hair care products. In: Aust LB (ed) Cosmetic claims substantiation. Marcel Dekker, New York, pp 21–68
5. Speakman JB (1927) J Textile Inst 18:T431
6. Reed RE, Den Beste M,Hummoler FL (1947) J Soc Cosmet Chem 12:133
7. Edman W, Marti M (1961) J Soc Cosmet Chem 12:133
8. Beyak R, Meyer CF, Kass GS (1969) J Soc Cosmet Chem 20:615
9. Wolfram LJ, Hall K, Hui 1 (1970) J Soc Cosmet Chem 21:875
10. Haefele JW, Broge RW (1961) Proc Sci Sect TGA 36:31
11. Deem DE, Rieger MM (1968) J Soc Cosmet Chem 19:395
12 . Khalil E (1986) Cosmet Toilet 101:51
13. Garcia ML, Nadgorny EM, Wolfram LJ (1990) J Soc Cosmet Chem 41:149
14. Mitchel TW, Feughelman M (1965) Textile Res J 35:311
15. Simpson W (1965) J.Textile Inst 51:675
16. Scott G, Robbins C (1969) Textile Res J 39:975
17. Bogaty H (1967) J Soc Cosmet Chem 18:575
18. Morton WE, Permanyer F (1947) J Textile Inst 38:T54
19. Wolfram LJ, Albrecht L (1985) J Soc Cosmet Chem 36:87
20. Schwartz A, Knowles DJ (1963) J Soc Cosmet Chem 14:455
21. Scott GV, Robbins CR (1980) J Soc Cosmet Chem 31:179
22. Stamm RF, Garcia ML, Fuchs C (1977) J Soc Cosmet Chem 28:571
23. Reich C, Robbins CR (1963) J Soc Cosmet Chem 44:221
24. Guiolet A, Garson JC, Leveque JL (1986) Study of the optical properties of human hair. Proc 14th IFSCC Congress, Barcelona 2:1019
25. Wolfram U, Albrecht L (1987) J Soc Cosmet Chem 38:179
26. Ambrose EJ, Elliott A (1951) Proc R Soc Lond Ser A206:206
27. Bendit EG (1966) Biopolymers 4:561
28. Bendit EG (1966) Biopolymers 4:539
29. Strassburger J, Breuer MM (1985) J Soc Cosmet Chem 36:61
30. Gomez N, Julia MR, Lewis DM (1995) J Soc Dyers Col 11:281

31. Pande CP (1997) J Soc Cosmet Chem 45:2 57
32. Nicholls CH, Pailthorpe MT (1976) J Textile Inst 67:397
33. Collins S, Davidson S,Greaves PH, Healey M, Lewis DM (1988) J Soc Dyers Col 104:348
34. Pande CP, Jachowicz J (1993) J Soc Cosmet Chem 44:109
35. Wolfram LJ (1981). The reactivity of human hair. A review. In: Orfanos Montagna, Stuttgen (eds) Hair research. Springer, Berlin Heidelberg New York, pp 479–500
36. Eckstrom MG (1950) J Soc Cosmet Chem 2:244
37. Valko El, Barnett G (1951) J Soc Cosmet Chem 3:108
38. Astbury WT, Woods HJ (1933) Phil Trans Proc R Soc 232A:336
39. Zahn H (1997) Hair sulfur amino acid analysis. In: Jollies P, Zahn H, Hocker H (eds) Formation and structure of human hair. Birkhauser, Basel, pp 239–258
40. Leach SJ (1960) Aust J Chem 13:520
41. Wolfram LJ, Lennhof M (1967) Textile Res J 37:145
42. Jenkins AD, Troth HG, Wolfram LJ (1965) An autoradiographic method for the determination of the distribution of reduction in keratin fibers. Proc 3rd Wool Research Textile Conference, Paris 2:53
43. Evans TA, Ventura TN, Wayne AB (1994) J Soc Cosmet Chem 45:279
44. Sandhu SS, Robbins CR (1993) J Soc Cosmet Chem 44:163
45. Harris M, Smith AL (1936) J Res Nat Bur Stand 17:577
46. Garcia ML, Diaz J (1976) J Soc Cosmet Chem 27:379
47. Kamath YK, Weigmann HD (1986) J Soc Cosmet Chem 37:111
48. Wedderburn DL, Prall JK (1973) J Soc Cosmet Chem 24:561
49. Hough PS, Huey JE, Tolgyesi WS (1976) J Soc Cosmet Chem 27:571
50. Garcia ML, Wolfram LJ (1978) Measurement of bulk compressibility and bulk resiliency of a hair mass. Proc 1Oth IFSCC Congress, Sydney, Australia 3:595
51. Weigmann HD, Kamath Y, Mark H (1985) Studies of the modification of human hair properties by surface treatment. Phase 11. Hair assembly behavior. Progress report No 2. Textile Research Institute, Princeton NJ
52. Clark J, Robbins CJ, Reich C (1991) J Soc Cosmet Chem 42:341
53. Wong MY, Diaz P (1983) J Soc Cosmet Chem 34:205
54. Bauer D, Beck JP, Monnais C, Vayssie C (1983) Int J Cosmet Sci 5:113
55. Jachowicz J, WisSurel G, Wolfram U (1984) Textile Res J 54:492
56. Lunn AC, Robert EE (1977) J Soc Cosmet Chem 28:549
57. Mills CM, Ester VC, Henkin H (1956) J Soc Cosmet Chem 7:466
58. Curtis RK, Tyson DR (1976) J Soc Cosmet Chem 27:411
59. Cooperman ES, Johnsen VL (1973) Cosmet Perfum 88:19
60. Jurdana LE, Leaver IH (1992) Polymer Inst 27:197
61. Swift JA, Brown AC (1975) J Soc Cosmet Chem 26:289
62. Garcia ML, Epps JA, Yare RS, Harik LD (1978) J Soc Cosmet Chem 29:1556
63. Shaw DA (1979) Int J Cosmet Chem 1:317
64. Smith JR (1997) J Soc Cosmet Chem 48:199
65. Corcuff P, Gremillet P, Jourlin M, Duvault Y, Leray F, Leveque JL (1993) J Soc Cosmet Chem 44:1
66. Jachowicz J, Williams C (1994) J Soc Cosmet Chem 45:309
67. Cassel B, Twombly B (1991) American Laboratory, January p 22

CHAPTER 15

Racial Differences in Skin Function: Related to Claim Support[1]

E. Berardesca, H.I. Maibach

Introduction

Racial variability in skin function is an area in which data are often conflicting. The understanding and quantifying of racial differences in skin function are of importance for skin care and the prevention and treatment of skin diseases. A key feature that characterizes race is skin color: is deeply pigmented skin (black or brown) different than fair skin in terms of responses to chemical and environmental insults? Is skin care the same? Is there a different risk among racial groups to develop a skin disease after exposure to the same insults? The issue is difficult to define and the interpretation of pathophysiologic phenomena should consider not only anatomical and functional characteristics of ethnic groups, but also socioeconomic, hygienic and nutritional factors. Indeed, even though it is well established that all humans belong to the same species, many physical differences exist among human populations. These differences, appeared during the latest stages of evolution, could be due both to genetic and environmental factors [1]. This paper reviews and discusses recent findings as relates to claim support.

Barrier Function

Stratum corneum is equally thick in black and white skin [2, 3]. However, Weigand et al. demonstrated that the stratum corneum in blacks contains more cell layers and requires more cellophane tape strips to remove than the stratum corneum of Caucasians [4]. They found great variance in values obtained from black subjects, whereas data from white subjects were more homogeneous. No correlation existed between the degree of pigmentation and the number of cell layers. These data could be explained by greater intercellular cohesion in blacks resulting in a increased number of cell layers and an increased resistance to stripping. This mechanism may involve lipids, because the lipid content of the stratum corneum, ranges from 8.5% to 14%, with higher values in blacks [5]. This result was confirmed by Weigand et al. who showed that delipidized specimens of stratum corneum were equal in weight in the two races [4]. Johnson and Corah found the mean electrical resistance of adult black skin to be twice that of adult white skin, suggesting an increased

Corcuff et al. [7] investigated the corneocyte surface area and spontaneous desquamation and found no evidence of differences between black, white and oriental skin.

---

[1] Modified with permission from [1]

However, an increased desquamation (up to 2.5 times) was found (p<0.01) in blacks (Table 1). They concluded that the differences may be related to a different composition of the intercellular cement of the stratum corneum. Sugino et al. [8] found significant differences in the amount of ceramides in the stratum corneum, with the lowest levels in Blacks followed by Caucasian, Hispanics and Asians. In this experiment ceramide levels were inversely correlated with TEWL and directly correlated with water content. These data may partially explain the controversial findings in the literature on the mechanisms of skin sensitivity.

Changes in skin permeability and barrier function have been reported: Kompaore et al. [9] evaluated TEWL and lag time after application of a vasoactive compound before and after removal of the stratum corneum. They found a significantly higher TEWL after stripping in Blacks and Asians than in Whites (Fig. 1). In particular, after stripping, Asians showed the highest TEWL and, at the same time, an increased permeability (compared to the other races) obtained immediately after a few strips.

Table 1. Racial differences in corneocyte surface area and spontaneous desquamation. Spontaneous desquamation is significantly increased in black subjects (p<0.001). (Modified from [7])

Racial group	Mean surface area (μm2±SE)	Desquamation (N/cm2±SE)
Black	911±20	26500±4900
White	899±22	11800±1700
Oriental	909±24	10400±2100

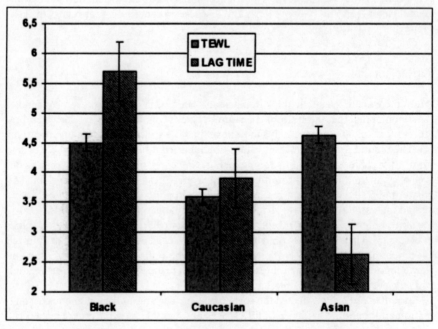

Fig. 1. TEWL (g/m2/h±SD) and Lag time (s/100 ±SD) in blacks, Caucasians and Asians. (Modified from [9].) See text for details

In contrast, Reed et al. [10] found differences in the recovery of the barrier between subjects with skin type II/III compared to skin type IV, but no differences between Caucasians in general and Asians. Darker skin recovered faster after barrier damage induced by tape stripping.

Reactions to Light

Light penetration into skin has been studied extensively. Despite structural differences in the stratum corneum, the total reflectance of light is between 4% and 7% for both blacks and whites, whereas spectral remittance over 300 to 800 nm shows a two- to threefold difference in blacks [11]. Pathak and Fitzpatrick compared the light transmission of the epidermis in blacks and fair-skinned Caucasians. Caucasian epidermis was more transparent to ultraviolet and visible wavelengths. At 300 nm, there was a considerable increase in transmission through Caucasian epidermis [12]. Everett et al. found light transmission through American Indian skin to be intermediate between that of white and black epidermis [13]. Kaidbey et al. measured the protection factor and the light transmission both for ultraviolet B and A in the stratum corneum and in the epidermis [14]. The mean UVB protection factor for black epidermis was 13.4 compared with 3.4 for white, whereas the transmission by black epidermis was 7.4% and 29.4% for white. The difference was less pronounced with stratum corneum specimens, in which the mean protection factor of black tissue was 3.3 and that of white 2.1. Hence, the mean UVB transmission by stratum corneum was 30.3% and 47.6% in blacks and whites, respectively (Fig. 2). Similar differences were detected using UVA sources. White stratum corneum is only slightly less protective than black. With stratum corneum specimens instead of a sunscreen, Kaidbey et al. found that black and white stratum corneum are indistinguishable, with a protection factor averaging about 2.2. On the basis of these data, the most striking difference in black epidermis is that it is three to four times more photoprotective than white epidermis at all wavelengths.

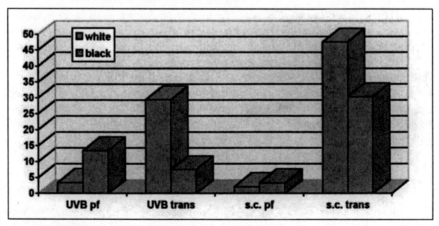

Fig. 2. Epidermal UVB protection factor and transmission (%)and stratum corneum protection factor and transmission (%) in white and black skin. (Modified from [14])

Thus, the light filtration properties appear primarily in the epidermis rather than in the stratum corneum, and melanin in the malpighian layer is effective mainly in photoprotection. When melanin in black skin reaches the stratum corneum, it apparently loses much of its protective capabilities. The melanosomes of the black are individually dispersed within the keratinocyte, whereas most Caucasian and Oriental melanosomes are in membrane-bound aggregates [15]. There appears to be a good correlation of skin color with the degree of melanosome aggregation. The larger and more melanized melanosomes of blacks adsorb and scatter more energy, thus providing a higher photoprotection. Despite these data showing three- to fivefold protection in vivo, the minimal erythema dose of blacks is 10–33 times that of whites [16, 17]. The reason for this discrepancy remains unclear.

Percutaneous Penetration

In vitro penetration of fluocinolone acetonide through skin samples obtained from amputated black and white legs revealed increased permeabilty in whites [18]. In contrast, in vitro water permeation through human skin did not reveal the sex and racial differences that had been reported by Bronaugh et al. [19].

In vivo studies show different patterns of penetration depending on the molecules tested [20]. Tritiated diflorasone diacetate does not have different pharmacokinetics in blacks and whites [21] while topical application of the local anesthetic EMLA showed less efficacy in Blacks [22]. Wedig and Maibach [23] applied C-labeled dipyrithione in different vehicles to stripped and unstripped skin of black and white volunteers and found 34% less absorption by blacks. A significantly lower penetration in blacks (47%) was also noted when a cosmetic vehicle (1:12:22:25:39 sodium lauryl-sulfate, propylene glycol, stearyl alcohol, white petrolatum, distilled water) was compared with methyl alcohol on the forehead and when the methyl alcohol vehicle was compared with the shampoo vehicle on the scalp. The penetration of intact versus stripped skin by either the cosmetic cream or the shampoo vehicle was not different.

Racial differences in methylnicotinate-induced vasodilatation in human skin were studied by Guy et al.; they induced vasodilatation by applying the substance to the skin and monitored the response with laser Doppler velocimetry [24]. They found statistically indistinguishable differences among the groups in the time to peak response, the area under the response-time curve, and the time from the response to 75% decay. Only the magnitude of the peak response revealed significant differences, with increased levels in young white subjects. No important differences seem to exist between black and white skin when tested with this chemical model [25]. Percutaneous penetration of nicotine via transdermal tape did not significantly differ in orientals and Caucasians [26].

Biophysical Parameters

Transepidermal water loss (TEWL), skin conductance and skin mechanical properties have been measured under basal conditions in whites, Hispanics and blacks to assess whether skin color (melanin content) could induce changes in skin biophysical properties [27]. Differences appear in skin conductance but are more marked in biomechanical features such as skin extensibility, skin elastic modulus and skin recovery. They differ in dorsal and ventral sites according to races and highlight the influence of solar irradiation on skin and the role of melanin in maintaining it unaltered.

No racial differences in TEWL exist either on the volar or dorsal forearms. However, water content is increased in Hispanics on the volar forearm and decreased in whites (compared only to blacks) on the dorsal forearm. These findings partially confirm previous observations [28, 29]. Skin lipids may play a role in modulating the relation between stratum corneum water content and TEWL resulting in higher conductance values in blacks and Hispanics.

Racial differences in skin conductance are difficult to interpret in terms of stratum corneum water content, because other physical factors, such as the skin surface or the presence of hair, can modify the quality of the skin-electrode contact. In all races significant differences exist between the volar and dorsal forearms [27]. These results are in apparent contrast with TEWL recordings. Indeed, increased stratum corneum water content, correlates with a higher TEWL [30]. The data may be explained on the basis of the different intercellular cohesion or lipid composition. A greater cell cohesion with a normal TEWL could result in increased skin water content.

Racial variability should be considered in terms of different skin responses to topical and environmental agents. Race provides a useful tool to investigate and compare the effects of lifetime sun exposure. It is evident that melanin protection decreases sun damage; differences between sun-exposed and sun-protected areas are not detectable in races with dark skin (Table 2).

Table 2. Differences between exposed and unexposed sites in three racial groups (expressed in p values) (from [27]). The differences increase as pigmentation decreases, making sun exposed areas more susceptible to damage

	Blacks	Hispanics	Whites
Conductance	0.02	0.05	0.01
Skin thickness	0.01	0.01	0.01
Extensibility	n.s.	0.01	0.01
Elastic modulus	n.s.	n.s.	0.01
Elastic recovery	n.s.	0.01	0.01
Viscoelasticity	n.s.	0.02	0.02
Elasticity	n.s.	n.s.	n.s.
TEWL	n.s.	n.s.	n.s.

However, transepidermal water loss studies are characterized by a large inter-individual variability and biased by environmental effects and eccrine sweating. To bypass these influences, an in vitro technique for measuring TEWL was used to compare TEWL in two racial groups (blacks and whites) [31]. Black skin had a significantly higher mean TEWL than white skin. In both groups a significant correlation between skin temperature and increased TEWL was found (p<0.01). The data confirm differences between races found in in vivo studies [28, 29].

Irritation

In 1919, Marshall et al. investigated cutaneous reactions to 1% dichloroethylsulfide in whites and blacks [32]. A drop on the forearm elicited erythema in 58% of white but only 15% of black subjects, suggesting a decreased susceptibility to cutaneous irritants in blacks. Weigand and Mershon studied patch test reactions to ortho-chlorobenzyli-dene malononitrile [33]. The results indicated that blacks were more resistant and required a significantly longer exposure to develop an irritant reaction. Subsequently, Weigand and Gaylor measured minimal perceptible erythema in blacks and whites after applying dinitrochlorobenzene to intact skin and to skin after the stratum corneum was largely removed by tape stripping [34]. The results confirmed that blacks were generally less susceptible to cutaneous irritants. However, this difference was not detectable when the stratum corneum was removed. They also observed that the range of reactions in normal skin in both races was wider than in stripped skin suggesting that the stratum corneum may modulate the different racial responses to skin irritants.

Irritation, as measured by TEWL [28, 29], revealed a different pattern of reaction in whites after chemical exposure to sodium lauryl sulfate. Blacks and Hispanics developed stronger irritant reactions after exposure.

Subjective (Sensory) Irritation

Stinging may occur in the nasolabial folds and on cheeks after an irritant is applied. Frosch and Kligman reported that the most "stingers" were light-complexioned persons of Celtic ancestry who sunburned easily and tanned poorly [35]. Later, however, Grove et al. found no skin-type propensity to stinging; they applied 10% lactic acid to the nasolabial folds and cheek of volunteers and noted that increased stinging was related mainly to the person's history of sensitivity to soaps, cosmetics, and drugs [36].

Allergic Contact Dermatitis

Conflicting findings have been reported on the incidence of allergic contact dermatitis in blacks. Kenney reported a decreased rate, (5% in black patients in his own private practice) [37]. Marshall and Heyl reported that the incidence of industrial contact dermatitis in South Africa is less in darkly pigmented blacks [38]. Bantus showed a 7.4% prevalence [39]. Scott noted that contact dermatitis was less frequent in Bantus handling detergents, waxes, and fuels [40]. Despite a previous report describing an increased sensitization rate in whites, Kligman and Epstein found no significant difference in the two races after testing many topical materials [41]. Fisher reported an approximately equal incidence of contact dermatitis in blacks and whites [42]. Para-phenylenediamine, nickel, and potassium bichromate appeared to be the most common allergens.

In Nigeria, nickel was the most frequent sensitizer, with an incidence of 12.3% [43] compared with 11% in North America. In Lagos, the female:male ratio is 1:1, whereas Fregert et al. recorded a ratio of 6:1 [44]. In North America, the ratio is 3:1 and in Stockholm, it is 7:3.

Clinically, acute contact dermatitis with exudation, vesiculation, or bullae is more common in whites, whereas blacks more commonly develop disorders of pigmentation and lichenification. Hypopigmentation has been described from contact with phenolic detergents [45], alkyphenols, and monobenzylether of hydroquinone [46]. Hyperpigmentation occurs more readily in black patients after contact with mild irritants. Keratolytics and other chemicals used in acne therapy often cause hyperpigmentation in blacks. The epidemiology studies are different to interpret for reasons related to exposure etc.

Studies of transdermal clonidine permitted identification of certain racial and sex-related differences in sensitization. The occlusive transdermal patch is applied for 1 week. The sensitization rate was as follows: Caucasian women, 34%; Caucasian men 18%; black women, 14%; black men, 8%. These differences are large and presumably biologically significant (unpublished data).

Effects of Topically Applied Products

A proneness of blacks to "pomade acne" has been suggested [25]. This eruption, consisting mainly of comedones on the forehead and temporal area, seems to be a peculiar response of black skin to topical agents, because this reaction can be detected in black children from 1 to 12 years of age [47]. Plewig et al. examined 735 blacks and found that 70% of long-term users of pomades had a form of acne [48]. The more elaborate formulations induced pomade acne more frequently and more intensively than simpler preparations such as mineral oil and petroleum jelly. The distribution of the lesions corresponded to the area of contact. Comparable data for whites are lacking.

Kaidbey and Kligman studied race-dependent cutaneous reactivity to topical coal [49]. There was a strikingly different response in the two groups: in whites, the response was primarily inflammatory, with development of papules and papulopustules in about 2 or 3 weeks, whereas in blacks the inflammatory response was largely absent and, after about 14 days, an eruption of small open comedones appeared. The follicles of white subjects responded early, with rupture of the wall and outpouring of follicular contents in the dermis, whereas in blacks, the first response was proliferative with production and retention of horny cells. That is, in blacks, the skin reacts to a comedogenic compound with hyperkeratoses rather than with disintegration of follicles, suggesting a greater resistance to irritants.

The postocclusive hyperemic reaction before and after a single 1-h application of clobetasol 0.05% was determined by laser Doppler velocimetry to elucidate different racial responses [50]. In black subjects there were a decreased area under the curve response, decreased peak response and a decreased decay slope after peak blood flow. These data are consistent with a different reactivity of blood vessels in black skin and possibly not related to the transcutaneous penetration of the chemical compound.

General Comment

How can these relatively sparse experimental data be used into a biological perspective? Tables 3 and 4 summarize the main differences between black and white skin. Since our earlier reviews [51, 52], more data have become available but much remains

Table 3. Main structural differences (blacks vs whites) in stratum corneum barrier function

Barrier function: differences in stratum corneum	Reference
Equal thickness	[2, 3]
Increased number of cell layers and resistance to stripping	[4]
Increased lipid content	[5]
Increased electrical resistance	[6]
Increased desquamation	[7]
Equal corneocyte size	[7]
Decreased amount of ceramides	[8]
Increased recovery after stripping	[10]

Table 4. Light penetration in blacks and whites

	Reference
Differences in light penetration	
Same reflectance in blacks and whites	[11]
Increased light transmission in whites	[12]
Increased photoprotection in blacks mainly due to epidermis rather than to the stratum corneum	[14]

to be done to understand the various mechanisms underlying the different clinical expressions.

Therefore, we still cannot answer the question "How resistant is black skin compared to white?". Much remains to be done to resolve these issues as related to claim support. We remain optimistic that further knowledge will lead to refined claim support and more appropriated formulation for race based skin care.

References

1. Shriver MD (1997) Ethnic variation as a key to the biology of human disease. Ann Intern Med 127:401–403
2. Freeman RG, Cockerell EG, Armstrong J et al. (1962) Sunlight as a factor influencing the thickness of epidermis. J Invest Dermatol 39:295–297
3. Thomson ML (1955) Relative efficiency of pigment and horny layer thickness in protecting the skin of European and Africans against solar ultraviolet radiation. J Physiol (Lond) 127:236
4. Weigand DA, Haygood C, Gaylor JR (1974) Cell layers and density of Negro and Caucasians stratum corneum. J Invest Dermatol 62:563–565
5. Rienertson RP, Wheatley VR (1959) Studies on the chemical composition of human epidermal lipids. J Invest Dermatol 32:49–51
6. Johnson LC, Corah NL (1963) Racial differences in skin resistance. Science 139:766–769
7. Corcuff P, Lotte C, Rougier A, Maibach H (1991) Racial differences in corneocytes. Acta Dermatol Venereol (Stockh) 71:146–148
8. Sugino K, Imokawa G, Maibach H (1993) Ethnic difference of stratum corneum lipid in relation to stratum corneum function. J Invest Dermatol 100:597
9. Kompaore F, Marty JP, Dupont Ch (1993) In vivo evaluation of the stratum corneum barrier function in Blacks, Caucasians and Asians with two noninvasive methods. Skin Pharmacol 6:200–207
10. Reed JT, Ghadially R, Elias PM (1994) Effect of race, gender and skin type on epidermal permeability barrier function. J Invest Dermatol 102:537
11. Anderson R, Parrish J (1981) The optics of human skin. J Invest Dermatol 77:13–17
12. Pathak MA, Fitzpatrick TB (1974) The role of natural photoprotective agents in human skin. In: Fitzpatrick TB, Pathak MA, Harber RC et al. (eds) Sunlight and man. University of Tokyo Press, Tokyo, pp 725–750

13. Everett MA, Yeagers E, Sayre RM et al. (1966) Penetration of epidermis by ultraviolet rays. Photochem Photobiol 5:533
14. Kaidbey KH, Poh Agin P, Sayre RM et al. (1979) Photoprotection by melanin-a comparison of black and Caucasian skin. Am Acad Dermatol 1:249
15. Szabo G, Gerald AB, Pathak MA (1969) Racial differences in the fate of melanosomes in human epidermis. Nature 222:1081
16. Hausser KW, Vahle W (1969) Sunburn and suntanning. In: Urbach F (ed) The biologic effect of ultraviolet radiation. Pergamon, London, pp 13–21
17. Olson RL, Gaylor J, Everett MA (1973) Skin color, melanin and erythema. Arch Dermatol 108:541–544
18. Stoughton RB (1969) Bioassay methods for measuring percutaneous absorption. In: Montagna W, Stoughton RB, Van Scott EJ (eds) Pharmacology of the skin. Appleton-Century-Crofts, New York, p 542
19. Bronaugh RL, Stewart FR, Simon M (1986) Methods for in vitro percutaneous absorption studies VII: use of excised human skin. J Pharm Sci 75:1094
20. Berardesca E, Maibach HI (1989) Physical antrolopgy and skin: a model for exploring skin function. In: Maibach HI, Lowe N (eds) Models in dermatology 4. Karger, Basel, pp 202–208
21. Wickema-Sinha WJ, Shaw SR, Weber OJ (1978) Percutaneous absorption and excretion ot tritium-labelled diflorasone diacetate, a new topical corticosteroid in the rat, monkey and man. J Invest Dermatol 71:372–377
22. Hymes JA, Spraker MK (1986) Racial differences in the effectiveness of a topically applied mixture of local anesthetics. Reg Anesth 11:11–13
23. Wedig JH, Maibach HI (1981) Percutaneous penetration of dipyrithione in man: effect of skin color (race). Am Acad Dermatol 5:433–438
24. Guy RH, Tur E, Bierke S et al. (1985) Are there age and racial differences to mrthyl nicotinate-induced vasodilatation in human skin? J Am Acad Dermatol 12:1001
25. Berardesca E, Maibach HI (1988) Contact dermatitis in blacks. Dermatol Clin 6:363–368
26. Lin S, Ho H, Chien YW (1993) Development of a new nicotine transdermal delivery system: in vitro kinetics studies and clinical pharmacokinetic evaluations in two ethnic groups. J Contr Rel 26:175–193
27. Berardesca E, de Rigal J, Leveque JL, Maibach HI (1991) In vivo biophysical characterization of skin physiological differences in races. Dermatologica 182:89–93
28. Berardesca E, Maibach HI (1988) Racial differences in sodium lauryl sulphate induced cutaneous irritation: Black and white. Contact Dermatitis 18:65–70
29. Berardesca E, Maibach HI (1988) Sodium lauryl sulphate induced cutaneous irritation. Comparison of white and Hispanic subjects. Contact Dermatitis 19:136–140
30. Rietschel RL (1978) A method to evaluate skin moisturizers in vivo. J Invest Dermatol 70:152–155
31. Wilson D, Berardesca E, Maibach HI (1988) In vitro transepidermal water loss: differences between black and white human skin. Br J Dermatol 119:647–652
32. Marshall EK, Lynch V, Smith HV (1919) Variation in susceptibility of the skin to dichloroethylsulfide. J Pharmacol Exp Ther 12:291–301
33. Edgewood Arsenal Technical Report (1970) The cutaneous irritant reaction to agent O-chlorobenzylidene malonitrile (CS). Quantitation and racial influence in human subjects. Edgewood Arsenal Technical Report 4332, February 1970
34. Weigand DA, Gaylor JR (1974) Irritant reaction in Negro and Caucasian skin. South Med J 67:548–551
35. Frosh P, Kligman AM (1981) A method for appraising the stinging capacity of topically applied substances. J Soc Cosmet Chem 28:197
36. Grove GL, Soschin DM, Kligman AM (1984) Adverse subjective reactions to topical agents. In: Drill VA, Lazar P (eds) Cutaneous toxicology. Raven, New York
37. Kenney J (1970) Dermatoses seen in American Negroes. Int J Dermatol 9:110—113
38. Marshall J, Heyl T (1963) Skin diseases in the Western Cape Province. S Afr Med J 37:1308
39. Dogliotti M (1970) Skin disorders in the Bantu: a survey of 2000 cases from Baragwanath Hospital. S Afr Med J 44:670
40. Scott F (1972) Skin diseases in the South African Bantu. In: Marshall J (ed) Essays on tropical dermatology. Excerpta Medica, Amsterdam
41. Kligman AM, Epstein W (1975) Updating the maximization test for identifying contact allergens. Contact Dermatitis 1:231
42. Fisher AA (1977) Contact dermatitis in black patients. Cutis 20:303–320
43. Olumide YM (1985) Contact dermatitis in Nigeria. Contact Dermatitis 12:241–246
44. Fregert S, Hjorth N, Magnusson B et al. (1969) Epidemiology of contact dermatitis. Trans St John's Hosp Dermatol Soc 55:17

45. Fisher AA (1976) Vitiligo due to contactants. Cutis 17:431–437
46. Kahn G (1970) Depigmentation caused by phenolic detergent germicides. Arch Dermatol 102:177–187
47. Verhagen AR (1974) Pomade acne in black patients. Arch Dermatol 110:465
48. Plewig G, Fulton JE, Kligman AM (1970) Pomade acne. Arch Dermatol 101:580
49. Kaidbey KH, Kligman AM (1974) A human model for coal tar acne. Arch Dermatol 109:212–215
50. Berardesca E, Maibach HI (1989) Cutaneous reactive hyperaemia: racial differences induced by corticoid application. Br J Dermatol 120:787–794
51. Andersen KE, Maibach HI (1979) Black and white human skin differences. J Am Acad Dermatol 1:276–282
52. Berardesca E, Maibach H (1996) Racial differences in skin pathophysiology. J Am Acad Dermatol 34:667–672

The In Vivo Biomechanical Testing of the Skin and the Cosmetological Efficacy Claim Support: A Critical Overview

L. Rodrigues

Introduction

In vivo skin mechanical assessment is one of the most complex matters within cutaneous research, directly depending from many different areas ranging from basic sciences (mathematics, physics statistics chemistry, biology and physiology) through computers, rheology and biomedical engineering, to pathology and clinical dermatology. A most important issue for all the scientific areas involving skin, it is particularly crucial for claim support and efficacy testing, specially if it helps to establish the extent to which topical or other treatments are able to assist in maintaining or restoring normal mechanical properties.

The development of several types of technological approaches and instruments giving birth to practical commercially available assessment tools, promoted the interest on this issue as revealed from the significant amount of papers produced specially over the last 20 years. In fact, a considerable amount of information reflecting multiple study perspectives on human skin biomechanical behavior is actually available covering a wide range of biomechanical related topics from normal skin's physiology [6, 8, 26, 37, 49, 50, 54, 56] through special physiopathological conditions such as aging [9, 21, 30, 34, 51, 55, 56], dermatological pathologies [11, 45, 56, 58, 61] or other dysfunction with cutaneous translation [12, 18, 44, 59], to the pharmacological efficacy of systemic [53, 57] or topical [4, 36, 46, 53, 57, 63] therapeutics.

But apparently these developments did not contribute to an advanced knowledge on in vivo skin mechanics since many of the complex emerging doubts remain unanswered, specially those regarding the nature and significance of the experimentally observed phenomena. Undoubtedly a major limiting factor results from these methods being applied on in vivo skin surface meaning that all measurements are affected by the skin and other tissue it is attached to, impairing any objective appreciation on a pure mechanical basis. In other words, the nature and significance of the variables obtained with these systems is unclear and, there's no way to relate the quantitative data obtained to particular structures of skin.

However and no matter the foreseeable difficulties, the interest and potential usefulness of this theme justifies a systematic approach even if simplified. The present chapter is then oriented to a practical approach overview, focusing on the critical aspects which limit and affect data interpretation, stressing those aspects which can contribute to optimize technological and methodological procedures.

Skin Biomechanics Fundamentals

Anisotropy is a is well defined characteristic of human skin, also applied to its mechanical properties. As a reflex of a particular structure of many different anatomical and biochemical elements, in vivo skin mechanical behavior has been related with Langer's (tension) lines, skin's microdepressionary network and cutaneous three-dimensional topography [2, 6, 21, 50, 56]. Relationships with age [14, 15, 26, 30, 34], sex [8, 15, 26, 50] and anatomical region [14, 15, 31, 37, 49] have also been established. It is clear that the mechanical characteristics of human skin result from the global contribution of connective tissue, dermis and hypodermis and, at least in some degree, from the epidermis [6, 13, 17, 47, 50, 54]. Fiber constituents qualities, their orientation, network structure and their relation with the interstitial medium are fundamental factors determining the overall properties of the entire organ [6, 50, 54, 58].

Flexibility is therefore a paramount characteristic of human skin, fundamental to allow movement without cracking, contributing to cutaneous overall cohesion and to barrier function maintenance, depending on elastic, plastic and viscous components which are responsible for an extremely complex mechanical behavior, far from the pure elastic or plastic materials [2, 6, 47–50, 60, 65].

Mathematical modelling is an often used alternative approach to describe skin mechanics. The most frequently used model involves stress–strain relationships [2, 47, 48, 50, 60], stress being a quantity that is proportional to the force causing a deformation (external force per unit cross-sectional area acting on an object) and strain a measure of the degree of deformation. For sufficiently small values the stress is proportional to the strain; the constant of proportionality depends on the material being deformed and on the nature of the deformation that is – the elastic modulus defined as the ratio of stress to strain. Therefore, living tissues deformation in its multiple forms, can be conceptualized through specific „modulus" such as the elastic modulus (Young's modulus), the most frequently referred parameter used for skin biomechanical description, referred to the resistance of a solid to its change in length [2, 34, 50]. Other moduli such as the shear modulus and the bulk modulus, referred respectively, to the resistance to motion of the planes of a solid sliding past each other and, the resistance offered by solids (or liquids) to changes in volume are not used. Several analogical models were also proposed to visualize the mechanical properties of normal and pathological human skin [6, 41, 50, 54] but its usefulness is limited and interpretation difficult to draw. More recently algebraic models were used to fit experimental data obtained from commercially available testing systems as an attempt to obtain parameters to better describe the occurring changes and relate them to skin structure and respective physiological events [60]. In spite of suggesting that mechanical studies of in vivo skin can be made more sensitive and understandable, it is clear that a rigorous mathematical representation of the mechanical properties of skin in vivo is an extremely complex task and the technological tools available cannot solve by itself the many limitations involved. Some of the measuring systems (see below) allow to obtain stress-strain curves but only in the first part of the curves for some specified experimental conditions [2, 25, 33, 50]. Nevertheless the range of values reported for the Young's modulus for normal skin lies within 10^4–10^8 N/m2 [2, 33, 50], a direct consequence of a wide variety of experimental protocols and devices used, which does not contribute to obtain comparable results and justifies the absence of normalised data.

The Technological Assessment: Methods and Parameters

Objective criticism can be pointed out regarding the different methods and techniques developed to non invasively assess in vivo skin mechanical properties, specially for two main reasons: (1) These are „contact-methods" often evaluating skin performance after inducing unphysiological movements through externally imposed loads, and (2) measurements always involve multiple cutaneous plus non-cutaneous elements.

However, in practical terms, these systems proved to be extremely useful in many different ways providing quantitative indicators of a change occurring independently from its nature and physiological significance. These technological tools are based on the measurement of changes induced by the application of external forces having different orientation on skin surface. Then, it is fundamental to attend to each method specification since according with the type and orientation of the external force used different physiological features will be revealed as a result of different predominant participation of structural components [24–29, 31, 40, 50, 65]. Moreover method's performance, including its discriminative capacity are known to depend critically on the specific measuring conditions including pre-conditioning (fixation) the skin, contact probe's and body positioning, load adjustment and load application time [2, 7, 13, 25, 60, 64]. Thus, different systems provide different information which stresses the need to evaluate potential advantages and opportunities for each system facing the predefined objectives of each study (see below). Detailed description of each system is out of the scope of this text. In most cases its physical principles and experienced applicability is already published and the reader can easily assess this information. For practical purposes, Table 1 resumes some of the most relevant references. Basically, these methods are grouped in two major classes according with the orientation of the imposed loads (Table 1).

Suction and torsional methods should be specially mentioned since most of the experimental data published around the in vivo biomechanical assessment of human skin, including the topical efficacy of cosmetic products, was obtained from the application of these systems and respective parameters. Of course this is a direct conse-

Table 1. Summary of different systems developed to assess in vivo skin biomechanical properties. Some of these systems are still used as prototypes (P) while others have been made commercially available (CA). Accordingly with system's specifications (most important reference papers are indicated), respective practical usefulness includes different applicability levels (I, basic biomedical research; II, clinical; III, topical efficacy)

Designation	Applicability status	References
Methods using perpendicular forces		
Elevation testing (levarometry) (P)	I, II	[39, 51, 58]
Indentation testing (indentometry) (P)	I, II	[38, 51, 58]
Impact testing (ballistometry) (P)	I	[1, 27]
Suction testing (CA)	I, II, III	[7, 20, 21, 42, 45, 61]
DPE (CA)	I, II	[10, 20]
Methods using parallel forces		
Stretching methods (P)		[24, 65]
Gas-bearing electrodynamometer (GBE) (P)	I, II	[28, 29, 36]
Torsional testing devices (CA)	I, II, III	[3, 21–23, 35, 48, 60]
Wave propagation (P)	I, II	[19]

quence of its commercial availability but also because, from a practical stand, these systems represent very „easy-to-use" practical tools allowing a low cost assessment of the phenomena under study.

Systems using a negative (suction) pressure applied through a specially designed chamber/probe to promote skin „elevation" are the most frequently used to assess in vivo skin biomechanical changes and certainly the more extensively applied and studied [7, 20, 25, 31, 40, 42, 48, 61].

Two systems based on this principle, are currently commercially available : the Dermaflex A (Cortex Technology, Hadsung, Denmark) and the Cutometer SEM474 (CK Electronic, Cologne, Germany). Technical information on its electronics, hardware and measuring principle have been published [7, 20]. Recently a new version of the Cutometer system, the SEM575 was developed. Although based on the same principle this system allegedly provides increased accuracy of measurement due to increased stability of the probe to temperature changes and new calibration procedures [16] but experimentally supported data is still inexistent.

From the practical perspective some differences between the Dermaflex A and the Cutometer SEM474 systems should be considered since they provide different information. A main difference concerns the measuring probe diameter. The standard Dermaflex A system presents a 10 mm chamber providing a so called „proportional" full-thickness strain [25] which means that it is particularly sensitive to mechanical properties of sub-epidermal structures and apparently considered to be specifically appropriated to clinical research. The Cutometer SEM474 uses in its standard version a 2-mm probe, providing a „disproportional" superficial strain, since it involves mostly the outer mechanical compartment of the skin epidermis, papillary dermis and, to a lesser degree deeper dermal layers and subcutis, being therefore specially appropriate for other uses, including cosmetological applications [25, 31, 43, 46]. However, according to the manufacturer specifications, this system can also operate with other probe's diameters (from 2 to 13 mm) being therefore able to provide a proportional strain, enlarging its applicability potential. For this system it has been demonstrated both by in vitro stripping of entire skin and in vivo measurements, that deformations resulting from bigger probe's aperture diameters will in fact involve more components from the deepest layers of the skin including infiltration of fat tissue [25, 40, 49].

Torsional testing of skin mechanics has been used and developed by several research groups over the last 30 years [3, 17, 22, 23, 35, 60, 64], giving birth to the commercial version Dermal Torque Meter (DTM) (Dia-Stron, Hampshire, UK). The technical principle consists in applying a disk glued on the skin with cyanoacrilate which can be rotated under control, loading the skin with a torque. This way the „twist" induces the elongation of the skin which can be refined by the introduction of a guardring concentrical to the disc delimiting an annular area and, according to some authors, limiting the sliding of the skin over the subcutis. The use of a non-rotating guard-ring secured to the skin surface and concentric with the rotating disc has been recognised as enabling the strain to be confined to a narrow annulus, assuring that the narrower this annulus the more the results depend from the most superficial structures which is a crucial aspect to allow its application to many different purposes, including cosmetic efficacy testing [17, 22, 33, 60].

Both technological systems use the angular deformation of skin to characterise its behavior through which all the classical deformation variables (Ue, Uf, Uv, Ua and Ur) described in the literature can be assessed [2, 4, 13, 25, 48–52, 59]. Stress-strain curves obtained with this systems are typically nonlinear except in the first part of the curves for some precise pressures interval where Young's modulus can be calculated [2, 25, 34, 50]. Skin stiffness or distensibility is represented by a value of skin elevation or strain at the end of the first load, while resilient distention corresponds to the residual skin

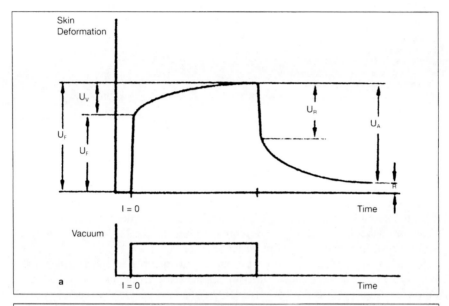

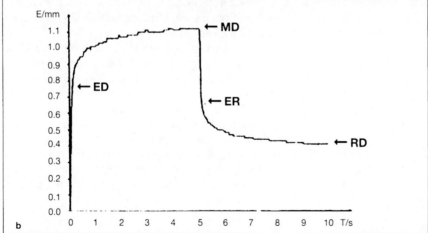

Fig. 1a, b. a An ideal suction curve obtained with the Cutometer. The upper curve represents deformation as a function of time while the lower curve represents the pressure on set and off during measurement. **b** A typical plot diagram obtained with a Cutometer, representing variation in the elevation of skin (E/mm) as a function of time (T/s) showing the equivalent parameters above. ED, elastic deformation of the skin; MD, maximum deformation of skin at the end of stress application; ER, elastic retraction of the skin; RD, residual deformation of the skin at the end of the pressure application cycle

Table 2. Biomechanical approximation of the most frequently used variables and parameters obtained by suction and torsion methods

Variables and parameters	Symbol	Units (suction/torsion)
Total (maximum) extensibility of skin	Uf	µm/deg.
Elastic deformation of the skin as a consequence of stress (suction or torsion)	Ue	mm/deg.
Viscoelastic creep occurring after elastic deformation	Uv	mm/deg.
Elastic deformation recovery after stress withdraw	Ur	mm/deg.
Total deformation recovery at the end of the stress-off period	Ua	mm/deg.
Deformation amount not recovered by the end of the stress-off period	R or Uf-Ua	%
Distention elastic deformation (as a consequence of stress)	Uf-Ur	mm/deg.

elevation after the release of the first load. In any case one should be aware that these curves will greatly vary according with several experimental conditionant factors (see below). In fact, recent history of stress affecting the skin before measurement seems to be a major factor affecting results, but skin's fixation (pre-conditioning), probe's and body positioning, probe's aperture diameter, pressure (load) adjustment and application time are additional factors which should always be considered for both systems.

Figure 1a,b shows an ideal graphic representation of typical strain-time and stress-strain curves obtained with the Cutometer SEM474.

Special care is needed for selecting the quantitative parameters considering the study objectives, and to its conclusive interpretation. Facing the impossibility to establish a direct relationship between the variables provided by those systems and any particular anatomical or physiological variable, these, taken by itself or arranged as external (indicative) indexes are oversimplifications and thus, should rather be considered as „experimental descriptors" of the observed phenomena.

Table 2 resumes the most important descriptors used and referred in literature as an approximation to the biomechanical changes observed. Ratios used as practical quantitative indicators [14, 21, 49, 52, 55] especially for comparative purposes are:

- The „viscoelastic ratio or extension phase during retraction" obtained from the ratio between the delayed (MD-ED) and immediate (ED) distensions
- The „relative elastic recovery" obtained from the ratio between the immediate elastic retraction (MD-ER) and the maximal distension (MD)
- The „biological elasticity" representing the relationship between the return to the resilient distention (MD-RD) and the maximal distension (MD)
- The „elastic function" obtained from the ratio between the immediate elastic retraction (MD-ER) and the immediate elastic distension (ED).

The Applicability Potential to Cosmetological Claim Support

Prior to all consideration around cosmetic claim support related with the biomechanical improvement of human skin and, apart from the questions concerning the nature and significance of the quantitative variables obtained from in vivo skin biomechanical characterisation, it is important to clarify the participation of the epidermis in the global mechanical behavior of the in vivo skin. The relatively few papers focusing this subject is a clear demonstration of the experimental difficulties faced. Nevertheless, epidermis and stratum corneum have been referred as presenting large flexibility and small extensibility with some resistance to shear stress and strain [13, 47] and recently, it was demonstrated that after stratum corneum stripping, the skin's mechanical modulus evaluated by a gas-bearing electrodynamometer, decreased almost to zero [28, 29]. These data suggest an effective contribution of this layer to the overall mechanical behavior of the skin and this is a particularly important aspect for the claim support issue since epidermis is the primary target of a topical intervention and ideally, any practical assessment under this scope must be suitable enough to identify these changes if present. Available data also suggests that the overall mechanical behavior of entire human skin can be influenced by the „plastization" effect induced by the epidermal hydration level [5, 13, 17, 32, 46, 63]. It was demonstrated that skin distensibility, resilient distensibility and hysteresis increase 20 min after epidermal hydration with tap water, while elasticity decreases (slightly) upon epidermal hydration [5, 13, 17, 32, 46]. Other similar study using tap water tried to confirm experimental relationship between biomechanical properties and hydration measured with an electrical capacitance system [32]. A good correlation between hysteresis and capacitance values was found, while elasticity decreased when capacitance increased. However, recently published papers focusing the sensitivity analysis of suction and torsion systems to stratum corneum hydration measured by other capacitance method [43] could not demonstrate a clear correlation between those data which probably reflects the relative influence of skin thickness on the measurements since there are reported differences in the depth into the skin which these instruments measure [21, 42, 43].

Complementary data focusing the experimental demonstration of the biomechanical benefits of normal or aged skin following the use of topical substances, is still poorly documented. Yet, industrial skin care marketing frequently refers a beneficial impact on the mechanical properties of the skin resulting from the regular use of their products. Packages and literature often present mechanical related adjectives ranging from general unprecise words („softness", „suppleness", „toughness", „firmness", and „slackness") to biomechanical designations („elasticity" and „flexibility") applied to any class of skin care formulation (including cleansing or hydrating emulsions). These claims provide a competitive advantage to these products by creating an additional efficacy expectation near the consumer. However, unlike other efficacy claims which can be objectively supported by experimental (rigorous, scientifically based) data, demonstration on the eventual benefits on mechanical behavior resulting from the use of these products is difficult to address and, as a consequence, is far from being entirely established. Nevertheless some papers have demonstrated the positive effect of emollients and moisturizer formulations following short-term and long-term application regimes, basically revealed by an increase in skin's extensibility [4, 17, 33, 46, 59, 63] which means the capacity to reinforce the distorsional capacity of the skin.

These examples are truly important indicators on the usefulness of the available technological systems applicability no matter the great and varied difficulties encountered. Technological improvement of the systems is expected but independently from this evolutionary perspective, more useful and comparable data can be obtained focusing on the optimization of the available experimental procedures.

Optimisation of Experimental Procedures

Usefulness of an objective correlation between the observational data and the phenomena quantitatively assessed with the non-invasive measurement systems is beyond
question, specially when comparative testing of skin and topical products is concerned. From a practical stand, considering the limitations and pitfalls stressed out in the
previous paragraphs, it is possible to optimize the experimental procedures (technological and methodological) in order to contribute to data valuation and results comparison, a necessary step to ensure objective advancements on this field. Fundamental
aspects to consider are discussed in the following sections.

Unattributability of Observed Phenomena

To accept that observed phenomena cannot be directly attributed to a specific cutaneous structure and, therefore have no direct correlation with the physical variables
used in mechanics or represent a pure biomechanical behavior of the entire organ. Physical complications, intra and inter-individual biological variabilities, and the practical
impossibility to individualise participation of each structure justify this perspective.

Study Design and Protocol

Another important aspect concerns study design and protocol, which should be con-
structed according with specific objectives and previously defined rationale for choice
of the method and measurement system, including relevance to meet the objectives.
General aspects regarding claim support study design are already published and the
reader will definitely benefit from this consultation [61].

General Aspects of Practical Guidance

General aspects of practical guidance which are recognised as basic variability sources
for biomechanical in vivo assessment should always be considered (briefly summarised in Table 3).

Table 3. Summary of the most important variability sources related to volunteers' panel definition and
laboratory operation procedures which should be considered for biomechanical experimental assessment

Regarding volunteers	Regarding operating procedures
Age	Laboratory environment (controlled temperature and humidity)
Sex	Seasonal variations
Race	Circadian and other cyclic rhythms
Anatomical site	Physical stress
General and specific skin condition (intrinsic and extrinsic aging indicators)	Standard experimental procedures (independently of the method used)
Concomitant therapeutics (topical or systemic)	

Measuring Systems

Choosing a measuring system is an extremely important task since, according with the specific purposes of the study (cosmetics efficacy or clinical assessment), several technical options should be considered [61] keeping in mind that relationship between the same variables obtained by different systems has not yet been establish. Therefore, it is important to:
- Consider accuracy, precision, repeatability, reproducibility, and suitability of the systems
- Consider calibration procedures and measuring standards
- Attend to and predefine other specific limiting factors which do affect results and its interpretation, such as body positioning, preconditioning of the skin to avoid lateral displacement, the force application mode, and the characterisation of the parameters chosen in order to ensure a precise interpretation of the results.

Optimising Suction/Torsion Data

Finally, suction/torsion being the most frequently used systems, its is also important to optimize the specific experimental operating procedures from which standardisation and results comparison depends. Particularly important aspects are:
- On set and off set time. Ideal suction curves (see Fig. 1) greatly differ when these parameters vary. These values must always be indicated
- Probe diameter aperture. Small apertures seem to be the most appropriated choice specially for cosmetological testing [14, 25, 40, 49]
- Pressure adjustment. Available information suggests to choose rather small deformations (300 mbar) for reduced periods of time [25, 35, 40]
- Repeated testing. According to the manufacturers this procedure provides hysterisis assessment. However, this information should be judge with some reserve since fatigue phenomena is, under these conditions, apparent.

Conclusion

The in vivo biomechanical assessment of human skin is a matter of extraordinary importance for all the sciences related to dermatology, from fundamental skin physiology to cosmetology and efficacy claim support. However, knowledge and practical application of this analysis still faces several complexities. These may be partially explained by the limited technological advancements made so far regarding the assessment tools available which cannot provide true mechanical characteristics of human skin on a pure physical basis. Also many of the available information is obtained from many different techniques, under different experimental methodologies which precludes the necessary comparison of results. Nevertheless, usefulness of these methods and respective quantitative descriptors have been demonstrated stressing the urgency to optimise experimental procedures in order to improve analysis quality. Encouraging standardised measurements is therefore a crucial step to maximise the potential application and usefulness of these methods and ultimately to allow results comparison and, by doing so, to contribute to a real advancement on the field.

References

1. Adhoute H, Berbis P, Privat Y (1993) Ballistometric properties of aged skin. In: Lévèque JL, Agache P (eds) Aging skin. Chap 4. Marcel Dekker, New York, p 39
2. Agache P, Monneur C, Lévèque JL, de Rigal J (1980) Mechanical properties and Young's modulus of human skin in vivo. Arch Dermatol Res 269:221–232
3. Agache P (1995) Twistometry measurement of skin elasticity. In: Serup J, Jemec GBE (eds) Handbook of non-invasive methods and the skin. Chap 14.1. CRC Press, Boca Raton, p 319
4. Aubert L, Antoine P, de Rigal J, Lévèque JL (1985) An in vivo assessment of the biomechanical properties of human skin modifications under the influence of cosmetic products. Int J Cosmet Sci 7:51–59
5. Auriol F, Vaillant L, Machet L, Diridollou S, Lorette G (1993) Effects of short-time hydration on skin extensibility. Acta Dermatol Venereol (Stockh) 73:344–347
6. Barbenel JC, Payne PA(1981) In vivo biomechanical testing of dermal properties. Bioeng Skin 3:8–38
7. Barel AO, Courage W, Clarys P (1995) Suction method for measurement of skin mechanical properties : The cutometer. In: Serup J, Jemec GBE (eds) Handbook of non-invasive methods and the skin. Chap 14.3. CRC Press, Boca Raton, p 335
8. Berardesca E, Gabba P, Farinelli N, Borroni G, Rabiosi G (1969) Skin extensibility time in women. Changes in relation with sex hormones. Acta Dermatol Venereol (Stockh) 69:431–433
9. Berardesca E, Maibach HI (1993) Mechanical properties and photoageing In: Lévèque JL, Agache P(eds) Aging skin. Chap 3. Marcel Dekker, New York, p 29
10. Bjerring P (1985) Skin elasticity measured by dynamic admittance. A new technique for mechanical measurements in patients with scleroderma. Acta Dermatol Venereol (Stockh) [Suppl] 120:83–90
11. Borroni G, Vignati G, Vignoli GP et al. (1989) PUVA induced viscoelastic changes in the skin of psoriatic patients. Med Biol Environ 17:663–671
12. Bramont C, Vasselet R, Rochefort A, Agache P (1988) Mechanical properties of the skin in Marfan's syndrome and Ehlers-Danlos syndrome. Bioeng Skin 4:217–227
13. Christensen MS, Hargens CW, Nacht S, Gans EH (1977) Viscoelastic properties of intact human skin, instrumentation, hydration, effect and the contribution of the stratum corneum, J Invest Dermatol 69:282–286
14. Couturaud V, Coutable J, Khaiat A (1995) Skin biomechanical properties: in vivo evaluation of influence of age and body site by a non-invasive method. Skin Res Technol 1:68–73
15. Cua AB, Wilhelm K-P, Maibach HI (1990) Elastic properties of human skin: relation to age, sex and anatomical region. Arch Dermatol Res 282:283–288
16. Cutometer SEM575 User's Manual (1997) CK electronics, Germany
17. de Rigal J, Leveque JL (1985) In vivo measurement of stratum corneum elasticity. Bioeng Skin 1:13–23
18. Deleixhe-Mauhin F, Piérard-Franchimont C, Rorive G, Piérard GE (1994) Influence of chronic haemodialysis on the mechanical properties of skin. Clin Exp Dermatol 19:130–133
19. Dorogi PL, Dewitt GM, Stone BR, Buras EM (1986) Viscoelastometry of skin in vivo using shear wave propagation. Bioeng Skin 3:59–70
20. Elsner P (1995) Skin elasticity. In: Berardesca E, Elsner P, Wilhelm KP, Maibach H (eds) Bioengineering of the skin: methods and instrumentation. CRC Press, Boca Raton, p 53
21. Escoffier C, de Rigal J, Rochefort A, Vasselet R, Lévèque JL, Agache P (1989) Age-related mechanical properties of human skin: an in vivo study. J Invest Dermatol 93:353-357
22. Finlay B (1970) Dynamic mechanical testing of human skin in vivo, J Biomech 3:557–568
23. Finlay B (1971) The torsional characteristics of human skin in vivo. J Biomed Eng 6:567–573
24. Fung YCB (1967) Elasticity of soft tissues in simple elongation. Am J Physiol 213:1532–1544
25. Gniadecka M, Serup J (1995) Suction chamber method for measurement of skin mechanical properties: the Dermaflex. In: Serup J, Jemec GBE (eds) Handbook of non-invasive methods and the skin. Chap 14.2. CRC Press, Boca Raton, p 329
26. Gniadecka M, Gniadecki R, Serup J, Sondergaard J (1994) Skin mechanical properties present adaptation to man's upright position. In vivo studies in young and aged individuals, Arch Dermatol Venereol (Stockh) 74:188–190
27. Hargens CW (1995) Ballistometry. In: Serup J, Jemec GBE (eds) Handbook of non-invasive methods and the skin. Chap 14.8. CRC Press, Boca Raton, p 359
28. Hargens CW (1981) The gas-bearing electrodynamometer (GBE) applied to measuring mechanical changes in skin and other tissues. In: Marks R, Payne PA (eds) Bioengineering and the skin. Chap 14. MTP Press, Lancester, UK, p 113

29. Hargens CW (1995) The gas-bearing electrodynamometer. In: Serup J, Jemec GBE (eds) Handbook of non-invasive methods and the skin. Chap 14.7. CRC Press, Boca Raton, p 353
30. Henry F, Pierard-Franchimont C, Cauwenbergh G, Piérard G (1997) Age-related changes in facial skin contours and rheology. J Am Geriatr Soc 45:220–222
31. Jemec GB, Gniadecka M, Jemec B (1996) Measurement of skin mechanics. A study of inter and intra-individual variation using the Dermaflex A. Skin Res Technol 2:164–166
32. Jemec GBE, Serup J (1990) Epidermal hydration and skin mechanics. The relationship between electrical capacitance and the mechanical properties of human skin in vivo. Acta Dermatol Venereol (Stockh) 70:245–247
33. Lévèque JL (1987) In vivo methods for measuring the viscoelastic properties of the skin. Bioeng Skin 3:375–382
34. Lévèque JL, Corcuff P (1984) In vivo studies of the evolution of physical properties of human skin with age. Int J Dermatol 23:322–329
35. Lévèque JL, de Rigal J, Agache P, Monneur C (1980) Influence of aging on the in vivo extensibility of human skin at a low stress. Arch Dermatol Res 269:127–135
36. Maes D, Short J, Turek BA, Reinstein JA (1983) In vivo measurement of softness using the gas-bearing electrodynamometer. Int J Cosmet Sci 5:189–200
37. Malm M, Samman M, Serup J (1995) In vivo skin elasticity of 22 anatomical sites. The vertical gradient of skin extensibility and implications in gravitational aging. Skin Res Technol 1:61–67
38. Manny-Aframian V, Dikstein S (1995) Indentometry. In: Serup J, Jemec GBE (eds) Handbook of non-invasive methods and the skin. Chap 14.6. CRC Press, Boca Raton, p 349
39. Manny-Aframian V, Dikstein S (1995) Levarometry. In: Serup J; Jemec GBE (eds) Handbook of non-invasive methods and the skin. Chap 14.5. CRC Press, Boca Raton, p 345
40. Masson P, Blin P, Urbaniack R, Mérot F (1994) Influence of operative procedures on cutaneous deformations following measurement of skin elasticity by vertical stretching. Proc 18th Int IFSCC Congress, Italy
41. Millington PF, Wilkinson R (1983) Skin. Cambridge University Press, Cambridge
42. Murray BC, Wickett RR (1996) Sensitivity of Cutometer data to stratum corneum hydration level. Skin Res Technol 2:167–172
43. Murray BC, Wickett RR (1997) Correlations between Dermal Torque Meter, Cutometer, and Dermal Phase Meter measurements of human skin. Skin Res Technol 3:101–106
44. Nikkels-Tassoudji N, Henry F, Letawe C, Piérard-Franchimont C, Lefébvre P, Piérard GE (1996) Mechanical properties of the diabetic waxy skin. Dermatology 192:19–22
45. Nikkels-Tassoudji N, Henry F, Piérard-Franchimont C, Piérard GE (1996) Computerized evaluation of skin stiffening in scleroderma. Eur J Clin Invest 26:457–460
46. Olsen LO, Jemec GBE (1993) The influence of water, glycerin, paraffin oil and ethanol on skin mechanics. Acta Dermatol Venereol (Stockh) 73:404–406
47. Park AC, Baddiel CB (1972) Rheology of stratum corneum; a molecular interpretation of the stress-strain curve. J Soc Cosmet Chem 23:3–12
48. Pichon E, de Rigal J, Lévèque JL (1990) In vivo rheological study of the torsional characteristics of the skin. Proc 8th Symp Bioengineering and the Skin, Stresa. Italy, p 70
49. Piérard GE, Nikkels-Tassoudji N, Piérard-Franchimont C (1995) Influence of the test area on the mechanical properties of skin. Dermatology 191: 9–15
50. Piérard GE (1989) A critical approach to in vivo mechanical testing of the skin. In: Lévèque JL (ed) Cutaneous investigation in health and disease. M Dekker, New York, Chap 10, p 215
51. Piérard GE (1993) Mechanical properties of aged skin: Indentation and elevation experiments. In: Lévèque JL, Agache P (eds) Skin aging: properties and functional changes. M Dekker, New York, p 49
52. Piérard GE, Henry F (1995) Essai de classement catégoriel des propriétés biomécaniques de la peau. Evaluations par la méthode de succion. Nouv Dermatol 14:630–636
53. Piérard GE, Henry F, Piérard-Franchimont C (1996) Comparative effect of short-term topical tretinoin and glycolic acid on mechanical properties of photodamaged facial skin in HRT-treated menopausal women. Maturitas 23:273–277
54. Piérard GE, Hermanns JF, Lapiére ChM (1974) Stéréologie de l'interface dermoépidermique. Observation de la plasticité de la membrane basale au microscopie électronique à balayage. Dermatologica 149:266–273
55. Piérard GE, Kort R, Letawe C, Olemans C, Piérard-Franchimont C (1995) Biomechanical assessment of photodamage: derivation of a cutaneous extrinsic ageing score. Skin Res Technol 1:17–20
56. Piérard GE, Lapière CM (1977) Physiopathological variations in the mechanical properties of skin. Arch Dermatol Res 260:231–239
57. Piérard GE, Letawe C, Dowlati A, Piérard-Franchimont C (1995) Effect of hormone replacement therapy for menopause on the mechanical properties of skin. J Am Geriatr Soc 43:662–665

58. Piérard GE, Piérard-Franchimont C, Lapiére ChM (1983) Altération des locis minoris resistentiae du derme dans la photosclérose. Dermatologica 167:121–126
59. Piérard-Franchimont C, Henry F, Crielaard JM, Piérard GE (1996) Mechanical properties of skin in recombinant human growth factor abusers among adult bodybuilders. Dermatology 192:389–392
60. Salter DC, McArthur HC, Crosse JE, Dickens AD (1993) Skin mechanics measured in vivo using torsion: a new and accurate model more sensitive to age, sex and moisturising treatment. Int J Cosmet Sci 15:200–218
61. Serup J, Northeved A (1985) Skin elasticity in psoriasis. In vivo measurement of tensile distensibility, hysteresis, and resilient distention with a new method. Comparison with skin thickness as measured with high-frequency ultrasound. J Dermatol 12:318–324
62. Serup J (1994) Bioengineering and the skin: from standard error to standard operating procedures. Acta Dermatol Venereol (Stockh) [Suppl]185:5-8
63. Vogel HG (1985) Age dependence of mechanical and biochemical properties of human skin modifications under the influence of cosmetic products. Int J Cosmet Sci 7:51–57
64. Wickett RR, Murray BC (1997) Comparison of Cutometer and Dermal Torque Meter for skin elasticity measurements. Skin Res Technol 3:101–106
65. Wijn P (1980) The alinear viscoelastic properties of human skin in vivo for small deformations, PhD Thesis, University of Nijmegen, The Netherlands, p 34

CHAPTER 17

Skin Gloss Metry

V. Wienert

Introduction

Unlike the determination of skin roughness, the determination of skin gloss has as yet been given little attention. Recent books on examination techniques for human skin contain nothing on this subject [1–4]. This may be connected with the fact that no methods exist for an objective assessment of skin gloss. Gloss measurement in industry, on the other hand, is an established and standardised procedure, particularly in the field of surface finishing [5–7].

Skin gloss plays an important role in both cosmetology and dermatology. The acceptance of external agents depends among other things on the question as to whether and how long after application they cause a cosmetically unacceptable greasy gloss. Numerous cosmetic powders are available which temporarily reduce skin gloss. There is a great demand for such products: a glossy skin, particularly in the face, is regarded as displeasing. The reason for this is an optical phenomenon: irregularities show up much more clearly on a glossy surface than on matt structures on account of light reflections. Moreover, a glossy skin is often instinctively associated with various skin diseases, for example acne vulgaris or the seborrhoea of patients suffering from Parkinson's disease. The increased skin gloss which accompanies these illnesses is either due to increased secretion from the sebaceous glands [8] or their larger number [9].

We developed a method which could objectively determine the intensity of skin gloss according to existing industrial standards. The system had to fulfil the following demands: it should function without contact and provide results within a few seconds. Moreover, a high resolution of measured values was required since skin gloss, unlike material surfaces in industry, only changes within a very narrow spectrum.

Measurement of Skin Gloss

A device was developed on the basis of DIN 67 530 [6] which permits the contactless determination of skin gloss by reflection optometry. The principle of measurement is based on an assessment of the light reflected by the skin from a tungsten filament lamp (2.5 V, 60 mA), recorded at an angle of 60° by a silicon photocell. The size of the elliptical measuring spot is 9×18 mm. The measurement set-up as well as subsequent signal evaluation are explained in Figure 1.

The measuring window is let into a 4.5×14.5 cm base plate to ensure that the measuring device remains stable on the examination surface. The power supply is from a 9-volt alkaline compound battery.

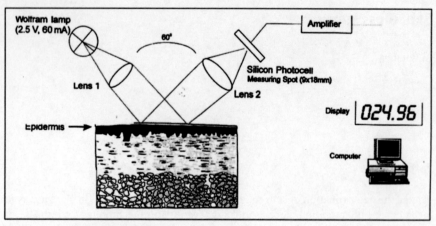

Fig. 1. Principle of skin gloss measurement

The results can be read off immediately on an integrated display (5-digit LCD) or transferred to a PC via a serial interface. The measuring range is 0.00–180.00 reflectometer units (RU) at a resolution of 0.01 RU and an accuracy of <1 RU between 0 and 100 RU. A measurement takes on average 3 s.

The device's measuring method complies with standards DIN 67 530 [6], ISO 2813 [7] and ASTM D-523 [5].

Instrumental Evaluation of the Method

The following measurements were performed on human skin in order to evaluate the equipment for skin physiology: the skin gloss on the forehead and lower arm of 30 test persons with healthy skin (10 women, 20 men, mean age 38.0 years, standard deviation (SD) 15.2 years) was initially determined.

A series of tests was then performed to test the suitability of the equipment for use in cosmetology, e.g. to assess external agents. The skin gloss on the lower arm of 10 test persons with healthy skin was determined before and then 1, 10, 20 and 30 min after application of four different cream bases. The development of skin gloss was recorded during the temporal course of a cream treatment.

The following standard bases from the German pharmacopoeia were used [10]: (1) Paraffinum perliquidum (purified mixture of liquid, saturated hydrocarbons from mineral oil) 10, p. 363. (2) Vaselinum album (mixture of purified, bleached, saturated hydrocarbons with ceresine) [10, p. 504]. (3) Eucerin cum aqua (mixture of wool alcohols, cetostearyl alcohols, with vaseline and water; water content 50%) [10, p. 535]. (4) Unguentum emulsificans aquosum (mixture of cetostearyl alcohol, viscous paraffin, white vaseline and water; water content 70% [10, p. 436]. Vaseline and viscous paraffin were chosen to investigate the influence of the various consistencies of external agents on the skin gloss.

Eucerin cum aqua and Unguentum emulsificans aquosum essentially differ from one another through their water content, though also by the fact that the first is based on wool wax, whereas the latter is based on mineral oil raffinates.

The quantity of 0.5 g in each case was standardised, i.e., it was rubbed evenly into an area of skin 4.5×14.5 cm, corresponding to the size of the base plate, and for a period of 30 s.

Statistics

The mean value and SD or only the mean value were specified in the descriptive statistics. We employed the t test when testing for significant differences between the individual groups, provided the data followed the normal distribution. If this was not the case, the Mann-Whitney ranking sum total test was used.

Results

The mean (±SD) skin gloss on the forehead of all test persons was 2.70 ±0.59 RU. The average value on the lower arm was 1.99 ± 0.28 RU and thus significantly lower (p<0.0001).

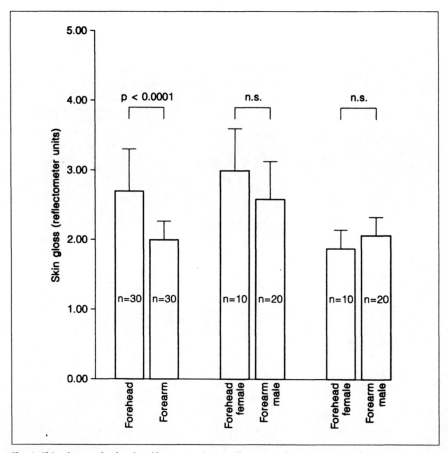

Fig. 2. Skin gloss on forehead and lower arm in overall group and incomparison of sexes

There were no sex-specific significant differences for either the forehead or the lower arm (forehead women 2.98 ±0.61 RU), forehead men 2.56 ±0.55 RU, lower arm women 1.86 ±0.27 RU, lower arm men 2.05 ±0.26 RU). The results are shown in Figure 2.

The water-free bases paraffin and vaseline increased skin gloss more than the aqueous emulsions following the application of external agents. Liquid paraffin displayed on average the highest gloss value 1 min after application, though this subsequently dropped relatively quickly to the value measured for Eucerin cum aqua. The development of skin gloss following the application of vaseline remained almost constant during the complete test period of 30 min. The two aqueous external agents displayed an initial rise with parallel curves and a slow decline over the 30-min period, Eucerin cum aqua resulting in a much greater skin gloss than Unguentum emulsificans aquosum. These findings are illustrated in Figure 3. The 1- and 30-min values for the various cream bases were compared in the statistical analysis. The individual results are compiled in Table 1; these show that the differences described above are generally very significant.

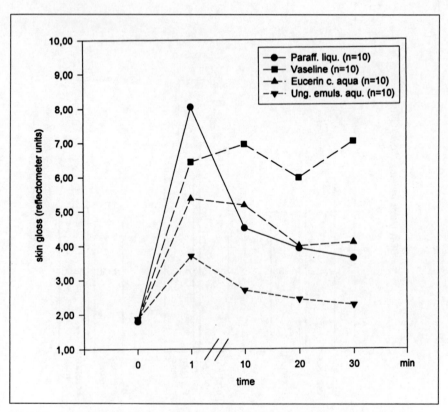

Fig. 3. Change in skin gloss before and during application of various cream bases (0.5 g each on 4.5×14.5 cm)

Table 1. Statistical analysis of the skin gloss effect of various external agents (1 and 30 min after application)

Comparison	Time	Significance level
Ung. emuls. vs Paraff. liqu.	1 min	p<0.016
Ung. emuls. vs vaseline	1 min	p<0.033
Ung. emuls. vs Eucerin c. aqua	1 min	n.s.
Paraff. liqu. vs vaseline	1 min	n.s.
Paraff. liqu. vs Eucerin c. aqua	1 min	n.s.
Vaseline vs Eucerin c. aqua	1 min	n.s.
Ung. emuls. vs Paraff. liqu.	30 min	p=0.0023
Ung. emuls. vs vaseline	30 min	p=0.0032
Ung. emuls. vs Eucerin c. aqua	30 min	p=0.0022
Paraff. liqu. vs vaseline	30 min	p=0.0190
Paraff. liqu. vs Eucerin c. aqua	30 min	n.s.
Vaseline vs Eucerin c. aqua	30 min	p=0.0191

Discussion

The different skin gloss values on the forehead and lower arm can be explained by the number of sebaceous glands per square millimetre, which, as is generally known, is higher in the face. An increase in sebaceous gland density leads to a higher overall quantity of sebaceous matter and consequently to higher mean skin gloss.

Sex-specific differences could not be detected during these first measurements of skin gloss, although we expected this to be higher for men than women on account of the higher density of sebaceous glands. The number of test persons, 10 women and 20 men, was relatively small and may not have been representative. Further tests will have to be carried out with larger groups.

One result of our series of tests which should be noted is that on average the liquid paraffin caused the most intensive skin gloss after 1 min on account of its 100% grease content. Most of the practically liquid material then spread over the surrounding area so that the skin gloss dropped significantly in a very short period of time. High values were also obtained with vaseline, whose consistency is more viscous, on account of the maximum grease content, even though the values for vaseline were on the whole lower than those recorded for paraffin due to the slightly uneven surface. Vaseline remained unchanged like a film on the skin and was practically not resorbed. This is why the quality of skin gloss did not change over time.

The high H_2O content of the aqueous bases appeared to cause less skin gloss. The reduction in skin gloss over time can be explained by the evaporation effect of the water and the simultaneous skin resorption of the cream base.

The results also make it very clear that the method of skin gloss measurement does essentially differ from contact measurement of sebaceous matter (e.g. Sebutape method). The main advantage of skin gloss measurements for the cosmetics industry will be the better possibility of assessing the acceptance of old and new preparations.

In dermatology it will be possible to make statements on resorption kinetics and the pharmacodynamics of external agents with a knowledge of the parameter skin gloss. We also believe that in the future the duration of the effects of cream preparations can be better classified by systematic skin gloss tests. The behaviour of various external preparations can be assessed much more easily, particularly in combination with other skin physiological test methods, e.g. measurement of the transepidermal water loss.

A final assessment of the possibilities opened up by this new method of contactless skin gloss measurement is at present impossible. However, a number of questions in the fields of both dermatopharmacology and cosmetology can now undoubtedly be answered with the aid of systematic skin gloss determination.

Summary

A new method for an objective assessment of the gloss of human skin is presented. The reflectometric measuring set-up complies with DIN 67530. The principle of this new method is based on a contactless determination of the skin's reflection of light from a tungsten filament lamp, recorded at an angle of 60° by a silicon photocell. In a comparative study with 30 test persons it was discovered that the forehead, with 2.70 standardised reflectometer units (RU; SD +/-0.59 RU), displayed a significantly higher gloss than the lower arm (1.99 RU, SD 0.28 RU, $p < 0.0001$). In an investigation into the influence of four different cream bases on the skin gloss it could be determined that the value depends on the percentage of grease, the water concentration and the consistency of the respective base. The method presented permits a fast, contactless, randomly repeatable objective assessment of skin gloss. Since the acceptance of cosmetics and pharmaceutical products depends not least on their skin gloss effect, this method can provide valuable information when estimating the success of old and new products.

References

1. Frosch PJ, Kligman AM (eds) (1993) Noninvasive methods for the quantification of skin functions. Springer, Berlin Heidelberg New York
2. Leveque JL (eds) (1989) Cutaneous investigation in health and disease. Dekker, New York.
3. Serup J, Jemec GBE (eds) (1995) Handbook of non-invasive methods and the skin. CRC Press, Boca Raton
4. Baran R, Maibach HJ (eds) (1994) Cosmetic dermatology. Dunitz, London
5. ASTM D-523 Standard test method for specular gloss
6. DIN 67530 Reflektometer als Hilfsmittel zur Glanzbeurteilung an ebenen Anstrich- und Kunststoff-Oberflächen
7. ISO 2813: Paints and varnishes: measurement of specular gloss of nonmetallic paint films at 20°, 60° and 85°
8. Plewig G, Kligman AM (1994) Acne and rosacea, 2nd edn. Springer, Berlin Heidelberg New York
9. Cunliffe WJ, Shuster S (1969) The rate of sebum excretion in man. Br J Dermatol 81:697–702
10. Deutsches Arzneibuch (1978) 8th edn. Deutscher Apotheker Verlag, Stuttgart

Safety

CHAPTER 18

Hypoallergenic Cosmetics

P.G. Engasser, H.I. Maibach

Introduction

In the early 1930s, several dermatologists guided a US cosmetics company, Almay, in designing cosmetics to be safer. This company was the first to apply the term "hypoallergenic" to cosmetics. Interpreted literally, this term indicates that these products theoretically have less ability to induce allergic reactions. In the early 1930s, however, the range of adverse reactions that can result from use of topical preparations was understood only primitively and incompletely. As we explore the word's present-day meaning, we discover that consumers, government regulators, and dermatologists interpret "hypoallergenic" more broadly than its literal translation warrants.

Ingredient labeling initially distinguished hypoallergenic cosmetics from other cosmetics; in 1978, however, this became mandatory for all retail cosmetics in the USA and is now required in Europe also, eliminating this distinction.

Consumers' Perceptions

Consumers interpret hypoallergenic to mean reducing or eliminating reactions which indicate physiologic intolerance to a cosmetic to the extent that it cannot be used safely or comfortablly. Cosmetic intolerance has been intensively explored and categorized in the past two decades (Table 1). Although type IV, cell-mediated reactions are the most thoroughly studied and understood [1], most problems of consumers relate to

Table 1. Cosmetic intolerance

Irritation syndrome	
Objective	*Subjective*
Acute or Corrosive Reaction	Sensory Irritation
Irritant Dermatitis	
Irritant Reaction	
Cumulative Irritation	
Mechanical Irritation	
Acneiform and Pustular Eruption	
Phototoxic Reaction (Photoirritation)	
Type IV Allergic Contact Dermatitis	
Photoallergic Reactions	
Contact urticaria	
Immunologic	
Non-immunologic⟩	

other reactions. These problems may include irritant dermatitis; sensory irritation which yields no visual clues (eg, elusive and mild discomfort "tautness" after using skin cleansers); dissimilar acneiform eruptions; and contact urticaria. A detailed discussion of cosmetic intolerance is beyond the scope of this chapter and has been presented elsewhere [10]. Consumers cannot be expected to understand the nuances of categorizing the mechanisms of adverse reactions, and they therefore assume that hypoallergenic products assure protection against the entire range of dermatologic problems.

Consumers who perceive that they are susceptible to adverse reactions from cosmetic usage describe their skin as "sensitive," and surveys of consumers disclose that most classify their skin this way [14]. Mindful of these perceptions, cosmetic chemists design hypoallergenic cosmetics by restricting use of ingredients which commonly induce allergy. Indeed, fragrance allergy affects 1% of consumers and causes 35% of adverse reactions to cosmetics [7]. Consumers generally perceive hypoallergenic cosmetics to be fragrance-free, but careful scanning of ingredient labels may reveal fragrance ingredients (ie, used to mask unpleasant odors) which ensnare unsuspecting consumers, who generally do not recognize the names of fragrance additives.

Preservatives – introduced into cosmetic formulations to prevent product degradation and contamination – frequently cause allergic contact dermatitis; however, these substances cannot be simply eliminated despite some consumers' wish that this be done. A preservative's tendency to induce allergy does relate to the chemical configuration and composition of the preservative, but incidence of allergic reactions in a regional population also depends on the concentration of the preservative used and on the frequency of its use [8]. As international marketing of cosmetics becomes more pervasive, manufacturers may no longer be able to adjust concentrations based on observations of adverse reactions in regional markets.

Published scientific literature and manufacturers' proprietary data aid cosmetic chemists in formulating acceptable cosmetic products, ingredient labeling of all cosmetics has proved invaluable, enabling consumers diagnosed as allergic to cosmetic ingredients to choose cosmetics which are "hypoallergenic" for them specifically. However, dermatologists must educate their patients about the official nomenclature used by manufacturers on cosmetic labels, because this terminology is often used variously throughout the literature. For example, on cosmetic labels, cinnamic aldehyde is listed as cinnamal; glyceryl monothioglycolate is listed as glyceryl thioglycolate; colophony is represented as rosin or one of its constituents (eg, abietic acid); and toluene sulfonamide/formaldehyde resin is listed as tolysamide/formaldehyde resin.

Regulatory Agencies' Perceptions

In 1975, the US Food and Drug Administration (FDA) proposed a regulation which would define as "hypoallergenic" only those cosmetics whose claim of hypoallergenicity was substantiated by comparison testing against standard products [11]. The regulation was contested and overturned [2], and there remains no official standard for defining hypoallergenicity in cosmetics. As part of the abovementioned litigation, however, an independent panel suggested standards for defining hypoallergenicity in cosmetics (Table 2). For products containing rubber, the FDA Medical Device Group

Table 2. Standard for Hypoallergenicity Utilized in Opposing FDA Proposal in 1977

Technique for Approach	Comment
Cumulative Irritancy Assay	Hypoallergenic would be no more irritating than the market leader
Draize Repeat Insult Patch Test (RIPT)	Negative in 200 subjects
Photoirritation and Photoallergy Assays for products applied to sun exposed areas	Negative
Documentation of Toxicologic and Dermatologic Profile	Similiar to 1999 European Union Cosmetic Legislature
Dermatoxicologic Consultation available from the company regarding adverse reactions in consumers	Available for physicians and consumers

has published for comment standards likely to reduce the incidence of type IV sensitivity [12]. This definition depends on predictive testing (ie, using the modified Draize Repeat Insult Patch Test) in subjects who have not been sensitized to rubber as well as in subjects sensitized to specific ingredients added to rubber. Should these proposed FDA guidelines be adopted, they would provide a conceptual and experimental precedent which might be the basis for claiming hypoallergenicity of cosmetics.

Dermatologists' Perceptions

In the 1980s dermatologist Earl Brauer, MD, who was then the medical director for a major US cosmetics company, Revlon, contended that widely sold cosmetics were all hypoallergenic, and he dismissed the need for that term. Brauer contended that broad market acceptance of a cosmetic product indicates that it causes few adverse reactions. (Ironically, Revlon now owns Almay, the first company to describe its cosmetic products as hypoallergenic.) In line with Brauer's reasoning, vigilant postmarketing surveillance must be conducted by any manufacturer who claims hypoallergenicity for a cosmetic product.

In addition to postmarketing surveillance, careful selection of ingredients and premarket product testing remain the foundation on which hypoallergenic cosmetics are designed. "Predictive" testing, the broadest category of premarket product testing currently used by cosmetic manufacturers, tests the product under exaggerated circumstances in limited numbers of subjects to predict its adverse reaction profile when used by the general public. In the past decade, many cosmetic firms doing predictive testing have abandoned live animal testing and have substituted in vitro and human testing [18, 19]. The choice of tests depends on the nature of the product and its intended use [15, 17]. For example, the "acnegenicity" of a facial cosmetic product was classically screened using albino rabbit ears [3], but now is often assessed by use testing in acne-prone panels or (in dark-skinned subjects) by occlusive application to the back for one month and subsequent examination of stratum corneum specimens obtained by cyanoacrylate biopsy.

Cosmetics intended for facial application should be screened for sensory irritation by selecting a panel of "stingers" – persons who perceive a stinging sensation when 5%–10% lactic acid is applied to the nasolabial fold [13] or to the malar area [5]. This panel is then used to screen facial cosmetics to ascertain if they induce this unpleasant sensation. Unfortunately, these subjects cannot be assumed to be uniformly or consistently more susceptible to other adverse reactions such as contact urticaria or other forms of irritation [6].

Various methods for assessing dermatologic irritation exist [17], but most commonly patch tests are reapplied daily to the back or upper arms for 10–21 days. As many as ten products can be screened simultaneously, but well-established positive and negative controls should always be used.

The Repeated Insult Patch Test, a test used to screen for delayed hypersensitivity, has several variations but usually uses a panel of 200 subjects who receive repeated occlusive patch tests for 10–14 days and are then given a rest period and a 48-h elicitation patch test [16].

Phototesting is added to the above protocols to identify and subsequently eliminate phototoxic and photoallergic reactions.

Leyden [15] recommended screening for nonimmunologic and immunologic urticaria during toxicologic evaluation by applying the cosmetic product to scarified skin before and after repeated exposure to the product in any of the contact dermatitis protocols. In addition, the cosmetic ingredients responsible for eliciting contact urticaria are becoming well delineated [4].

At present, use testing combined with feedback from members of the test panels is also extensively used [19].

To assess dermatologists' understanding of the word hypoallergenic, Draelos and Rietschel [9] mailed a questionnaire to all members of the American Academy of Dermatology regarding their evaluation of hypoallergenicity claims. Of the dermatologists polled (10% responded), most believed that hypoallergenicity pertains to irritant, allergic, and subjective (burning, stinging, itching) symptoms. Respondents said that they recommend hypoallergenic cosmetics to patients who are atopic and those who have specific allergies to fragrances and preservatives.

Many dermatologists who have a historical perspective rely on manufacturers of hypoallergenic cosmetics to cooperate in diagnosing adverse reactions to cosmetics. These companies provide information, advice regarding substitutes for allergenic products, and supplies for patch testing patients.

Conclusion

Regrettably, a universally understood definition of hypoallergenicity as applied to cosmetics and skin care products has not been agreed upon. Consumers and dermatologists would benefit from achieving a consensus on this issue.

Acknowledgment. The Medical Editing Department, Kaiser Foundation Research Institute, provided editorial assistance.

References

1. Adams RM, Maibach HI (1985) A five-year study of cosmetic reactions. J Am Acad Dermatol 13: 1062–1069
2. Almay v. Califano, 569 F 2d 674, 187 US App DC 19 1977
3. American Academy of Dermatology Invitational Symposium on Comedogenicity (1989) J Am Acad Dermatol 20(2 Pt 1):272–277
4. Amin S, Maibach HI (1995) Contact urticaria syndrome: 1996. Cosmet Toilet 110 Aug:29–33
5. Christensen M, Kligman AM (1996) An improved procedure for conducting lactic acid stinging tests on facial skin. J Soc Cosmet Chem 47:1–11
6. Coverly J, Peters L, Whittle E, Basketter DA (1998) Susceptibility to skin stinging, non-immunologic contact urticaria and acute skin irritation; is there a relationship? Contact Dermatitis 38[2]: 90–95
7. de Groot AC, Frosch PJ (1997) Adverse reactions to fragrances: a clinical review. Contact Dermatitis 36(2):57–86
8. Dillarstone A (1997) Cosmetic preservatives. Contact Dermatitis 37[4]:190 (letter)
9. Draelos ZD, Rietschel RL (1996) Hypoallergenicity and the dermatologist's perception. J Am Acad Dermatol 35(2 Pt 1):248–251
10. Engasser PG, Maibach HI (1999) Cosmetics, skin care and dermatologic practice. In: Freedberg IM et al. (eds) Fitzpatrick's dermatology in general medicine, 5th edn. McGraw-Hill, NY 2772–2782
11. Federal Register (June 6, 1975) 40(110):24450–24451
12. Federal Register (May 4, 1998)63(85):24559–24560
13. Frosch PJ, Kligman AM (1977) A method for appraising the stinging capacity of topically applied substances. J Soc Cosmet Chem 28:197
14. Jackson EM (1993) Hypoallergenic claims. Am J Contact Dermatitis 4:108–110
15. Leyden JJ (1993) Risk assessment of products used on the skin. Am J Contact Dermatitis 4:158–162
16. Marzulli FN, Maibach HI (1996) Test methods for allergic contact dermatitis in humans. In: Marzulli FN, Maibach HI (eds) Dermatotoxicology, 5th edn. Taylor and Francis, Washington DC, pp 477–483
17. Patil SM, Patrick E, Maibach HI (1996) Animal, human, and in vitro test methods for predicting skin irritation. In: Marzulli FN, Maibach HI (eds) Dermatotoxicology, 5th edn. Taylor and Francis, Washington DC, pp 411–436
18. Rougier A, Goldberg AM, Maibach HI (eds) (1994) In vitro skin toxicology: irritation, phototoxicity, sensitization. Alternative methods in toxicology, vol 10. Mary Ann Liebert, New York
19. Sparacio RM (1996) Noninvasive evaluations of cosmetic products. Cosmet Toilet 111 Nov:47–51

CHAPTER 19

The Use of Sensitive Skin Panels to Substantiate Cosmetic Claims

E. M. Jackson

Cosmetic Claims

Definition

A cosmetic claim is a benefit that can be perceived by a consumer when using either a decorative cosmetic or a skin care product. The legal classification of what cosmetics are and the regulatory definition vary in various parts of the world. Regardless, cosmetic claims must be substantiated which means that they must have what is called a reasonable basis to support the claim a cosmetic is making.

Substantiation

There are two ways to substantiate a cosmetic claim (1) by testing the cosmetic to demonstrate that customers experience the cosmetic benefit claimed, and (2) by expert analysis and opinion which typically involves a review of already published information on a cosmetic ingredient or product type.

Tests are the most frequently employed means of substantiating a cosmetic claim. These include human patch testing and controlled human use testing. There are numerous types of prognostic patch tests available to substantiate cosmetic claims [2, 9–12]. Lanman's 21-day cumulative irritancy patch test has been modified [1,4]. The Berger and Bowman modification [1] reduces the number of patch test days and the Jackson [4] modification adds a challenge phase after a two week rest period after the induction phase.

The controlled use test [6] is the other type of test used to substantiate a cosmetic claim. In this test a statistically significant number of consumers or patients use the cosmetic product as instructed for a period of one to four weeks. Evaluations by scientists, physicians or the panelists themselves can be made before during and after the use of the cosmetic product.

Sensitive Skin Use Tests

Both the patch test and controlled use test described above have routinely used panelists with normal skin. The reason for this has been the historical perception on the part of both scientists and physicians that testing on sensitive skin individuals would yield results that were uninterpretable.

However, in the late 1980s panels of individuals with sensitive skin began to be used in testing. [5] These sensitive skin types are listed in Table 1. The reason sensitive skin

Table 1. Types of sensitive skin populations. Expanded from [8]

Defined sensitive skin panels
Fragrances
Preservatives
Nickel
Pathological condition panels
Atopics
Acne
Psoriatics
Diabetics
Ethnic panels
Chronological panels
Newborns
Elderly
Treatment/medicated panels
Vitamin A
AHAs
Environmentally stressed panels
Low humidity/low temperature
Sun exposed
Occupational panels
Frequent hand washing
Solvent exposed

panels have now been used is twofold. First, our scientific and clinical knowledge of what sensitive skin is with its various subsets, has increased dramatically [3]. Second, consumer surveys in the 1990s demonstrate that between 50% and 75% of those surveyed perceive their skin to be sensitive. This percentage is markedly higher than the surveys of the 1980s which showed that only 25–33% of consumers perceived their skin to be sensitive. Therefore, substantiating a cosmetic claim in panelists who have defined sensitive skin can provide strong support for various cosmetic claims including a hypo-allergenic cosmetic claim.

The balance of this section will describe actual tests on cosmetics conducted in various types of sensitive skin individuals.

Diabetic Sensitive Skin

A skin protectant cream and lotion product was assessed for its healing properties in diabetics. Diabetics were chosen to test the skin protectant cream and lotion because the cutaneous manifestations of diabetes mellitus include dry skin, susceptibility to skin infections, a higher reaction rate to specific treatments and various other complications. Diabetics therefore use moisturizers two to three times the rate of nondiabetic individuals. Diabetics use moisturizers the most frequently on their hands, elbows and feet in that order. Despite this only 0.3% of diabetics see dermatologists for their skin problems [7].

Fifty-eight (58) diabetic panelists completed a 4-week clinical, controlled use study. Eighty-five percent (85%) of the panelists were non-insulin dependent diabetics (diabetics controlled by diet and exercise) and fifteen percent (15%) were either insulin dependent or on oral antidiabetic medication An initial evaluation of all panelists was made by a board certified dermatologist.

Of the 58 diabetics in the controlled use test 20 were also patch tested to the cream or lotion on their skin according to a modified cumulative patch test [4]. Finally, all

Table 2. Evaluation parameters

Clinical evaluation of dry skin of the hands
  Erythema
  Fissuring
  Scaling
Patch test evaluation
  Induction phase (ICD)
  Challenge phase (ACD)
Instrumental evaluation of dry skin on the legs
  Dermal phase meter (cutaneous moisture content)
  D-Squame tape (degree of flakiness)
Post-study panelist/patient questionnaire
  Mildness (objective or subjective irritation)
  Effectiveness in decreasing dry skin

58 diabetics had the cream or lotion applied to the ventral side of a randomly assigned leg, the opposite leg serving as a control. The use test, patch test and instrumental analyses are listed in Table 2. In addition to these evaluation parameters, a poststudy questionnaire was completed by the diabetics to determine their personal assessment of the mildness and efficacy of the cream and lotion moisturizers.

The results from the use test phase of this study clinically demonstrated that the cream and lotion moisturizer were (1) safe since there were no product related reactions (2) efficacious since all the diabetics began to improve with the first usage of the cream and lotion moisturizer.

The use test phase of the test demonstrated that the cream and lotion moisturizer did not cause either irritant contact dermatitis (ICD) or allergic contact dermatitis (ACD) under occlusive patch test conditions and were therefore hypoallergenic.

Instrumental analyses of the right arm, left arm and randomized leg site showed a statistically significant decrease ($p<0.05$) in erythema and scaling between baseline and completion of the study. Decrease in fissuring also occurred at all test sites but were only statistically significant at the test leg site.

Atopic and Adhesive-Sensitive Skin

Four currently marketed adhesive bandages were tested against a new sensitive skin bandage that uses a proprietary formulated adhesive to eliminate the allergic contact dermatitis (ACD) for adhesive sensitive individuals and to eliminate the irritant contact dermatitis (ICD) that sensitive individuals often experience from the mechanical trauma involved in bandage removal. Positive and negative control bandages were chosen by the test facility from their internal test records and their experience in routinely conducting patch testing [8].

Fifty-nine (59) panelists completed a use study with the test, control and new sensitive skin bandage. This use test panel was composed of individuals with a history of wound bandage and adhesive sensitivity (70%), normal skin (20%) and atopy (10%). All panelists underwent patch testing according to a modified cumulative patch test [4]. In addition, all panelists were instrumentally evaluated on the volar aspect of the ventral surface of their forearms for damage to the stratum cornem. A panelist questionnaire was also completed at the end of the study by each participant to obtain their personal assessment of the bandage.

The new sensitive skin bandage was clinically and participant evaluated to be the mildest of the test bandages evaluated, including the control bandages. No ICD or ACD was produced by the new sensitive skin bandage in the cumulative patch test phase of the study, and the cumulative irritation score and classification of the new sensitive skin bandage were equivalent to the negative control bandage. Damage to the stratum corneum from bandage removal was instrumentally evaluated and again the new sensitive skin bandage was equivalent to the negative control bandage. Upon completion of the study the study participants rated the sensitive skin bandage as the most comfortable, most soft and most flexible of all bandages evaluated as well as the easiest bandage to remove.

Conclusions

There are also many studies using treatment medicated panels, and nickel sensitive individuals. Preservative sensitive (paraben, formaldehyde) panels have the longest history of use dating back some 10 years.

Clearly, evaluating products for safety and efficacy as well as specific claims such as hypoallergenic, will continue to the test populations of choice into the twenty-first century.

References

1. Berger RS, Bowman JP (1982) A reappraisal of the 21-day cumulative irritation test in many. J Cutan Ocul Toxicol l:109–115
2. Brunner MJ, Smilianic B (1952) Procedure for the evaluation of the skin sensitizing power of raw materials Arch Dermatol 66:703
3. Jackson EM (1993) Hypoallergenic claims. Am J Contact Dermatitis 4:108–110
4. Jackson EM (1994) A modified cumulative patch test to substantiate hypoallergenic claims. Cosmet Dermatol 7/8:44–46
5. Jackson EM (1996) The use of sensitive skin populations to test Hypoallergenic Products. Cosmet Dermatol supplement 9/11:22–23
6. Jackson EM, Robillard NF (1982) The controlled use test in a cosmetic product safety substantiation program. J Cutan Ocul Toxicol 1:117–132
7. Jackson EM, Stephens TJ, Goldner R (1994) The use of diabetic panels to test the healing properties of a new skin protectant cream and lotion. Cosmet Dermatol 7/10:44–48
8. Jackson, EM, Stephens, TJ, Rizer RL, Herndon JR (1994) The use of atopics and adhesive sensitive panelists to assess a new sensitive skin bandage. Cosmet Dermatol 7/11:52–58
9. Lanman BM, Elvers WB, Howard CS (1968) The role of human patch testing in a product development program. Proceedings of the Joint Conference of Cosmetic Scientists, The Toilet Goods Association (now called The Cosmetic Toiletry and Fragrance Association), Washington, D.C., April 21–23
10. Schwartz L, Peck SM (1944) The patch test and contact dermatitis. Public Health Rep 59:2
11. Shelanski HA, Shelanski MV (1953) A new technique of human patch test. Proceedings of the Scientific Section of the Toilet Goods Association (now called The Cosmetic, Toiletry and Fragrance Association), vol 19:46 ff
12. Traub EF, Tussing TW, Spoor HJ (1954) Evaluating dermal sensitivity, Archives of Dermatology, 69:399

CHAPTER 20

Fragrances Between Allergic, Hypoallergic, and Irritant: In Vitro Studies

S. Sieben, B. Blömeke, H.F. Merk

Introduction

Fragrances are ubiquitously used to refine cosmetic, hygiene and household products such as soaps, shampoos, lotions, facial and toilet tissues, household cleansers and detergents but also medicaments, food, plastics, paper, or paints (Tables 1 and 2) [25, 27, 34, 37, 49, 53, 74, 83]. Until the last century, natural extracts from plants and animal secretions have been the only source of raw materials for fragrances. Today, approximately 3000 synthetic and 300–400 natural fragrances are used in fragrance industry [6]. Natural fragrances are commonly extracted from essential plant oils and animal secretions (isolates), tree bark (balsams), or are obtained by solvent extraction from plant materials (concretes, absolutes [33]). Well known examples of isolates are eugenol from cloverleaf, citral from lemmon grass and menthol from peppermint oil [65]. In general, many fragrances are viscous, oily substances. However, they are very heterogeneous regarding their chemical structures. Fragrances can be classified for example as terpenes, aromatics, aliphatics, as well as alicyclics and heterocyclics [38, 65].

The ubiquitous use of fragrances leads to an unavoidable exposure. Hence, possible adverse effects need to be investigated. According to the guidelines of the International Fragrance Association (IFRA) and the Research Institute of Fragrance Materials (RIFM), routine toxicological tests, such as acute oral and dermal toxicity, irritation, sensitization and phototoxicity testings are recommended to evaluate the safety of fragrances [17–19].

Table 1. Perfume concentrations of various products (in %) [26, 77]

Aerosol freshner	0.5–2
Bathroom cleaners	≤5
Colognes	2–5
Compressed powders	0.5
Dishwashing liquid	0.1–0.5
Facial make-up	1
Hair pomade	0.5
Hair spray	0.1–0.3
Laundry powder	0.1–0.3
Lipstick	1
Liquid detergents	0.1–1
Masking perfume	≤0.1
Perfume	12–40
Shower and bath formulations	0.5–4
Skin care products (emulsions)	0.3–0.5
Soap	0.5–2
Toilet water	5–30

Table 2. Most commonly found fragrances in cosmetic and toiletry products

Fragrances found in 300 products in the Netherlands[a] [6]		Fragrances found in 400 products in the USA[a] [17, 18]	
Fragrance	Percentage	Fragrance	Percentage
Linalool	90	Linool	91
Phenylethyl alcohol	82	Phenylethyl alcohol	79
Linalyl acetate	78	Benzyl acetate	78
Benzyl acetate	74	Limonene	71
Benzyl salicylate	74	Citronellol	71
Coumarin	68	Linalyl acetate	67
Terpineol	66	γ-Methylionone	63
Hedione	56	Terpineol	52
Hexylcinnamic aldehyde	51	β-Pinene	51
γ-Methylionone	51	Geraniol	50
Terpinyl acetate	50	Hydroxycitronellal	49
Lilial	49	Benzyl benoate	49
Lyral	46	Hexylcinnamic aldehyde	48
Geraniol	43	Lilial	48
Heliotropin	43	Coumarin	44
Galaxolide	41	Benzyl salicylate	43
Acetyl cedrene	41	Benzyl alcohol	42
Musk ketone	38	Eugenol	36
Citronellol	38	α-Pinene	35
Amyl salicylate	32	Geranyl acetate	35
Eugenol	26	α-Amylcinnamic aldehyde	35
Vertenex	25	Musk ketone	34
Isobornyl acetate	23	Caryophyllene	33
α-Amylcinnamic aldehyde	21	Lyral	33
hydroxycitronellal	21	Camphor	31

[a] Percentage of products containing the fragrances listed.

Nevertheless, adverse effects of fragrances such as contact urticaria, photodermatitis, irritation and depigmentation can be observed [23, 35, 36, 39, 40, 60, 78]. However, the most common reaction to fragrances is allergic contact dermatitis [24, 54].

Allergic contact dermatitis is a typical example of a delayed-type hypersensitivity reaction [20] meaning that inflammatory symptoms develop approximately 12 h after exposure and peak after 24–72 h. The reaction has two main phases: sensitization and elicitation phase. During the sensitizing phase (afferent phase) allergens (mostly low molecular weight compounds) penetrate the skin, where they act as haptens by covalently binding to carrier proteins to become immunogenic [52]. The necessity to form a complete antigen by binding to a high molecular weight compound has been generally accepted, however, it requires – at least in most cases – a chemical activation of the compound. Metabolizing enzymes such as cytochrome P450 isoenzymes and transferases are involved in this process. Both are mainly present in the liver, but are also expressed in the skin and immuno-competent cells [3, 61]. Langerhans cells which are DC of the skin [81] are believed to process and transport the hapten-carrier complex to the regional lymph nodes. The T-lymphocytes located in the regional lymph nodes recognize the antigen in association with major histocompatibility complex (MHC) class II molecules on the surface of the DC. Activated T-lymphocytes, which are retained in the draining lymph nodes develop to specific memory and effector T-cells. Upon a renewed contact, specific effector T-cells, present at or attracted to the site of application, are stimulated by the antigenic complex (eliciting phase). They induce a cascade of inflammatory events, causing varying degrees of erythema, edema and vesiculation of the skin. The sensitization to a single fragrance may cause tedious problems as many fragrances cross-react [24]. This may lead to an increased susceptibility to further products emphasizing the importance to trace out the responsible sensitizers.

In order to diagnose for example an allergic response to fragrances patch-testing is used. An 8% fragrance mix is used in the European standard series including eight fragrances (α-amyl-cinnamic aldehyde, cinnamic alcohol, cinnamic aldehyde, eugenol, geraniol, hydroxycitronellal, isoeugenol, oak moss, 1% each fragrance). In most surveys of patch test results during the last years the fragrance mix is usually the second most often observed allergen after nickel sulfate in most countries, reflecting the relevance of allergic contact dermatitis due to fragrance materials [24]. It is estimated that the fragrance mix detects approximately 70%–80% of patients with fragrance allergy [54]. Overall, highest scores were observed for oak moss, isoeugenol and cinnamic aldehyde [24]. Patch-testing represents a reliable and easy method to test many components at the same time. However, discrepancies may occur, when reactions to the mix and its constituents are compared. In some studies only 40%–60% of fragrance mix positive patients showed positive reactions to one or more of the tested single components of the mix [29, 58]. Additionally, the results may not always correlate with the clinical symptoms or history of the patient. The reasons for these discrepancies are only speculative and are still under investigation. A further drawback of this method is that the procedure may cause active sensitization of previously nonallergic patients, thus may represent a risk for the patient.

In Vitro Studies

These problems have initiated the development of rapid and reproducible in vitro tests, enabling us to predict the allergenic potential of xenobiotics. In the past decades several in vitro methods, such as the migration inhibition assay, the procoagulant assay and the lymphocyte transformation test (LTT) have been developed in order to evaluate hypersensitivity reactions. The migration inhibition assay examines cell migration of lymphocytes influenced by cytokins, such as the migration inhibition factor or the leukocyte inhibition factor, which are produced by stimulated lymphocytes [46, 75, 82]. In contrast, the procoagulant activity assay uses the procoagulant activity of lymphocytes, which increases in lymphocytes following antigenic stimulation, as a means to evaluate hypersensitivity reactions [2]. The LTT has been applied to measure lymphocyte transformations to blast cells due to antigenic stimulation [12, 87]. However, in a comparative study the LTT gave more sensitive results than the migration inhibition assay [84, 86]. This is why many investigators have focused on the LTT.

The Lymphocyte Transformation Test

The transformation of lymphocytes to large blast cells due to cocultivation with mitogens such as phytohemagglutinin (PHA) has already been observed in 1960 [67]. The transformation of cells culminates in increased mitosis [69] and is associated with increased cytokine formation and release [8, 85], RNA and DNA levels [21, 56]. In general, the uptake of the radiolabelled baseanalogue 3H-thymidine [13] or the non-radioactive 5'-Bromo-2-deoxy-uridine [11, 57] into proliferating cells correlates well with lymphocyte proliferation, and represents one possibility to quantitate mitogenic or antigen-specific induced transformation. In the past, the LTT has been proven to be a reliable method to study dose response relationships of contact sensitizers such as nickel, chromate, urushiol and p-phenylenediamine [12, 31, 87]. Therefore, we used the LTT as a diagnostic tool to investigate allergic skin reactions to fragrances. A total of 20 patients with a positive patch test reaction to the fragrance mix and to at least one single component of the mix and eight controls were tested. To perform the LTT we isolated peripheral blood mononuclear cells (PBMC) by high density gradient centrifugation, incubated them in the presence or absence of fragrances (components of the fragrance mix) for 7 days and measured the proliferation of lymphocytes either by the uptake of 3H-thymidine or BrdU. A test was considered positive if the proliferation of the stimulated cells was twice as high as of the non-treated control cells (stimulation index ≥2).

We first investigated the bioavailability and toxicity of the fragrances, as well as the influence of different culture conditions. In general, fragrances are highly viscous substances, may form micelles and possess a poor solubility in water and media [38], which may cause an insufficient bioavailability of these substances. Other investigators have tried to overcome this problem by using water-soluble forms of the allergen [55], or hapten-derivatized leukocytes or by introducing protein conjugated haptens [51]. In our case, we decided to test the fragrances in an unmodified way and observed significant fragrance induced proliferations of PBMC from patch test positive patients (Table 3). Figure 1 shows the dose-dependency of this reaction, indicating the bioavailibility of fragrances for PBMC.

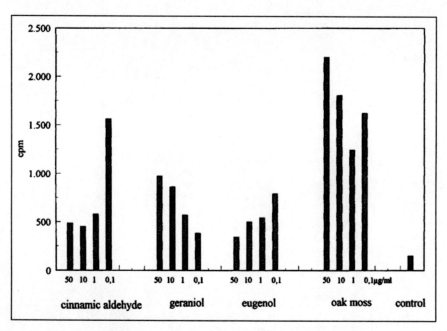

Fig. 1. Dose-dependent proliferation of lymphocytes to fragrances

Table 3. A total of 20 patients and 8 controls were tested in vitro using the LTT

Patients/controls	Fragrances tested	LTT SI	Patch test reaction
Patients			
1	Oak moss	7.2	++
2	Hydroxycitronellal	12	++
3	Oak moss	21	+
	Geraniol	10	–
	Cinnamic aldehyde	6.5	–
4	Eugenol	7.3	++
	Geraniol	2.1	++
5	Oak moss	3.6	+++
	Geraniol	3.2	+
6	Oak moss	3.2	+
7	Oak moss	9.1	++
8	Isoeugenol	8.2	++
9	Eugenol	2.0	++
	Isoeugenol	2.0	+
10	Oak moss	–	++
	Cinnamic aldehyde	–	+
	Cinnamic alcohol	–	+
11	Oak moss	–	+
	Isoeugenol	–	+
12	Cinnamic alcohol	–	+
13	Geraniol	–	+
14	Oak moss	–	++
15	Oak moss	–	+
16	Isoeugenol	–	+
17	Oak moss	–	+
18	Eugenol	–	++
	Cinnamic alcohol	–	+
19	Isoeugenol	–	++
	Eugenol	–	++
20	Isoeugenol	–	+
	Eugenol	–	+
Controls			
1	Cinnamic alcohol	3.2	–
	Isoeugenol	–	–
	Hydroxycitronellal	4.5	–
2	Cinnamic alcohol	–	–
	Isoeugenol	–	–
	Hydroxycitronellal	3.5	–
3	Eugenol	15.0	–
	Geraniol	20.0	–
4	Cinnamic aldehyde	2.5	–
	Oak moss	8.0	–
5	Eugenol	6.0	–
	Oak moss	14.0	–
6	Cinnamic alcohol	–	–
	Isoeugenol	–	–
	Hydroxycitronellal	–	–
7	Cinnamic alcohol	–	–
	Isoeugenol	–	–
	Hydroxycitronellal	–	–
8	Cinnamic alcohol	–	–
	Isoeugenol	–	–
	Hydroxycitronellal	–	–

The stimulation index (SI) equates to the proliferation of treated peripheral blood mononuclear cells divided by untreated peripheral blood mononuclear cells.
SI ≥ 2 defines a significant proliferation.

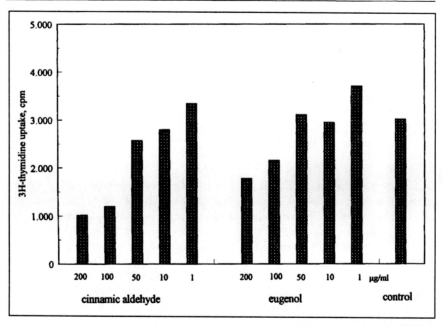

Fig. 2. Toxicity testings of fragrances

Secondly, we assessed the toxicity of fragrances by measuring the inhibition of PHA-induced lymphocyte proliferation. Cells were co-stimulated with PHA (0.5%) and different concentrations of the fragrances ranging from 0.01 to 250 µg/ml. In average, PHA-induced cell proliferation was reduced by the majority of fragrances at concentrations higher than 50 µg/ml. In contrast, cinnamic aldehyde and cinnamic alcohol already exerted toxic effects at concentrations higher than 10 µg/ml (Fig. 2). Therefore, fragrances were adjusted to final concentrations ranging from 0.1–50 µg/ml and 0.01–10 µg/ml, respectively.

Growth of cells requires optimal culture conditions. Most basal cell culture media need supplements such as amino acids, vitamins, growth factors and sera to supply cells with substances they may not synthesize by themselves, thus being crucial for cell proliferation and maintenance. In general, in vitro culture conditions should try to mimic the in vivo situation [14]. Therefore, we compared the use of autologous serum (AS) versus commercially available pooled human serum (PHS) in six parallel assays (Table 4). The generation of AS is fairly simple and inexpensive as it is gained by density gradient centrifugation of peripheral blood. It only needs to be heat inactivated at 56°C for 30 min and centrifuged at 1000 g for 10 min prior to use in the LTT. It was speculated that the use of AS may improve culture conditions and reduce background stimulation. However, as shown in Table 4 only in two assays the application of autologous serum increased T-cell proliferation, whereas PHS gave better results in four out of six cases. Thus, in our case supplementation of culture media with PHS was more advantageous and in addition gave standardized culture conditions.

Most cells exhibit a marked reduction of proliferative activity due to a cell-to-cell contact or are adversely affected by a density-dependent inhibition (diminished nutri-

Table 4. The influence of different sera on lymphocyte proliferation was tested using the LTT

Antigen	PHS stimulation index	AS stimulation index
Geraniol 50 μg/ml	1.0	2.1
Geraniol 10 μg/ml	1.1	3.2
Oak moss 50 μg/ml	7.2	5.3
Oak moss 10 μg/ml	3.6	0.9
Cinnamic aldehyde 50 μg/ml	3.2	0.7
Cinnamic aldehyde 10 μg/ml	6.5	3.2

PHS, pooled human serum; AS, autologous serum.

ent supply or release of cell derived factors including waste products). Thus, appropriate cell densities are crucial to successfully culture cells [59]. Therefore, we investigated the influence of cell densities on fragrance induced PBMC proliferation in the LTT. In preliminary experiments growth conditions seemed optimized when cells were seeded in lower cell densities (10^5 cells instead of 2×10^5 cells per well) after stimulation with the mutagen PHA. However, cells which were treated with different fragrances showed two times higher proliferation indices if 2×10^5 cells per well were used (Fig. 3). This improvement may be attributable to an increased number of fragrance specific T-cells and indicates that higher cell densities are needed to optimize fragrance induced cell proliferation.

The usefulness of the LTT has been subject of many controversial discussions since its development in the 1960s. Recently, Cederbrant et al. [16] came to the conclusion that the LTT cannot be used to accurately diagnose contact allergies to metals such as gold, palladium and nickel because of its low specificity and sensitivity. Moreover,

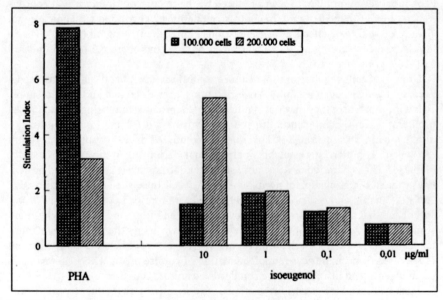

Fig. 3. The influence of different cell-densities on T-cell proliferation

Hoffmann et al. [42], who investigated allergies to cow's milk, considered the LTT as neither predictive nor diagnostic due to high in vitro responses of control patients. These results contradict several other studies, in which the LTT was proven to be a useful diagnostic test to evaluate drug allergies [68] or to distinguish between nickel allergic and non-allergic patients [31, 70].

We tested the usefulness of the LTT as a diagnostic tool to evaluate fragrance induced hypersensitivity reactions in vitro. A total of 20 patients with positive patch test results and eight controls were tested (Table 3). Overall, 45% (nine patients) of the tested patients had also positive reactions in vitro, thus 55% of the results were false negative, if ones takes the patch test result as a golden standard. In contrast, the stimulation of control PBMC from patch test negative patients revealed that 50% of the controls reacted in vitro.

These data indicate that positive patch test results are mediated by T-lymphocyte dependent immunological responses and that the LTT represents a useful tool to examine the cellular basis of these hypersensitivity reactions to fragrances. Further studies must be performed to recognize its value for the diagnosis of allergic contact dermatitis.

T-Cell Cloning

Sometimes skin reactions to fragrances in the patch test are considered to be irritant. Thus, the question arises whether these reactions are cell-mediated (allergic) or not (irritant). This prompted us to clone antigen-specific T-lymphocytes and to study their reactivity to fragrances. It has been shown earlier that antigen-specific T-lymphocytes are involved in the cellular response of allergic contact dermatitis to different antigens such as urushiol [47], nickel [80] or para-phenylenediamine [48]. T-cell cloning may also represent a useful tool to elucidate the pathogenesis of fragrance induced skin reactions as this method allows to describe the cell-types, mediators (cytokines) and mechanisms involved in the reaction.

A T-cell clone is a population of cells which are all descended from a single parental T-cell. The purpose of cloning is to minimize the degree of genetic and phenotypic variation within a cell population. For example, primary stimulated T-cells are very heterogeneous in terms of cytokine expression levels [50]. In contrast, repeated stimulation of T-cells in vitro leads to increasingly polarized T-cell subsets [22, 66].

T-cell cloning is performed by isolation and subsequent expansion of a single cell. Most often the limiting dilution technique is applied. In limiting dilution, cells are plated at dilutions which give a reasonable probability that any colony growing subsequently has been derived from a single cell. T-cell cloning by limiting dilution can be performed on bulk cultures after a single restimulation in vitro or on T-cell lines.

Fragrance-specific T-cell clones were established of epidermal punch biopsies from patch-test positive skin lesions. Epidermal cell suspensions were derived from punch biopsies to eugenol and cultured in the presence of X-irradiated autologous PBMC and appropriate concentrations of the antigen. After seven days, T-cell blasts were cloned by limiting dilution. T-cell blasts were adjusted to a final concentration to 0.6 cells per well and cultured in the presence of heterologous X-irradiated feeder cells and 20 U/ml recombinant interleukin-2 (IL-2). The growing T-cell clones were maintained by repeated stimulations with the antigen. T-cells were cultured with autologous,

X-irradiated B-lymphoblastoid cell lines (B-LCLs) and proliferation was determined by the uptake of ^{3}H-thymidine. Nine epidermal T-cell clones were established from a patch test reaction to eugenol. Four showed significant proliferations in the presence of autologous B-cells as antigen-presenting cells and eugenol, supporting the concept that the pathogenesis of hypersensibility reactions to fragrances is mediated by fragrance-specific T-lymphocytes.

The presentation of allergen by MHC class II molecules requires additional cellular adhesion molecules (CAM) to modulate the binding between antigen-presenting cells and T-cells and to activate T-cells. CAMs of interest are for example the CD4 molecule on T-cells, which pocesses a high affinity to the MHC class II molecule of antigen-presenting cells, the leukocyte function associated antigen (LFA-1) on T-cells and its binding structure ICAM-1, present on DC. Further co-stimulatory signals are provided by the CD2/LFA-3 and the CD28/B7 complex.

Co-stimulatory signals required for stimulating fragrance-specific T-cell clones were tested by the addition of blocking antibodies to the LTT. The addition of anti-HLA-DR and anti-ICAM-1 inhibited the proliferation of T-cell clones, whereas anti-LFA-1 inhibited the reaction only by 39%. Thus, co-stimulatory requirements of fragrance specific T-cell clones were in accordance with those typically observed [7, 10 41, 43].

Mosmann et al. [63] demonstrated that mouse CD4+ T-cell clones can be classified in a Th1 and a Th2 subpopulation depending on the cytokine profiles which they produce. Th1 cells produce IL-2, interferon (IFN)-γ and tumor necrosis factor (TNF)-β and Th2 cells produce IL-4, IL-5, IL-6, and IL-13. It was postulated that Th1 like cells lead to cell mediated allergic reactions such as contact dermatitis and Th2 cells to IgE dependent allergic reactions [9, 62]. However, different cytokine profiles produced by T-cells have been found including mixed cytokine profiles (Th0) in early phases after leukocyte stimulation. Therefore, phenotypic characteristics of our established fragrance-specific T-cell clones, such as cell surface marker and cytokine-expression patterns, were determined by flow cytometric analysis and ELISA techniques, respectively. Fluorescence activated cell sorting (FACS) analysis revealed that the fragrance-specific T-cell clones were CD3$^+$, CD4$^+$, CD13$^-$, CD8$^-$, thus were CD4 positive T-helper cells. Culture supernatants were harvested after T-cell stimulation to determine released cytokines. The established T-cell clones produced significant amounts of IL-2 and (IFN)-γ. Immunoreactive IL-4 and IL-10 were not detectable, suggesting that the clones are Th1-like cells.

In summary, T-cell cloning of fragrance sensitized T-lymphocytes was successful. The characterization of fragrance-specific T-cell clones revealed that clones were CD4 positive and had a Th1 like cytokine expression pattern. Antigen-presentation could be inhibited by common co-stimulatory signals such as ICAM-1 and LFA-3. Thus, our data demonstrate that the hypersensitivity reaction to fragrances is a T-cell mediated antigen-specific phenomenon rather than a non-specific irritative reaction.

Dendritic Cells for In Vitro Prediction of Sensitizing Fragrances

Aiba and Katz [1], who established LC suspensions from ear skin of naive mice painted with various haptens and irritants, observed an increase in LC size and an upregulation of MHC class II molecules 24 h after treatment with allergens but not with irritants. Enk and Katz [30], who were interested in different mRNA expression of epidermis-derived cytokines following the application of allergens and irritants, observed a nonspecific upregulation of TNF-α and IFN-γ mRNA levels, whereas mRNA levels of IL-1β, IL-1α, macrophage inflammatory protein (MIP)-2 and inflammatory protein (IP)-10 were upregulated only after treatment of contact sensitizers. IL-1β levels increased as early as 15 min after treatment. According to cell depletion assays IL-1β was almost entirely attributable to LC. It was concluded that LC derived IL-1β may have a crucial role in the course of allergic contact dermatitis and may induce a cascade of cytokines [64]. Consequently, the IL-1β expression may be used as a screening assay for allergens. However, the isolation of DC has been hampered because of their sparse distribution in human tissues. In human blood less than 0.1% of white cells are DC [81]. Therefore, methods were established to develop DC from proliferating precursors such as CD34+ cells from bone marrow and blood [15, 28, 71]. However, the low frequency of CD34+ cells in peripheral blood make these methods less applicable if small samples of human blood are only available. A major progress was made by the development of DC from cultured CD2 and CD19 depleted PBMC fractions in GM-CSF and IL-4 supplemented media [72, 73, 76]. These cells can be stimulated in vitro with allergens. The upregulation of IL-1β mRNA from these monocyte-derived DC may represent a useful tool to screen the allergenic potential of xenobiotics. Evidence exists that this system may function as a screening method [44] because only small amounts of IL-1β mRNA signals were detected in untreated DC, whereas IL-1β mRNA signals were upregulated after treatment with contact allergens.

To study the allergenic potential of fragrances we examined the effects of fragrances on DC IL-1β mRNA expression. Immature DC were generated according to a protocol described by Jonuleit et al. [45] and Romani et al. [72] and DC-precursors were transferred to a well-defined cytokine cocktail described elsewhere [45] to induce maturation of DC precursors, providing a tool to investigate the integrity of immature DC. On day 5 of culture, DC were co-incubated with non-toxic concentrations of fragrances for 15–45 min at 37°C and mRNA levels of control and treated DC were examined using RT-PCR. The established immature DC precursors were CD3-, CD4-, CD8-, CD56-, CD19-, CD14-, CD80-negative and HLA DR-, CD54-, and CD58-positive, as indicated by FACS analysis (Fig. 4). Maturation of DC precursors was successful, revealed by upregulation of CD80 and CD83 surface markers. In general, IL-1β mRNA expression levels of treated and untreated DC were very high. First studies with fragrances using this cell system revealed no clear result with regard to the sensitization potency of fragrances. Among other reasons the metabolism of fragrances may play a role.

Role of Metabolism in Fragrance Allergy

Many haptens require the binding to high molecular weight compounds which often requires their chemical activation. In the case of fragrances their metabolism has already been demonstrated in different systems. Cinnamic alcohol for example is converted to the aldehyde via the action of alcohol dehydrogenases [4]. The role of cytochrome P450 1A1 in the metabolic activation of eugenol and isoeugenol into reactive haptens is under study using cytochrome P450 1A1 knock-out mice. It has been shown that these knock-outs cannot be sensitized to eugenol in opposite to the wild type [5].

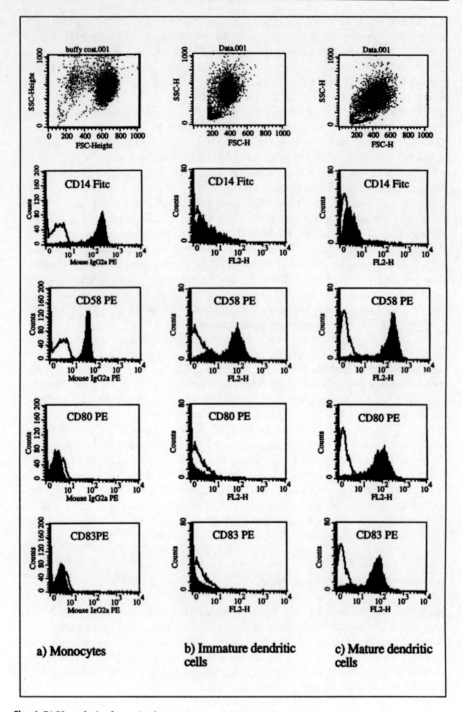

Fig. 4. FACS-analysis of examined monocytes and dendritic cells

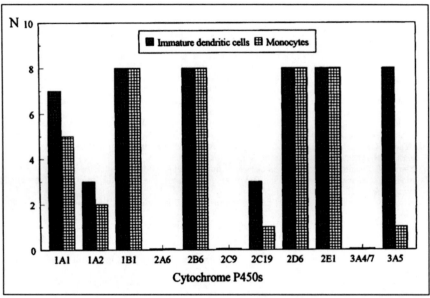

Fig. 5. Expression of cytochrome P450 isoenzymes in immature dendritic cells and monocytes from eight different individuals ($n=8$)

In general, the cytochrome P450 isoenzymes, particularly the four enzyme families: cytochrome P450 1, 2, 3, and 4 are involved in the metabolism of xenobiotics and represent in many cases the first receptor in this process. The resulting metabolites may react with proteins and/or DNA to become immunogenic and/or genotoxic, respectively. The processing and metabolic activation of allergens may be performed by antigen presenting cells such as monocytes, dendritic cells or keratinocytes. Therefore we characterized the P450 isoenzymes of keratinocytes and monocytes on their catalytic, protein and m-RNA level [3, 61, 79].

Moreover, we investigated the expression of P450 isoenzymes of dendritic cells and monocytes from eight different donors to elucidate the metabolizing capacity of these cells by RT-PCR (Fig. 5). All donors of immature DCs and monocytes expressed the CYP 1B1, 2B6, 2D6 and 2E1. The CYP 1A1, 1A2 and 2C19 was almost equally expressed in DCs and monocytes. In contrast to monocytes, more DCs expressed CYP 3A5. CYPs 2A6, 2C9 and 3A4/7 were not found in both cell types. These data indicate that DCs as well as monocytes express a broad range of P450 isoenzyms, suggesting that they possess the potential to metabolize xenobiotics, such as fragrances and encouraged our laboratory to continue the evaluation of the involvement of DC in the metabolism of fragrances.

Acknowledgements. This work was supported by a grant from the BMBF (07ALL006). We thank Elke Wölfle and Tames Al Masaoudi for their excellent technical assistance.

References

1. Aiba S, Katz SI (1990) Phenotypic and functional characteristics of in-vivo activated Langerhans cells. J Immunol 145:2791–2796
2. Aldridge RD, Milton JI, et al. (1985) Leukocyte procoagulant activity as an in-vitro index of nickel contact hypersensitivity. Int Arch Allergy Appl Immunol 76:350–353
3. Baron JM, Merk HF, et al. (1998) Cytochrome P450 1B1 is a major P450 isoenzyme in human blood monocytes and macrophage subsets. Biochem Pharmacol (in press)
4. Basketter DA (1992) Skin sensitisation to cinnamic alcohol: the role of skin metabolism. Arch Derm Venerol 72:264–265
5. Basketter DA, Pendlington RU, et al. (1996) The role of P450 1 A in the activation of prophaptens in skin sensitization. J Invest Dermatol 106:915
6. Bauer K, Garbe D, et al. (1990) Common fragrance and flavor materials: preparation, properties and uses. VCH Verlagsgesellschaft, Weinheim, Germany
7. Bierer BE, Burakoff SJ (1988) T cell adhesion molecules. FASEB J 2:2584–2590
8. Bloom BR, Bennett B (1966) Mechanism of a reaction in vitro associated with delayed hypersensitivity. Science 153:80–82
9. Bottomly K (1988) A functional dichotomy in CD4+ T lymphocytes. Immunology Today 9(9): 268–274
10. Breitmeyer JB (1987) Lymphocyte activation. How T cells communicate. Nature 329:760–761
11. Brüning T (1994) A nonradioactive lymphocyte proliferation assay for diagnostics of cellular immune defects in a clinical laboratory. Klin Lab 40:917–927
12. Byers VS, Epstein WL, et al. (1979) In vitro studies of poison oak immunity. I. In vitro reaction of human lymphocytes to urushiol. J Clin Invest 64:1437–1448
13. Caron GA, Sarkany I, et al. (1965) Radioactive method for the measurement of lymphocyte transformation in vitro. Lancet II:1266–1268
14. Cartwright T, Shah GP (1994) Culture media. In: Davis JM (ed) Basic cell culture. A practical approach. Oxford University Press, New York, pp. 57–91
15. Caux C, Massacrier C, et al. (1995) Human dendritic Langerhans cells generated in vitro from CD34+ progenitors can prime naive CD4+ T cells and process soluble antigen. J Immunol 155:5427–5435
16. Cederbrant K, Hultman P, et al. (1997) In vitro lymphocyte proliferation as compared to patch test using gold, palladium and nickel. Int Arch Allergy Immunol 112(3):212–217
17. Cooke MA (1991) IFRA and the dermatologist. Contact Dermatitis 25:209–210
18. Cooke MA, Cadby PA, et al. (1989a) Databases in the perfumery industry. Semin Dermatol 8:85–87
19. Cooke MA, Cadby PA, et al. (1989b) Data generation from perfume ingredient safety evaluation. In: Frosch PJ (ed) Current topics in contact dermatitis, Springer-Verlag, Heidelberg, 122–126
20. Coombs RRA, Gell PGH (1975) Classification of allergic reactions for clinical hypersensitivity and desease. In: Gell PGH, Coombs RRA, Lachman R (eds) Clinical aspects of immunology. Oxford Blackwell Scientific, London, pp. 761–781
21. Cooper HL, Rubin AD (1965) RNA metabolism in lymphocytes stimulated by phytohemagglutinin: initial responses to phytohemagglutinin. Blood 25:1014–1027
22. Croft M, Swain SL (1995) Recently activated naive CD4 T cells can help resting B cells, and can produce sufficient autocrine IL-4 to drive differentiation to secretion of T helper 2-type cytokines. J Immunol 154:4269–4282
23. De Groot AC, Liem DH (1983) Contact urticaria to rouge. Contact Dermatitis 9:322
24. De Groot AC, Frosch PJ (1997) Adverse reactions to fragrances. Contact Dermatitis 36:57–86
25. De Groot AC, Baar AJM, et al. (1991) Contact allergy to moist toilet paper. Contact Dermatitis 24:135–136
26. De Groot AC, Weyland JW, et al. (1994) Unwanted effects of cosmetics and drugs used in dermatology. Amsterdam, Elsevier
27. Dooms-Goossens A, Dubelloy R, et al. (1990) Contact and systemic contact-type dermatitis to spices. In: Adams RM, Nethercott JR (eds) Dermatologic Clinics. Contact Dermatitis. WB Saunders Company, Philadelphia, pp. 89–93
28. Egner W, Hart DNJ (1995) The phenotype of freshly isolated and cultured human bone marrow allostimulatory cells: possible heterogeneity in bone marrow dendritic cell populations. Immunology 85:611
29. Enders F, Przybilla B, et al. (1991) Patch testing with fragrance-mix and its constituents: discrepancies are largely due to the presence or absence of sorbitan sesquioleate. Contact Dermatitis 24:238
30. Enk AH, Katz SI (1992) Early molecular events in the induction phase of contact sensitivity. Proc Natl Acad Sci USA 89:1398–1402
31. Everness KM, Gawkrodger DJ, et al. (1990) The discrimination between nickel-sensitive and non-nickel-sensitive subjects by an in vitro lymphocyte transformation test. Br J Dermatol 122:293–298

32. Fenn RS (1989) Aroma chemical usage trends in modern perfumery. Perfumer and Flavorists 14:3–10
33. Fischer T (1995) Perfumed products. In: Guin JD (ed) Practical contact dermatitis. McGraw-Hill, New York, pp. 355–371
34. Fisher AA (1973) Allergic reactions to feminine hygiene sprays. Arch Dermatol 108:801–803
35. Giovinazzo VJ, Harber LC, et al. (1981) Photoallergic contact dermatitis to musk ambrette. Histopathological features of photobiologic reactions observed in a persistent light reactor. Arch Dermatol 117:344–348
36. Gonçalo S, Gil J, et al. (1991) Pigmented photoallergic contact dermatitis from musk ambrette. Contact Dermatitis 24:229–230
37. Guin JD (1981) Contact dermatitis to perfume in paper products. J Am Acad Dermatol 4:733–734
38. Hausen B (1996) Lexikon der Kontaktallergene. Ecomed Verlag, Landsberg, Germany
39. Hayakawa R, Matsunaga K, et al. (1987) Airborne pigmented contact dermatitis due to musk ambrette in incense. Contact Dermatitis 16:96–98
40. Hayakawa R, Hirose O, et al. (1991) Pigmented contact dermatitis due to musk moskene. J Dermatol 18:420–421
41. Hirschberg H, Braathen LR, et al. (1982) Antigen presentation by vascular endothelial cells and epidermal Langerhans cells: the role of HLA-DR. Immunol Rev 65:57–77
42. Hoffman KM, Ho DG, et al. (1997) Evaluation of the usefulness of lymphocyte proliferation assays in the diagnosis of allergy to cow's milk. J Allergy Clin Immunol 99(3):360–366
43. Jenkins MK, Johnson JG (1993) Molecules involved in T-cell costimulation. Curr Opin Immunol 5:361–367
44. Jonuleit H, Müller G, et al. (1996) IL-1-β upregulation in dendritic cells by contact sensitizers: generation of an in vitro test system for contact allergens (Abstr.). Arch Dermatol Res 288:279
45. Jonuleit H, Kühn U, et al. (1997) Pro-inflammatory cytokines and prostaglandins induce maturation of potent immunostimulatory dendritic cells under fetal calf serum-free conditions. Eur J Immunol 24: (in press)
46. Jordan WP, Dvorak J (1976) Leukocyte migration inhibition assay (LIF) in nickel contact dermatitis. Arch Dermatol 112:1741–1744
47. Kalish RS, Morimoto C (1989) Quantitation and cloning of human urushiol specific peripheral blood T-cells: isolation of urushiol triggered suppressor T-cells. J Invest Dermatol 92:46–52
48. Kapsenberg ML, Res P, et al. (1987) Nickel-specific T lymphocyte clones derived from allergic nickel-contact dermatitis lesions in man: heterogeneity based on requirement of dendritic antigenpresenting cell subsets. Eur J Immunol 17:861–865
49. Keith L, Erich W, et al. (1969) Toilet paper dermatitis. JAMA 209:269
50. Kelso A (1995) Th1 and Th2 subsets: paradigms lost? Immunology Today 16(8):374–379
51. Kimber I, Quirke S, et al. (1991) Lymphocyte transformation and thiuram sensitization. Contact Dermatitis 24:164–171
52. Landsteiner K, Jacobs JL (1936) Studies on the sensitization of animals with simple chemicals. J Exp Med 64:625-639
53. Larsen WG (1979) Allergic contact dermatitis to the perfume in Mycolog cream. J Am Acad Dermatol 1:131–133
54. Larsen WG (1985) Perfume dermatitis. J Am Acad Dermatol 12(1):1–9
55. Levis WR, Whalen JJ, et al. (1976) Specific blastogenesis and lymphokine production in DNCB-sensitive human leucocyte cultures stimulated with soluble and particulate DNP-containing antigens. Clin Exp Immunol 23:481–490
56. Mackinney AA, Stoklman F, et al. (1962) The kinetics of cell proliferation in cultures of human peripheral blood. Blood 19:349–358
57. Magaud J-P, Sargent I, et al. (1988) Detection of human white cell proliferative responses by immunoenzymatic measurement of bromodeoxyuridine uptake. J Immunol Meth 106:95–100
58. Malanin G, Ohela K (1989) Allergic reactions to fragrance mix and its components. Contact Dermatitis 21:62–63
59. McAteer JA, Davis J (1994) Basic cell culture technique and the maintenance of cell lines. In: Davis JM (ed) Basic cell culture. A practical approach. Oxford University Press, New York, pp. 93–148
60. McDaniel WR, Marks JG (1979) Contact urticaria due to sensitivity to spray starch. Arch Dermatol 115:628
61. Merk HF (1996) Skin metabolism in allergic contact dermatitis: the molecular basis. Springer Verlag, Berlin, Heidelberg, New York, pp 86–80
62. Mosman TR (1989) Th1 and Th2 cells: different patterns of lymphokine secretion lead to different functional properties. Annu Rev Immunol 7:145–173
63. Mosmann TR, Cherwinski H, et al. (1986) Two types of murine helper T cell clone. I. Definition according to profiles of lymphokine activities and secreted proteins. J Immunol 136(7):2348–357

64. Müller G, Knop J, et al. (1996) Is cytokine expression responsible for differences between allergens and irritants? Am J Contact Dermatitis 7(3):177–184
65. Muller PM, Lamparsky D (1991) Perfumes: art, science, and technology. Elsevier, New York
66. Murphy E, Shibuya K, et al. (1986) Reversibility of T helper 1 and 2 populatoins is lost after long-term stimulation. J Exp Med 183:901–913
67. Nowell PC (1960) Phytohemagglutinin, an initiator of mitosis in cultures of normal human leucocytes. Cancer Res 20:462–466
68. Nyfeler B, Pichler WJ (1997) The lymphocyte transformation test for the diagnosis of drug allergy: sensitivity and specificity. Clin and Exp Allergy 27:175–181
69. Oppenheim JJ (1969) Immunological relevance of antigen and antigen antibody complex induced lymphocyte transformation. Ann Allergy 27:305–315
70. Räsänen L, Tuomi M-L (1992) Diagnostic value of the lymphocyte proliferation test in nickel contact allergy and provocation in occupational coin dermatitis. Contact Dermatitis 27:250–254
71. Reid CDL, Stackpoole A, et al. (1992) Interactions of tumor necrosis factor with granulocyte-macrophage colony-stimulating factor and other cytokines in the regulation of dendritic cell growth in vitro from early bipotent CD34+ progenitors in human bone marrow. J Immunol 149:2681
72. Romani N, Gruner S, et al. (1994) Proliferating dendritic cell progenitors in human blood. J Exp Med 180:83–93
73. Romani N, Reider D, et al. (1996) Generation of mature dendritic cells from human blood. An improved method with special regard to clinical applicability. J Immunol Meth 196:137–151
74. Rothenborg HW, Hjorth N (1968) Allergy to perfumes from toilet soaps and detergents in patients with dermatitis. Arch Dermatol 97:417–421
75. Rytter M, Hausten U-F (1982) Hapten conjugation in the leukocyte migration inhibition test in allergic chromate eczema. Br J Dermatol 106:161–168
76. Sallusto F, Lanzavecchia A (1994) Efficient presentation of soluble antigen by cultured human dendritic cells is maintained by granulocyte/macrophage colony-stimulating factor plus interleukin 4 and downregulated by tumor necrosis factor a. J Exp Med 179:1109–1118
77. Scheinmann PL (1996) Allergic contact dermatitis to fragrance: a review. Am J Contact Dermatitis 7:65–76
78. Serrano G, Pujol C, et al. (1989) Pigmented contact dermatitis caused by fragrances. J Am Acad Dermatol 21:1057–1060
79. Sieben S, Al Masaoudi T, et al. (1998) Phase I and II enzyme expression in human monocytes, dendritic cells and keratinocytes (abstract 358). 12th International Symposium in Microsomes and Drug Oxidation, July 20–24, Montpellier
80. Sinigaglia F, Scheidegger D, et al. (1985) Isolation and characterization of Ni-specific T cell clones from patients with Ni-contact dermatitis. J Immuno 135:3929–3932
81. Steinman RM (1991) The dendritic cell system and its role in immunogenicity. Annu Rev Immunol 9:271–296
82. Tio D (1976) A study on the clinical application of a direct leukocyte migration test in chromium contact allergy. Br J Dermatol 94:65–70
83. Veien NK, Hattel T, et al. (1987) Dietary restrictions in the treatment of adult patients with eczema. Contact Dermatitis 17:223–227
84. Von Blomerg-van der Flier BME, Bruynzeel DP, et al. (1988) Impact of 25 years of in vitro testing in allergic contact dermatitis. In: Frosch PJ, Dooms-Goossens A, Lachapelle J-M, et al. (eds) Current topics in contact dermatitis. Springer-Verlag, Berlin Heidelberg New York, pp. 569–577
85. Wheelock EF (1965) Interferon-like virus inhibitor induced in human leukocytes by phytohemagglutinin. Science 149:310–311
86. Williams WR, Williams WJ (1982) Comparison of lymphocyte transformation and macrophage migration inhibition tests in the detection of beryllium sensitivity. J Clin Pathol 35:684–687
87. Yamada M, Niwa Y, et al. (1972) Lymphocyte transformation in allergic contact dermatitis. Jpn J Dermatol 82:94–97

CHAPTER 21

Contact Urticaria Syndrome and Claims Support

S. J. Bashir, H. I. Maibach

Introduction

Contact urticaria syndrome (CUS) was first defined by Maibach and Johnson [28], and since then numerous reports of contact urticaria to a variety of compounds such as foods, preservatives, fragrances, plant and animal products, metals and others, continue to be reported. Therefore, it is important to determine, in a scientific manner, whether or not a particular substance causes contact urticaria, and in what dose. Accurate experimental models are required to document urticaria-inducing properties of a substance; we also propose protocols to quantify efficacy of formulations that putatively inhibit CUS.

In this chapter, we outline current scientific knowledge and approaches to experimental methodology.

Symptoms and Signs

Immediate contact reactions, such as contact urticaria, appear within minutes or up to about 1 hour after exposure of the urticariant to the skin. The patient may complain of local burning, tingling or itch, and swelling and redness may be seen (wheal and flare). Symptoms may extend extracutaneously, inducing, for example, bronchial asthma. In the most severe cases, anaphylactoid reactions may occur. A staging system of CUS has been described (see Table 1).

Table 1. Staging of contact urticaria [3]

Cutaneous reactions only		Extracutaneous reactions	
Stage 1	Localized urticaria (redness and swelling)	Stage 3	Bronchial asthma (wheezing)
	Dermatitis (eczema)		Rhinitis, conjunctivitis (runny nose, watery eyes)
	Nonspecific symptoms (itching, tingling, burning)		Orolaryngeal symptoms (lip swelling, hoarseness, difficulty of swallowing) Gastrointestinal symptoms (nausea, vomiting, diarrhea, cramps)
Stage 2	Generalized urticaria	Stage 4	Anaphylactoid reactions (shock)

Epidemiology

Kanerva et al. [16, 17] gathered statistical data on occupational contact urticaria in Finland. The incidence more than doubled from 89 reported cases in 1989 to 194 cases in 1994. From 1990 to 1994, 815 cases were reported in total. The most common causes were, in decreasing order, cow dander, natural rubber latex (NRL) and flour/grains/feed. These three groups comprised 79% of all cases. Reflecting this, the most affected occupations (per 100, 000 workers) were bakers, preparers of processed food and dental assistants, in decreasing order.

Contact urticaria, therefore, is a common problem which may affect many people in the course of their daily lives.

Mechanisms of Contact Urticaria

CUS can be described in two broad categories: non-immunologic contact urticaria (NICU) and immunologic contact urticaria (ICU). The former does not require pre-sensitization of the patient's immune system to an allergen, whereas the latter does. There are, however, contact urticaria reactions of unknown mechanism, which are unclassified.

Nonimmunologic Contact Urticaria

Nonimmunologic contact urticaria (NICU) is the most frequent immediate contact reaction [20] and occurs, without prior sensitization, in most exposed individuals. The symptoms may vary according to the site of exposure, the concentration, the vehicle, the mode of exposure and the substance itself [18].

The mechanism of NICU is not well understood. It was previously assumed that histamine was released from mast cells in response to exposure to an eliciting substance. However, the H-1 antihistamines, hydroxyzine and terfenadine, do not inhibit NICU to benzoic acid, cinnamic acid, cinnamic aldehyde, methyl nicotinate in prick tests, although they do inhibit reactions to histamine itself [18, 19]. Therefore, mechanisms that do not involve histamine may mediate NICU for these substances.

Evidence suggests that prostaglandins may mediate NICU. Oral and topical non-steroidal anti-inflammatory drugs (NSAIDs) inhibit non-immunologic reactions (see [21] for review). Lahti et al. [19] used laser doppler flowmetry to demonstrate a reduction in NICU induced erythema in subjects pretreated with NSAIDs. This group believed that inhibition of prostaglandin metabolism may explain this effect.

Supporting this, Morrow et al. [30] demonstrated an increase in plasma PGD_2 following the topical application of 1% sorbic acid to the human forearm. The time course of PGD_2 peaks correlated temporally with the observed intensity of cutaneous vasodilatation. Notably, histamine and PGE_2 levels at peak erythema were not significantly higher than pretreatment levels. This suggests that the release of vasodilatory prostaglandins induced by sorbic acid was selective for PGD_2, and that histamine is not involved in sorbic acid contact urticarial reactions. The release of PGD_2 was a dose dependent effect, increasing with greater concentrations of sorbic acid, until reaching a plateau at between 1–3%. Pre-treating the subjects with oral aspirin (325 mg b.d., for 3 days) attenuated the observed cutaneous vasodilatation and inhibit release of PGD_2. In later studies, based on the same model, this group demonstrated similar results with benzoic acid and nicotinic acid-induced contact urticaria (see [14, 29] for reviews).

These studies add evidence to the argument that prostaglandin metabolism is significant in the pathophysiology of CUS. Also, they not only suggest that NSAIDs are useful as a treatment but also that experimental subjects should avoid these drugs when participating in a contact urticaria study.

Ultraviolet A and B light also inhibits immediate non-immunologic contact reactions. Notably this effect can last for two weeks after irradiation, and inhibits skin sites which were not directly irradiated [21]. The authors suggest that there may therefore be a systemic effect rather than simply a local one, however the mechanism by which ultraviolet light inhibits NICU is not known.

Immunologic Contact Urticaria

This is less frequent in clinical practice than the NICU form. It is a type 1 hypersensitivity reaction mediated by IgE antibodies, specific to the eliciting substance (see [3] for review). Therefore, prior immune (IgE) sensitization is required for this type of contact urticaria.

This sensitization can be at the cutaneous level, but also via mucous membranes, for example in the respiratory or gastrointestinal tracts. Notably, ICU reactions may spread beyond the site of contact and progress to generalized urticaria and, most severely, to anaphylactic shock.

People with an atopic background (personal or family background of eczema, hayfever or asthma) are predisposed toward the immunologic form of contact urticaria.

A well studied example of ICU is allergy to natural rubber latex (NRL), which is found in a wide variety of products, such as balloons, condoms, and importantly, surgical or protective gloves. ICU to NRL is a major occupational hazard in occupations which wear such gloves, for example, the health care profession.

Typically, latex gloves cause a wheal and flare reaction at the site of contact. This can affect either the person wearing the gloves or the person being touched by the wearer: in a study of 70 German patients with contact urticaria, 51% suffered rhinitis, 44% conjunctivitis, 31% dyspnea, 24% systemic symptoms and 6% severe systemic reactions during surgery [15]. In addition to direct skin contact, allergy may be caused by airborne NRL (for review see [35]). Clearly, sensitized, yet undiagnosed, individuals are therefore at risk when contacting ICU allergens.

Cross allergy can also induce ICU reactions: the patient may be sensitized to one protein and reacts to other proteins which contain the same or similar allergenic molecule. In the example of latex allergy, patients may also experience symptoms from banana, chestnut and avocado [13]. This phenomenon places ICU patients at further risk.

Site Specificity of Contact Urticaria Reactions

Characteristics of the skin and also of its sensitivity to urticariants varies from site to site. This is an important consideration in experimental design, discussed below, and in diagnosis. Schriner and Maibach [32] used laser doppler flow to map the regions of the human face most sensitive to NICU induced by benzoic acid: the neck was the most sensitive area, followed by the perioral and naso-labial folds. The least sensitive are was the volar forearm. The authors conclude that the neck or naso-labial or perioral areas are the most sensitive to test for potential NICU to this agent. Lahti [18] found that the back was more sensitive than the hands, ventral forearms or the soles of the feet, in his study of benzoic acid sensitivity at various body sites.

Human Experimental Protocols

Human subjects are suitable in determining the potential for a product to cause CUS in the human population. The protocols for ICU and NICU are the same, although ICU requires volunteers who are pre-sensitized to the product. Subject selection, dosing, test site, application methods and analysis are discussed in this section.

Subject Selection

To test a product for use in the general population, it is desirable that a random pool of volunteers be recruited. However, this may introduce several confounding factors such as age, skin disease, atopic tendency and medication such as NSAIDs which may alter the results. Therefore subjects must be chosen with particular regard to the aim of the study and screened carefully for inclusion and exclusion criteria, and for possible confounding factors.

Spriet et al. [34] suggest that subjects can be considered in three categories: serious sufferers; symptomatic volunteers and healthy volunteers. It is likely that the latter is most suitable for testing new products, whereas the former two groups may be better suited to ICU studies or investigating claims that a product already in use causes CUS.

Ideally, subjects should be representative of the population at which the product is aimed.

Site Selection

In the diagnostic investigation of a patient, one may test the site affected in the patient's history. However, in the design of a trial to test a new product the site studied is preferably that at which the product is to be used. This may not be convenient, though, for the volunteers, and so concealed sites may be chosen, such as the volar aspect of the forearm or the upper back. Importantly, the site selected should be consistent in patients and controls, as different areas of the skin may demonstrate differing sensitivities to the urticariant, thereby distorting comparability of the data. As noted above, different areas of the skin have varying capacity to induce urticaria, which should be considered when a site is chosen. Even in ICU, different skin sites may vary in their ability to elicit contact urticaria [27].

A history of skin disease may also affect the result. A test that is negative in nondiseased skin may in fact be positive in previously diseased or currently affected skin 23. It may be desirable, if the initial studies are negative, to select subjects who are symptomatic and use the affected sites to test the substance.

Paired Comparison Studies

Paired comparison studies allow rapid comparison between treated and untreated groups. Randomized matched pairs can be grouped for treatment and control, or one can use the subject as their own control by applying the test substance and controls on separate sites. The latter is preferred, because each subject may have several doses applied to their skin, providing more data from a smaller pool of subjects. Further, this decreases inter-subject variation and confounding, providing better control.

Serial Doses

Performing studies at different doses of the product will allow the investigator to build a dose response profile. This may indicate a minimum dose which causes a threshold response in the study group and also the dose at which a maximum response is seen. Extrapolating this data to the general population may give manufacturers an indication of a safe concentration for an ingredient to be included in a product. Dose response analysis may also demonstrate that there is no safe concentration for that ingredient, or, indeed, that there is relatively little risk.

Examples of concentrations that have been used in dilution series in alcohol vehicles are 250, 125, 62, 31 mM for benzoic acid and 50, 10, 2, 0.5 mM for methyl nicotinate [21].

Application Techniques

Commonly used topical application techniques in both immunologic and non immunologic contact urticaria are the open test and the chamber test. A use test can be employed in known sufferers. A positive reaction comprises a wheal and flare reaction and sometimes an eruption of vesicles.

1. In the *open test*, 0.1 ml of the test substance is spread over a 3×3 cm area on the desired site. Lahti [21] suggests that using alcohol vehicles, and the addition of propylene glycol to a vehicle enhances the sensitivity of this test compared with previously used petrolatum and water vehicles. The test is usually read at 20, 40 an 60 minutes, in order to see the maximal response. Immunologic contact urticaria reactions appear within 15 to 20 minutes, and nonimmunologic ones within 45–60 min after application [3].

2. The *chamber test* is an occlusive method of applying the substance to be tested. These are applied in small aluminum containers (Finn Chamber, Epitest, Hyrylä, Finland) and attached to the skin via porous tape. The chambers are applied for 15 min, and the results read at 20, 40 and 60 min. The advantages of this method are that occlusion enhances percutaneous penetration, and therefore possibly the sensitivity of the test, and also a smaller area of skin is required than in an open test. For unexplained reasons, this occlusion may provide less responsivity than in the open test.

3. The *use test* is a method in which a subject known to be affected uses the substance in the same way as when the symptoms appeared, for example wearing surgical gloves on wet hands provokes latex ICU.

Other techniques used in the assessment of ICU are the prick test, the scratch test and the chamber prick test. RAST can be used to determine cross-reactivity (see 3, 35 for reviews).

CUS Inhibition

The above models can be employed to test the capability of a substance to inhibit CUS. This may be by topical application or by systemic means. Topical putative inhibitors can be studied by the paired comparison method, using multiple test sites and a control on the same subject. This allows serial dosing, with either the urticariant or the inhibitor, to identify its protective potential against a known urticariant. In systemic studies, for example of an oral putative CUS inhibitor, subjects can be randomized into matched pairs for treatment and control. Following systemic administration, a known urticariant can be applied topically in various doses, as outlined above, and the response assessed.

Clinical Assessment and Quantitative Methods

Previously, dermatological studies of the skin scored the degree of urticaria by means of visual assessment by an experienced observer, usually a dermatologist. There are several advantages and disadvantages to this technique. Advantages are that it is inexpensive, visual scoring is rapid, the subjects are regularly assessed so that the study can curtailed if adverse reactions are severe, that unexpected findings can be handled by the investigator. However, simple observation may introduce error, inter- and intra-observer variation. This is especially important in larger studies, which may involve a team of investigators.

Also, visual observations are often graded on an ordinal (nonlinear) scale, for example rating reactions as weak, moderate or severe. As this data is not in a linear numeric form, the statistical analysis is not as powerful as that for quantitative data. In many studies, subjects report symptoms, also on an ordinal scale; this again is a subjective analysis, prone to variation error.

In contrast, a quantitative analysis may provide linear numerical data, that is easily reproducible and accurate, in standardized conditions. Rather than providing a score, measured data allows for statistical comparison such as mean values and standard deviations. This adds to our understanding of the properties of the test substance. Thus, objective measurements can clearly benefit dermatology studies.

Visual Scoring of Contact Urticaria

Contact urticaria can be graded visually by marking the degree of erythema and edema on an ordinal scale. Examples are shown in Tables 2 and 3.

Measurement of Erythema

Erythema, redness of the skin, is part of the skin inflammatory response which reflects localized increase in capillary blood flow elicited. Therefore, erythema can be measured by both the redness and the blood flow in the inflamed area.

Table 2. Scale for use in scoring erythema [11]

Score	Description
1+	Slight erythema, either spotty or diffuse
2+	Moderate uniform erythema
3+	Intense redness
4+	Fiery redness with edema

Table 3. Scale for use in scoring edema [12]

Score	Description
1	Slight edema, barely visible or palpable
2	Unmistakable wheal, easily palpable
3	Solid, tense wheal
4	Tense wheal, extending beyond test area

Measuring Color

Two techniques have been used to measure color: remittance spectroscopy and tristimulus chromametry. Detailed descriptions of the two techniques can be found elsewhere[4, 10]. Essentially, both methods detect light remitted from illuminated skin. Remittance spectroscopy employs multiple sensors to "scan" the light over the whole visible spectrum, producing a spectrogram. This differs from a tristimulus chromameter, in which the remitted light is transmitted to three photodiodes, each with a color filter with a specific spectral sensitivity: 450 nm (blue), 550 nm (green), 610 nm (red). The data from a colorimeter is expressed as a color value.

Remittance spectroscopy has been used to measure erythema in contact urticaria [5, 6]. Berardesca's group evaluated remittance spectroscopy compared to visual scoring in the assessment of urticarial prick test reactions. They found that there was a significant difference between negative and positive reactions, and between positive and strong positive reactions (+/++). Baseline skin had an erythema index of 36, compared to 72 for a positive reaction. Negative skin sites had a slightly, but not significantly, raised erythema index, resulting from a dermographic reaction related to the procedure of the test itself. Notably, remittance spectroscopy was not as effective discerning between the stronger reactions (++/+++) possibly because of the reduction of blood flow and hemoglobin content associated with the whitening of the center of the lesion and also because the blood flow may already have been maximized.

Laser-Doppler Blood Flowmetry (LDF)

Several studies have identified a reliable correlation between skin blood flow measured by laser-Doppler blood flowmetry (LDF) and cutaneous inflammation [8, 9, 26, 31, 36]. Bircher [7] reviews the use of LDF to study the role of various mediators in altering cutaneous blood flow.

The LDF technique measures the Doppler frequency shift in monochromatic laser light backscattered from moving red blood cells. This shift is proportional to the number of erythrocytes times their velocity in the cutaneous microcirculation. This non-invasive technique measures a surface area of 1 mm^2 and a depth of 1–1.5 mm.

The 1 mm depth will therefore measure the upper horizontal plexus, consisting of arterioles, capillaries, and postcapillary venules. LDF does not measure the deep horizontal plexus which lies at the subcutaneous dermal junction. Detailed review of the principles, techniques and methodology can be found in [6].

The changes in blood flow can be expressed in two ways. Either as the net change in cutaneous blood flow over the time of the experiment, which is given by the area under the curve (AUC), or as the maximal increase in flow over the baseline value (PEAK). Following a measurement of baseline blood flow, the product can be applied and post treatment flow can be measured. The change in blood flow provides an indication of the degree of inflammation caused.

Measurement of Edema

Ultrasound has been used to quantify measure the edema component of urticaria.

Agner and Serup [2] demonstrated a significant difference in skin thickness compared to controls in irritant reactions to sodium lauryl sulfate, nonanoic acid and hydrochloric acid. Serup et al. [33] used ultrasound to quantify edema in patch tests, expressed in millimeters. Agner [1] suggests that A-mode ultrasound scanning is a simple, reproducible method of measuring skin thickness. One disadvantage, however, is that the technique is dependent on an experienced operator, potentially introducing observer error.

Animal Experimental Protocols

Animal models are potentially useful to identify putative contact urticariants.

Nonimmunologic Contact Urticaria

The guinea pig ear lobe resembles human skin in its reaction to contact urticariants [21] (review), [22] and is an established model for NICU. A positive reaction is seen as erythema and swelling of the ear, which can be quantified by measuring the thickness of the ear.

Immunologic Contact Urticaria

Laurema et al. [25] considered a possible animal model for ICU, topically presensitizing mice to trimellitic anhydride (TMA), known to cause IgE mediated reactions. Topical TMA was applied to the dorsum of the mice ears 6 days after they had been sensitized, eliciting a biphasic ear swelling response. However, further studies are required to validate this model.

Conclusion

In conclusion, study of contact urticaria is possible with both human and animal subjects, in whom a combination of subjective and objective analysis can identify potential immunologic and non-immunologic contact urticariants.

References

1. Agner T (1995) Ultrasound A mode measurement of skin thickness. In: Serup J, Jemel GBE (eds) Handbook of non-invasive methods and the skin, chap 12.5. CRC Press, Boca Raton
2. Agner T, Serup J (1989) Skin reactions to irritants assessed by non-invasive bioengineering methods. Contact Dermatitis 20:352–359
3. Amin S, Maibach HI (1997) Immunologic contact urticaria definition. In: Amin S, Lahti A, Maibach HI (eds) Contact urticaria syndrome, chap 2. CRC Press, Boca Raton
4. Andersen PH, Bjerring P (1995) Remittance spectroscopy: hardware and measuring principles. In: Berardesca E, Elsner P, Maibach HI (eds) Bioengineering of the skin: cutaneous blood flow and erythema, chap 17. (CRC series in dermatology) CRC Press, Boca Raton
5. Berardesca E (1995) Erythema measurements in diseased skin. In: Berardesca E, Elsner P, Maibach HI (eds) Bioengineering of the skin: cutaneous blood flow and erythema, chap 20. (CRC series in dermatology) CRC Press, Boca Raton
6. Berardesca E, Gabba P, Nume A, Rabbiosi G, Maibach HI (1992) Objective prick test evaluation: non-invasive techniques. Acta Derm Venereol, 1992 Aug 72(4):261-263
7. Bircher AJ (1995) Skin Pharmacology, In: Berardesca E, Elsner P, Maibach HI (eds) Bioengineering of the Skin: Cutaneous blood flow and erythema, chap 6. CRC Press Boca Raton
8. Bircher AJ, Guy RH, Maibach HI (1990) Skin pharmacology and dermatology. In: Shepherd AP, Oberg PA (eds) Laser-Doppler blood flowmetry. Kluwer Academic, Boston, pp 141–174
9. Blanken R, van der Valk PGM, Nater JP (1986) Laser-doppler flowmetry in the investigation of irritant compounds on the human skin. Dermatosen Beruf Umwelt 34:5–9
10. Elsner P (1995) Chromametry: hardware, measuring principles, and standardisation of measurements. In: Berardesca E, Elsner P, Maibach HI (eds) Bioengineering of the skin: cutaneous blood flow and erythema, chap 19. (CRC series in dermatology) CRC Press, Boca Raton
11. Frosch PJ, Kligman AM (1979) The soap chamber test. J Am Acad Dermatol 1:35
12. Gollhausen R, Kligman AM (1985) Human assay for identifying substances which induce non-allergic contact urticaria: the NICU test. Contact Dermatitis 13:98–105
13. Hannuksela M (1997) Mechanisms in contact urticaria. Clin Dermatol 15:619–922
14. Jackson Roberts L II, Morrow JD (1997) Prostaglandin D2 mediates contact urticaria caused by sorbic acid, benzoic acid, and esters of nicotinic acid. In: Amin S, Lahti A, Maibach HI (ed) Contact urticaria syndrome, chap 8. CRC Press, Boca Raton
15. Jaeger D, Kleinhans D, Czuppon AB, Baur X (1992) Latex specific proteins causing immediate type cutaneous, nasal, bronchial and systemic reactions. J Allergy Clin Immunol 89:759
16. Kanerva L, Toikkanen J, Jolanki R, Estlander T (1996) Statistical data on occupational contact urticaria, Contact Dermatitis, 35:229-233
17. Kanerva L, Jolanki R, Toikkanen J, Estlander T (1997) Statistics on occupational contact urticaria. In: Amin S, Lahti A, Maibach HI (eds) Contact Urticaria Syndrome Eds., CRC Press, Boca Raton, Florida:57-70
18. Lahti A (1980) Nonimmunologic contact urticaria. Acta Derm Venereol 60: Suppl 91:1–49
19. Lahti A (1987) Terfrenadine (H1-antagonist) does not inhibit nonimmunological contact urticaria. Contact Dermatitis 16:220
20. Lahti A (1995) Immediate contact reactions. In: Rycroft RJG, Menné T, Frosch PJ (eds) Textbook of contact dermatitis, chap 2.3. Springer, Berlin Heidelberg New York
21. Lahti A (1997) Nonimmunologic contact urticaria. In: Amin S, Lahti A, Maibach HI (eds) Contact urticaria syndrome, chap 3. CRC Press, Boca Raton
22. Lahti A, Maibach HI (1984) An animal model for nonimmunologic contact urticaria. Toxicol Appl Pharmacol 76:219–224
23. Lahti A, Maibach HI (1986) Immediate contact reactions (contact urticaria syndrome). In: Maibach HI (ed) Occupational and industrial dermatology, 2nd edn. Year Book Medical, Chicago, pp 32–44
24. Lahti A, Väänänen A, Kokkonen EL, Hannuksela M (1987) Acetylsalicylic acid inhibits non-immunologic contact urticaria. Contact Dermatitis 16:133–135
25. Laurema AI, Maibach HI (1997) Model for Immunologic Contact Urticaria. In: Amin S, Lahti A, Maibach HI (eds) Contact Urticaria Syndrome Eds., CRC Press, Boca Raton, Florida:57-70
26. Li Q, Aoyama K, Matsushita T (1992) Evaluation of contact allergy to chemicals using a laser doppler flowmetry (LDF) technique. Contact Dermatitis 26:27–33
27. Maibach HI (1986) Regional variation in elicitation of contact urticaria syndrome (immediate hypersensitivity syndrome). Shrimp. Contact Dermatitis 15:100
28. Maibach HI, Johnson HL (1975) Contact urticaria syndrome: contact urticaria to diethyltoluamide (immediate type hypersensitivity). Arch Dermatol 111:726–730
29. Morrow JD (1995) Prostaglandin D2 and contact urticaria. In: Berardesca E, Elsner P, Maibach HI (eds) Bioengineering of the skin: cutaneous blood flow and erythema, chap 8. (CRC series in dermatology) CRC Press, Boca Raton

30. Morrow JD, Minon TA, Awad JA, Roberts LJ II (1994) Release of markedly increased quantities of prostaglandin D2 from the skin in vivo in humans following the application of sorbic acid. Arch Dermatol 130:1408
31. Pershing LK, Heuther S, Conklin RL, Krueger GG (1989) Cutaneous blood flow and percutaneous absorption: a quantitative analysis using a laser doppler flow meter and a blood flow meter. J Invest Dermatol 92:355–359
32. Schriner DL, Maibach HI (1996) Regional variation of nonimmunologic contact urticaria. Functional map of the human face. Skin Pharmacol 9:312–321
33. Serup J, Staberg B, Klemp P (1984) Quantification of cutaneous edema in patch test reaction by measurement of skin thickness with high frequency pulsed ultrasound. Contact Dermatitis 10: 88–93
34. Spriet A, Dupin-Spriet T, Simon P (1994) Selection of subjects. In: Spriet A, Dupin-Spriet T, Simon P (eds) Methodology of clinical drug trials, chap 3. Karger, Basel
35. Turjanmaa K, Mäkinen-Kiljunen S, Ruenala T, Alenius H, Palosuo T (1995) Natural rubber latex allergy: the European experience. Immunol Allergy Clin North Am 15:71–88
36. Wilhelm KP, Surber C, Maibach HI (1989) Quantification of sodium lauryl sulfate irritant dermatitis in man: Comparison of four techniques: skin colour reflectance, transepidermal water loss, laser Doppler flow measurement and visual scores. Arch Dermatol Res 281:293–295

CHAPTER 22

Photoreactions

N.J. Neumann, B. Homey, H.W. Vohr, P. Lehmann

Definitions

Photoreactions may result from interaction of a chemical with ultraviolet or/and visible light in the skin. A chemical that absorbs UV irradiation (visible light) and leads to a biologic response is called a photosensitizer. As far as reactions between exogenous chemical agents, UV light and human skin are concerned, the term "photosensitization" includes phototoxic and photoallergic reactions.

Phototoxic reactions are defined as reactions caused by a single exposure to a photoreactive chemical plus UV-irradiation or visible light and start immediately or delayed (up to 48 h) after irradiation. Phototoxic reactions caused by topically applied agents are also called photoirritative reactions.

Photoallergic reactions are defined as immunologically mediated reactions. In contrast to phototoxic reactions no skin reactions are detectable after the first exposure to a photoallergen and UV light. After an induction period of approximately 1 week a second exposure leads to a typical delayed skin reactivity.

Since this article refers to UV-induced short-term skin reactions, genotoxic effects, e.g. photomutagenicity and photocarcinogenicity, will not be characterized.

Epidemiology and Pathogenesis

Based on clinical experiences phototoxic reactions are much more common than photoallergic reactions, but exact data regarding the incidence and the prevalence of photoreactions are not available.

Jung and Mauer classified 4% out of all positive test reactions they observed in their dermatological center between 1960 and 1965 as photoallergic reactions [23–26,45,46]. In 1966 only 1% of all contact reactions were diagnosed as photoallergic. Taken a presumed overall prevalence of 1% for contact allergic reactions in a given population into account, the prevalence of photoallergy, therefore, could be predicted as 0.01% (1 case out of 10.000 people).

The evaluation of our own data from 1984–1994 revealed 6,402 positive epicutaneous test reactions (clinically relevant contact allergies) and 82 positive photopatch test reactions (photoallergies). Thus, 1.3% of all relevant reactions were classified as photoallergic. Although this rate is in accordance with other reports, an incidence of photoallergy of 1% remains questionable. In contrast to the standardized epicutaneous test widely used by dermatologists all over the world, the photopatch test is a special procedure employed only in few dermatological centers [17, 32]. Therefore, it seems reasonable to assume the incidence of photoallergy lower than 0.01%.

From 1964–1971 Magnus (in [43]) retrospectively analyzed photoreactions caused by systemically applied drugs. Following his results, 1 out of 212.000 prescriptions led to a photoreaction. Focusing on the subgroups of protriptylin, desmethylchlortetracylin and nalidixin acid, out of 14.000 prescriptions 1 photoreaction was observed. These photoreactions were predominantly classified as phototoxic.

Many photosensitizers are able to cause both [49, 50] phototoxic and photoallergic reactions and often an exact clinical and histopathological discrimination is impossible.

Photoallergy is considered to be a T cell mediated delayed hypersensitivity reaction. Via complex interactions UV-light modifies a prohapten to become a hapten. Afterwards, the hapten reacts with skin proteins building a hapten-protein conjugate. Langerhans cells take up this complex, mature and migrate to local draining lymph nodes. There, relevant antigen determinants are presented via MHC-molecules (signal 1) to T cells and to co-stimulatory molecules (ICAM-1,B7–1,B7–2) and induce T cell proliferation and memory T cell formation [5].

In contrast to a contact dermatitis, UV irradiation is a prerequisite to elicit a photoallergy. Regarding the action spectrum, UVA plays a predominant role.

A phototoxic reaction is based on a non-immunological (non-antigen-specific) inflammatory skin reaction. Phototoxic agents are inactive without UV light. Thus, only the combination of the phototoxic substance and UV light (subsequently applied) leads to a phototoxic reaction. Therefore, a possible mechanism could be the absorption of a photon leading to a short-living, now electronically excited photosensitizer in a singlet or mainly in a triplet state. In general, phototoxicity is elicited in two different ways:

a) Free radicals built by electron or hydrogen transfer (type I)
b) Singlet oxygen species built by energy transfer (type II)

The chemical structure of the photosensitizer and the substrate conditions determine the phototoxic reaction. However, both reaction types can cause cytotoxic damage to keratinocytes and Langerhans cells. Furthermore, phototoxicity induces proinflammatory cytokines in keratinocytes [47], which, in turn, may activate Langerhans cells, macrophages and T cells. Moreover, a marked increased expression of ICAM-1 on endothelial cells and keratinocytes has been reported during chemical-induced phototoxicity. In addition, TNF-α may induce the differentiation, proliferation, and degranulation of mast cells.

Clinical Characteristics

Similar to contact dermatitis, photoallergic reactions show the typical symptoms of eczema. Starting with erythema and infiltration, papulovesicles or even bullae develop in skin areas exposed to UV light. Following prolonged exposure to a photoallergen and UV-irradiation, a chronic actinic dermatitis may be induced with a lichenoid scaly dermatitis even in skin areas not exposed to UV-irradiation. Both acute and chronic photoallergic dermatitis are often combined with vigorous itching. Occasionally the discrimination between an airborne contact dermatitis (e. g. caused by compositae) and a photoallergy might be a problem. In these cases dermatitis-free areas behind the ears, under the chin and in wrinkles at the neck (less sun exposed areas) might be helpful to support photoallergy (Fig. 1).

The clinical manifestation of phototoxic reactions depend on the kind and the concentration of the photosensitizer as well as on the intensity, wavelength and duration of the irradiation. Predominantly, phototoxic reactions appear as an exaggerated sunburn dermatitis (Fig. 2) comprised of erythema, edema (infiltration), and a burning

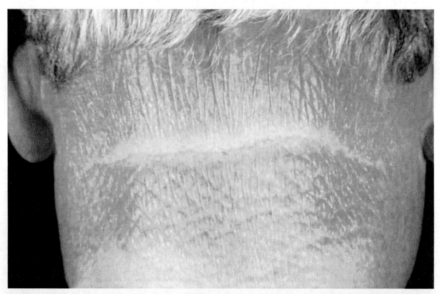

Fig. 1. Olaquindox-induced photoallergy. Wrinkles located in the neck-area are dermatitis free

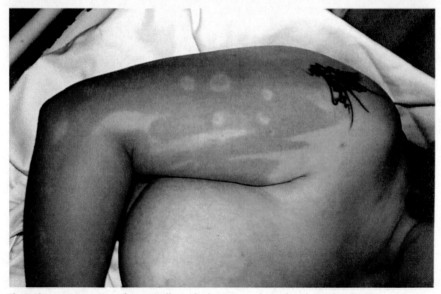

Fig. 2. Phototoxic reaction after topically applied 8-MOP and overdosed UVA irradiation

pain up to 24 h after irradiation followed by a persistent hyperpigmentation. This type of reaction is mostly induced by tar, dyes, benaxoprofen, and amidodarone in combination with relative high doses of UVA light.

Psoralen [contained in several plants, e.g. amni majus, (phytophotocontact dermatitis, Fig. 3)] or bergaptene [contained in diverse perfumes (berloque dermatitis, Fig. 4)] lead to a typical delayed painful erythema often observed with additional bullae. Later on, an intensive long-lasting hyperpigmentation was reported frequently.

Photo-onycholysis is a special form of a phototoxic reaction (Fig. 5), mostly described after systemic application of 8-methoxypsoralen, benoxaprofen, or tetra-

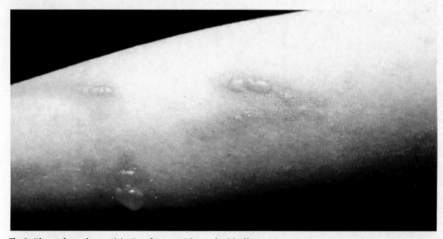

Fig. 3. Phytophotodermatitis. Erythema with marked bullae

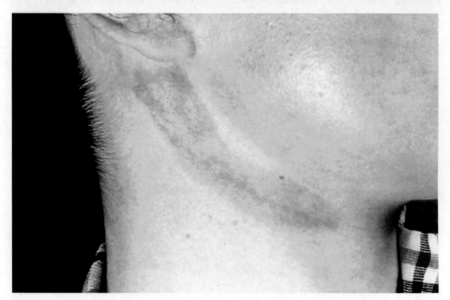

Fig. 4. Berloque dermatitis. The erythema phase (often followed by a long-lasting hyperpigmentation)

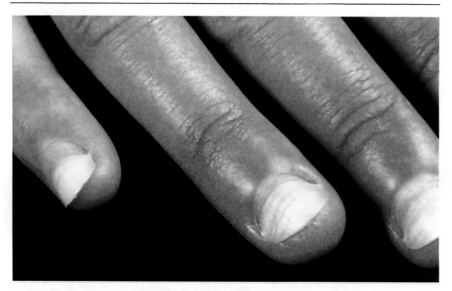

Fig. 5. Photo-onycholysis after oral intake of tetracycline and sun-light exposure

cycline. Photo-onycholysis starts from the distal part of the nail bed mainly after a protracted time of substance application.

Patients suffering from porphyria cutanea tarda characteristically develop bullae with clear fluid, milia, and pain from easily traumatized and fragile skin predominantly on the fingers. In contrast, the erythropoietic protoporphyria (EPP) induces acute phototoxic symptoms like burning pain in combination with erythema and edema shortly after UV irradiation. Cumulative phototoxic skin damage can cause hyalinosis cutis-like lesions, which are typical for juvenile EPP patients [38].

Diagnostic Procedures

The diagnosis of photoreactions is based on medical history, clinical and histological findings, and especially on photodiagnostic test procedures [16, 32–37]. Stephan Epstein early emphasized the eminent role of photopatch testing for the identification of photosensitizers, followed by numerous publications about methodological problems [6–9]. Nevertheless, until the early 1980s the photopatch test procedure was not standardized and varied between different countries and dermatological centers according to test tray, substance concentrations, vehicles as well as to the readings and the classification of test reactions [15]. The first standard method for photopatch testing was defined by the Scandinavian Photodermatitis Research Group (SPDRG) in 1982 [22]. Guided by the SPDRG, 45 dermatological centers from Austria, Germany, and Switzerland founded the Austrian, German, and Swiss Photopatch Test Group (Arbeitsgemeinschaft Photopatch-Test: DAPT) in 1984. Their new standardized test procedure is summarized in Tables 1 and 2 a, b. Additionally, the test substances are listed in Table 3 a, b. Systemically applied substances predominantly revealed false-

Table 1. Photopatch test

*	Application of test substances in Finn-Chambers
*	24 h occlusive to the back
*	Irradiation 10 J/cm^2 UV-A (320-400 nm)
*	Controls: Un-irradiated patch-test
	UVA-irradiated skin without patch-test

Table 2a. Photopatch test gradings

0	No reaction
1+	Erythema
2+	Erythema and infiltrate
3+	Erythema and papulovesicles
4+	Erythema, bullae or erosions

Table 2b. Classification of test reaction

Contact reaction
Every positive reaction in the control area without 1 +
immediately after removal of the test tray

Phototoxic Reaction
1+ or 2+, immediate or delayed, as decrescendo reaction

Photoallergic reaction
3+ or 4+, delayed, as crescendo reaction as well as the reaction
0, 1+, 2+, 3+

negative photopatch test results, because metabolites are probably the relevant photo-sensitizers instead of topically applied test substances. Therefore, the systemic photo-provocation might be a helpful test procedure [37, 59, 60]. After the first irradiation of test areas (preferably located on the back) the supposed photoallergic drug should be

Table 3a. List of substances : Photopatch test 1985-1990

Substances	Concentrations (%)	Substances	Concentrations (%)
1. Tetrachlorosalicylanilide	0,10	17. •Fragrance Mix	8,00
2. Monobromsalicylchloranilide	1,00	18. •6-Methylcumarine	1,00
3. Tribromsalicylanilide	1,00	19. Paraaminobenzoic acid	5,00
4. Buclosamide	5,00	20. Hydrochlorothiazide	1,00
5. Fenticlor	1,00	21. •Furosemide	1,00
6. Hexachlorophen	1,00	22. 2-hydroxy-4-methoxybenzophenone	2,00
7. Bithionol	1,00	23. 3-(4-methylbenzyliden)-Campher	5,00
8. Triclosan	2,00	24. 4-isopropyldibenzoylmethane	5,00
9. Sulfanilamide	5,00	25. •Cyclamate	1,25
10. Chlorpromazine	0,10	26. •Saccharin	0,40
11. Promethazine	1,00	27. •Wood tar	3,00
12. Carprofen	5,00	28. •Colophony	20,00
13. •Tiaprofenic acid	5,00	29. Balsam of Peru	25,00
14. Quinidine	1,00	30. Compositae Mix	6,50
15. Moschus Ambrette	5,00	31. •Tolbutamid	5,00
16. •Moschus Mix	5,00	32. •Thiourea	0,10

•Substances were discharged from the test tray in 1990, since they only caused a few or no relevant photo-reaction or since they are supposed to provoke a photoallergy via test procedure.

Table 3b. List of substances : Photopatch test 1991-1997

Substances	Concentrations (%)	Substances	Concentrations (%)
1. Tetrachlorosalicylanilide	0,10	15. Hydrochlorothiazide	1,00
2. Monobromsalicylchloranilide	1,00	16. Balsam of Peru	25,00
3. Tribromsalicylanilide	1,00	17. Compositae mix	6,50
4. Buclosamid	5,00	18. Paraaminobenzoic acid	
5. Fenticlor	1,00	19. 2-hydroxy-4-methoxybenzophenone	2,00
6. Hexachlorophene	1,00	20. 3-(4-methylbenzyliden)-campher	5,00
7. Bithionol	1,00	21. 4-isopropyldibenzoylmethane	10,00
8. Triclosan	2,00	22. •4-tert-butyl-4'methoxydibenzol-	
10. Chlorpromazine	0,10	methane	10,00
11. Promethazine	0,10	24. •2-ethylhexyl-p-methoxycinnamate	10,00
12. Carprofen	5,00	25. •Phenylbenzimidazolsulphonic acid	10,00
13. Chinidinsulfat	5,00	26. •p-methoxy-isoamyl-cinnamate	10,00
14. Moschus Ambrette	5,00		

•Substances newly integrated in the test tray in 1991.

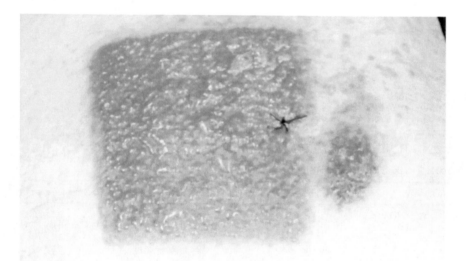

Fig. 6. Quinidine-induced photoallergy (positive test reaction after systemic provocation)

applied orally if possible twice the dose normally used. With consideration of the pharmacokinetics additional skin areas should be exposed subsequently to 10 J/cm² UVA, e.g. at 1, 2, 3, 5, 8, and 12 h after the drug application. The readings should be performed immediately, and 24, 48, and 72 h after first irradiation. An example of a positive photoreaction (after systemic quinidine application) is depicted in Figure 6 [59, 60].

Photosensitizing Agents

Although photoallergy might be a rare phenomenon, the diagnosis of chemically induced photoallergy is very important to prevent severe forms of chronic actinic dermatitis and to detect new photosensitizers. The increasing use of cosmetics and toilet items as well as the topical or systemic application of newly developed pharmaceutical products determine the potential risk for consumers to be exposed to unknown photosensitizers. An outstanding example was the epidemic appearance of a photoallergy due to tetrachlorosalicylanilide (TCSA), which had been used as disinfectant in soaps and other toilet items in England 1960–1993. Furthermore, moschus ambrette, a synthetic fragrance and preservative used worldwide in cosmetic products, is proved to be an important photosensitizer. Following the results of a Scandinavian multicenter study [62] moschus ambrette caused the highest rate of photosensitizations out of all test substances. Restrictive guidelines of the "International Fragrance Association" in 1985, concerning the use of moschus ambrette in cosmetics, led to a remarkable decrease of the photosensitization rate. Recently released photopatch test trays incorporate moschus ambrette only as a "historical photoallergen" [57].

The DAPT studies revealed that non-steroidal anti-inflammatory drugs, disinfectants, sunscreens, phenothiazines and fragrances contemporarily are the most relevant photosensitizers (Tables 4, 5).

Table 4. Ranking List of phototoxic reactions (1985-1990)

Substances	Frequencies (%)	Substances	Frequencies (%)
1. Tiaprofenic acid	30,41	6. Wood tar	5,16
2. Promethazine	21,33	7. Hexachlorophene	4,36
3. Carprofen	8,50	8. Balsam of Peru	3,38
4. Chlorpromazine	8,00	9. Fenticlor	3,29
5. Fragrance Mix	5,54	10. Triclosan	2,93

Table 5. Ranking List of photoallergic reactions (1985-1990)

Substances	Frequencies (%)	Substances	Frequencies (%)
1. Tiaprofenic acid	3,15	6. Promethazine	0,54
2. Fenticlor	1,60	7. Tetrachlorosalicylanilde	0,54
3. Carprofen	1,34	8. Moschus Ambrette	0,54
4. 4-isopropyldibenzoylmethane	0,89	9. Fragrance Mix	0,37
5. 2-hydroxi-4-methoxybenzo-phenone	0,71	10. Moschus Mix	0,36

In general, detected and proven photosensitizers will promptly be eliminated from the market, e.g. salicylanilides, musk ambrette, phenothiazines, triacetyldiphenolisantin, tetracycline derivatives as well as special non-steroidal anti-inflammatory drugs [54].

Besides these synthetic photosensitizers, there are also exogenous or endogenous natural phototoxic agents e.g. in plants: leguminaceae, moraceae, rotaceae and umbiliferae. Furthermore, porphyrins are important photosensitizers, which accumulate in several tissues and cells in case of distinct enzymatic defects, leading to clinical relevant phototoxic skin reactions if irradiated with UV light [38, 51].

Predictive Test Procedures

Concerning the risk evaluation of contact allergic or contact irritant reactions, the OECD recommended several test systems (e.g. Buehler's test, optimization test, guinea pig test, mouse ear swelling test, local lymph node assay) [28, 53]. Although official guidelines for the risk assessment of the phototoxic potency of newly developed substances are still lacking, the European Community demanded procedures to determine the potential photoallergic and phototoxic risk of skin care products in 1997[1]. Since UV-absorbing filters (if applied to the skin and irradiated subsequently with UV light) are able to cause severe phototoxic and photoallergic reactions, the authorities especially requested procedures for the safety assessment of sunscreens. Moreover, almost simultaneously they appealed to abandon animal testing.

A variety of biological systems were employed to evaluate phototoxicity. In general, phototoxic effects can be investigated by in vitro or in vivo test procedures (Table 6).

Table 6. In vitro test systems for phototoxicity

- Photohemolysis-test with erythrocytes
- Photo-basophils-histamin-releasing test
- Fibroblasts-indol-red-uptake test
- Candida albicans-inhibition test
- Paramecium aurelia-lethality test
- Photo Hen's Egg Test

In 1900, initial studies to investigate photosensitizers were performed by Raab using freshwater ciliate protozoans (paramecia) [55]. Since then this model has been employed by numerous investigators. The paramecia test procedure is inexpensive and relatively easy to perform and, therefore, may serve as a phototoxicity model for large test series.

Another phototoxicity test procedure based on Candida albicans was introduced by Daniels in 1965 [2]. He exposed Candida albicans on Sabouraud´s medium to a photosensitizer and UVA as a screening model for phototoxicity. Based on the phototoxic inhibition of growth, the Candida albicans test is a very simple, inexpensive, and effective method, which was especially useful in testing the phototoxic properties of psoralen [14, 31]. However, the well-known phototoxic agents sulfanilamide and demethylchlortetracycline elicited no phototoxic reactions in the "Candida inhibition test system."

In 1909 Hasselbach investigated photohemolysis using dyes. Erythrocytes are cells with no nucleus or cytoplasmatic organelles. Thus, erythrocytes provide the opportunity to investigated cell membrane damages caused by phototoxicity [27]. The experimental conditions are inexpensive and easy to perform. Induction of photohemolysis of 5% indicates a phototoxic reaction. Erythrocytes received from one individual only and exposure to a phototoxic agent showed a wide range of different results. So, pooled erythrocytes gained from different individuals are necessary for

---

[1] Commission of the European Communities, Scientific Committee on Cosmetology, 6th Amendment to the Cosmetics Directive (EC); Guidelines for Safety Assessment of a Cosmetic Product 1997

testing. However, well known potent phototoxic substances (e.g. psoralen) elicited no adequate phototoxic reaction in this test system.

Further in vitro test systems are based on cell cultures to test phototoxic agents [10, 43]. Gained from healthy skin samples, fibroblasts have to be cultured up to confluency or keratinocytes until multilayers will be developed. The highest nontoxic concentration of a test chemical has to be added to cell cultures for an incubation period of 24 hours. Afterwards, some cell cultures are additionally exposed to UVA light. As controls serve cell cultures incubated only with the test chemical without additionally applied UVA irradiation and cell cultures irradiated only with UVA light alone. Subsequently, after an incubation period of 24 hours, the morphological changes of the cells have to be analyzed microscopically, and the cell viability can be detected e.g. via neutral red uptake-assay [41a]. The results obtained by this in vitro test procedure correlated excellent with the in vivo data and were good reproducible. Taking these findings into account, the Scientific Committee on Cosmetic and Non-Food Products (SCCNFP) suggested the neutral red uptake-assay (3T3 NRU PT) as a standard test procedure to test UV light absorbing cosmetics ingredients in 1998 [1a].

The Photo Hen's Egg Test

In search of photobiological test systems more advanced than cell cultures [10] but replacing animal models, Neumann et al. developed the extra embryonal vasculature of the incubated hen's egg in combination with UV irradiation as a screening model for phototoxicity of different chemicals [50, 52]. A similar test was originally introduced by toxicologists as a screening model for mucocutaneous toxicity as an alternative to the Draize test [3] (rabbit's eye test) [4, 56].

First, a nontoxic effect level of the test substance and a nontoxic UVA-dose have to be defined. Therefore, the first step of the photo hen's egg test (PHET) is similar to the classic hen's egg test. Preliminary studies showed that 5 J/cm^2 UVA do not induce any visible pathological effects on the yolk sac blood vessel system (YS).

The second part of the PHET has a 2×2 factorial test design with the factors "irradiation" and "substance application" and the levels "yes" and "no."

During a period of 24 h, the following parameters were evaluated: embryolethality, membrane discoloration and hemorrhage (Fig. 7-9, Table 7).

Fertile white Leghorn eggs (Shaver Starcross 288 A, Lohmann, Cuxhaven, Germany) were incubated in a horizontal position using a commercial incubator at 37.5°C and 65% relative humidity. After 3 days of incubation, all eggs were candled in order to discard those that were defect. Without damaging the shell membrane a hole was drilled into the shell, through which 5 ml of egg white were sucked out to lower the embryo and its surrounding YS. Afterwards a 1.5×2.5 cm window was sawn out of the

Table 7. Photo hen's egg test classification of membran discoloration (MD) and hemorrhage (HE)

Level 0 (no)	No visible MD / HE
Level 1 (slight)	Just visible MD / HE
Level 2 (moderate)	Visible MD / HE, structures are covered partially
Level 3 (severe)	Visible MD / HE, structures are covered totally

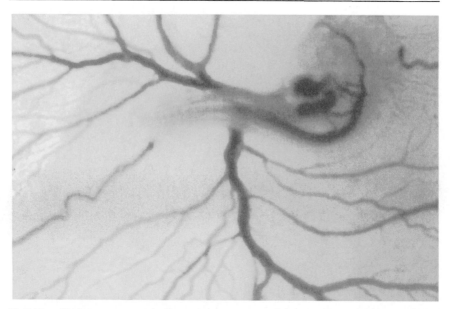

Fig. 7. Photo hen's egg test. Normal yolk sac blood vessel system (YS) at day 3 of incubation

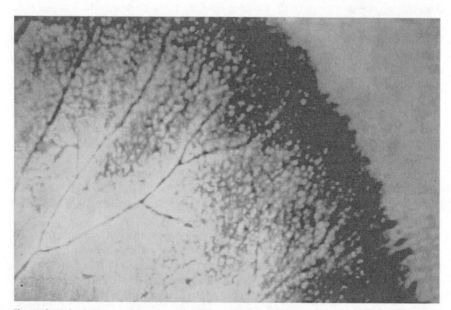

Fig. 8. Photo hen's egg test. Severe hemorrhage 24 h after application of 8-MOP and 5 J/cm^2 UVA irradiation

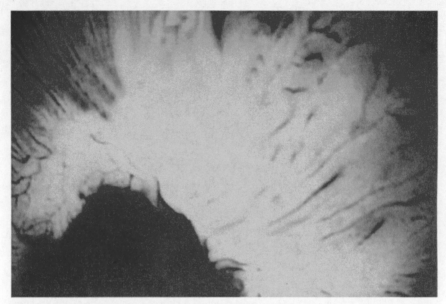

Fig. 9. Photo hen's egg test. Membrane discoloration 24 h after application of promethazine and 5 J/cm² UVA irradiation

shell. The eggs were covered with a wax sheet and placed back into the incubator. At day 4 of incubation, only eggs with normally developed embryos and blood vessel systems were used for testing.

Since we are interested in plain phototoxic reactions, in the PHET the embryo´s yolk sac blood vessel system is exposed to a proven nontoxic concentration of a test substance and to a nontoxic UVA dose simultaneously.

At day 4 of the incubation period, group 1 (each group consisted of 12 eggs) is exposed to a test substance, immediately followed by an irradiation with 5 J/cm² UVA (320–400 nm, Philips TL 09/40 W, Hamburg, Germany). Isotonic sodium chloride solution (NaCl) is normally used as vehicle. Serving as controls, two additional groups are exposed only to NaCl and 5 J/cm² UVA or to NaCl or to the test substance alone. Readings are performed 24 h after irradiation. During this observation period, the morphological parameters such as membrane discoloration (MD), hemorrhage (HR) [monitored and graded following a four point scale using a macroscope (M 420, Leitz, Wetzlar, Germany)] and the embryo lethality are assessed.

The test parameters MD and HR as well as embryo lethality can be summarized in a morphology and lethality index (Table 8). Employing these indices, the relative phototoxic potential of an assumed photosensitizer compared to other well known photosensitizers are easily to obtain. 8-Methoxypsoralen (8-MOP), a classic severe phototoxic substance (with no known photoallergic potential) is the leading phototoxic agent. On the other side, olaquindox, a well-known photoallergen, revealed no phototoxic effect in the PHET (Table 9).

Table 8. Photo hen's egg test factors

Relative lethality factor:	lethality rate of the interaction group (Li) minus the average lethality rate of controls $LC = (l_{c1}+l_{c2}+l_{c3}) / 3$ rel. lethality factor $L = L_i-L_c$ rel. lethality factor $L (\%) = \dfrac{L \times 100}{12}$
Relative morphology factor:	sum of the morphological gradings (m+h) from the interaction group (Mi) minus the sum of the avarage morphological gradings (m+h) of controls (Mc). $M_c = [(m_{c1}+h_{c1})+(m_{c2}+h_{c2})+(m_{c3}+h_{c3})] / 3$ rel. morphology factor $M = M_i-M_c$ rel. morphology factor $M (\%) = \dfrac{M \times 100}{12}$
Test period:	24 hours after substance application

Table 9. Phototoxicity-Ranking list based on the photo hen's egg test

Substances	Rel. Lethality factor (%)	Rel. Morphology factor (%)
1. 8-MOP	100,00	67,60
2. Promethazine	94,50	54,64
3. Protoporphyrine IX	94,50	64,82
4. Sparfloxacin	58,33	50,90
5. Acridine	58,33	49,54
6. TCSA	44,50	32,42
7. Hematoporphyrine	41,67	58,81
8. Lomefloxacin	30,58	35,67
9. Ciprofloxacin	0,00	62,50
10. Tetracyclin	0,00	2,79
11. Olaquindox	< 0	< 0

In summary, the PHET is an easily and quickly to perform test procedure, which represents an inexpensive, valid new screening model for phototoxicity, helping to reduce animal tests.

But focused on immunological sensitizing properties of photosensitizers, we assume, that animal tests cannot be replaced. Therefore, the UV-depended lymph node test (UV-LLNA) is proven to be an excellent test procedure.

In order to investigate the photoallergenicity of chemicals in the 1960s erythema tests with an induction and a challenge phase (in vivo test systems) were developed [64]. The erythema tests were later improved with special pre-treatments, leading to increased penetration rates, higher immunological reactivity, and a better photosensitivity of the skin. These pretreatments included: mechanical skin irritation (brushing), injection of an adjuvant (e.g. Freund's adjuvant), or application of irritants (e.g. natriumlaurylsulfat). Using these improved test systems, even very weak photoallergens were detected. On the other hand, these techniques are very laborious, time consuming (up to 63 days) and expensive [42, 44]. Moreover, large numbers of animals are needed and subjective criteria are used to classify test reactions (erythema scores).

The first test system based on objective criteria was the MEST, the "mouse ear swelling test" [11–13]. A relatively short test period (8 days), a low number of animals, and an objective test parameter (the thickness of the ear) are major advantages of the MEST. Unfortunately, the ear swelling test is unspecific, and does not provide a differentiation between phototoxic and photoallergic reactions.

The UV-dependent Lymph Node Assay

Recently, a local lymph node assay (LLNA) was described as a predictive assay for identifying the contact sensitizing potential of chemicals in mice [29,30]. In comparison with the widely used Buehler's occluded patch test [1] and other guinea pig test data [39–41, 63], the LLNA is proved to be a rapid and cost effective alternative method for the detection of at least moderate to strong contact sensitizers. In contrast to guinea pig models and the mouse ear swelling test (MEST), the LLNA is based upon the detection of a primary immune response as a function of auricular lymph node activation following topical application of chemicals on the dorsal surface of ears. Mainly in vivo ^{3}[H]-thymidine incorporation was measured as a function of LNC proliferation and activation. Recently we described a modified LLNA based on the detection of increases in lymph node weight and cell counts as a non-radioactive alternative to the original LLNA. Furthermore, additional UVA irradiation allowed the identification of photoreactive compounds [65].

Although the LLNA was first described to selectively detect allergic skin immune responses, recent studies showed that (photo)irritant test compounds also induce lymph node cell proliferation in vivo [18–21, 48, 58, 61, 64].

Previous studies showed that optimal sensitization and hapten-induced activation of skin-draining lymph node cells were obtained after sensitizer treatment on 3 consecutive days [11, 29, 64]. Therefore, 5 female NMRI mice per group were topically treated on the dorsal surfaces of both ears with 25 µl of photoallergic (e.g. TCSA) or phototoxic (e.g. 8-MOP) standards or vehicle alone on three consecutive days. For the induction of photocontact allergy and photoirritancy, mice were irradiated with 10 J/cm^2 UVA immediately after topical treatment. On day 0 and day 3, ear thickness was measured using a spring-loaded micrometer (Oditest; Kroeplin, Schluechtern, Germany) and mean ear swelling was calculated. Furthermore, mice were sacrificed and auricular lymph nodes from each animal were removed and pooled (for each individual mouse) on day 3. Lymph node cell proliferation was determined after automatic counting of lymph node cells per mouse (Coulter Counter ZM, Coulter, Heidelberg, Germany) and calculation of lymph node cell count indices. Lymph node cell count indices (LN index) were defined as the ratio of mean lymph node cell counts from mice treated with the test compound to corresponding results of vehicle-treated control groups. Positive test reactions were defined as either significant ear swelling or significant increase in lymph node cell counts.

The principle findings concerning the differentiation of photoallergic and phototoxic skin reactions are as follows:

1. Photocontact allergens as well as photoirritants induce skin-draining lymph node cell activation

2. Photoirritants predominantly induce skin inflammation which in turn induces draining lymph node proliferation
3. Induction of photocontact allergy causes only marginal skin inflammation, but a vigorous activation of skin-draining lymph nodes.

Referring to the mechanisms of phototoxic and photoallergic skin reactions, the results of the LLNA show that the development of an integrated model may provide accurate criteria to distinguish between a phototoxic and photoallergic potential of a compound by comparing local draining lymph node activation with skin inflammation.

In this context, validation studies with both LLNA and MEST have resulted in recognition from the OECD. These tests have been classified to be suitable for screening chemicals for sensitizing activity as the first stage of an assessment process. Chemicals may be designated as potential photosensitizers if a positive response is recorded in these assays.

In conclusion, the modified LLNA provides a non-radioactive method to differentiate between chemical-induced allergic and irritant skin reactions. Compared with guinea pig tests this model is objective and measures immunological relevant end points, is markedly less expensive, less vivarium space is required, the duration of the test is shorter (4 days), less test substance is utilized, and colored materials may be tested [11, 12, 30]. Furthermore, the monophasic treatment protocol offers the chance to skip the assessment of minimal phototoxic or maximal non-irritant doses of a test compound.

References

1a. Anon. (1998) Statement on the scientific validity of the 3T3 NRU PT test (an in vitro test for phototoxic potential). ATLA 26:7-8
1. Bühler EV (1965) Delayed contact hypersensitivity in the guinea pig. Arch Dermatol 91:171
2. Daniels F (1965) A simple microbiological method for demonstrating phototoxic compounds. J Invest Dermatol 44:259-263
3. Draize HJ (1959)Intracutaneous sensitization test on guinea pigs. In: Apraisal of the Safety of Chemicals in Food, Drugs and Cosmetics. Association of Food and Drug Officials of the United States, Austin, Texas
4. Duffy PA (1989) Irritancy testing-a cultured approach. Toxic In Vitro 3:157-158
5. Enk AH, Katz SI (1995) Contact sensitivity as a model for T-cell activation in skin J Invest Dermatol 105:80
6. Epstein S (1939) Photoallergy and primary photosensitivity to sulfanilamide. J Invest Dermatol 2:43-51
7. Epstein S (1963) "Masked" photopatch tests. J Dermatol 41:369-370
8. Epstein S (1964) The photopatch test. Its technique, manifestations, and significance Ann Allergy 22:1-11
9. Epstein S (1966) Simplified photopatch testing. Arch Dermatol 93:216-220
10. Freeman RG, Murtishaw W, Knox JM (1970) Tissue culture techniques in the study of cell photobiology and phototoxicity. J Invest Dermatol 54:164-169
11. Gad SC (1994) The mouse ear swelling test (MEST) in the 1990s. Toxicology 93:33
12. Gad SC, Dunn BJ, Dobbs DW, Reilly C, Walsh RD (1986) Development and validation of an alternative dermal sensitization test: the mouse ear swelling test (MEST). Toxicol Appl Pharmacol 84:93
13. Gerberick GF, Ryan CA (1990) A predictive mouse ear swelling model for investigating topical photoallergy. Food Chem Toxicol 28 (5):361
14. Gibbs NK (1987) An adaption of the Candida albicans phototoxicity test to demonstrate photosensitizer action spectra. Photodermatol 4:312-316

15. Hölzle E, Neumann N, Hausen B, Przybilla B, Schauder S, Hönigsmann H, Bircher A, Plewig G (1991) Photopatch testing: The 5-year experience of the German, Austrian, and Swiss Photopatch Test Group J Am Acad Dermatol 25:59-68
16. Hölzle E, Plewig G, Hofmann C, Braun-Falco O (1985) Photopatch testing. Results of a survey on test procedures and experimental findings. Zbl Hautkr 151:361-366
17. Hölzle E, Plewig G, Lehmann P (1987) Photodermatoses - diagnostic procedures and their interpretation. Photodermatol Photoimmunol Photomed 4: 109-114
18. Homey B, Neubert T, Arens A, Schuppe HC, Vohr HW, Ruzicka T, Lehmann P (1997) Sunscreen and Immunosuppression. J Invest Dermatol 109:395
19. Homey B, Schuppe HC, Assmann T, Vohr HW, Lauerma AI, Ruzicka T, Lehmann P (1997) A local lymph node assay to analyse immunosuppressive effects of topically applied drugs. Eur J Pharmacol 325:199
20. Homey B, Vohr HW, Schuppe HC, Kind P (1995) UV-dependent local lymph node reactions: photoallergy and phototoxicity testing. In Curr Probl Dermatol eds. C. Surber, P. Elsner, A.L. Bircher 22:44
21. Ikarashi Y, Tsukamoto Y, Tsuchiya T, Nakamura A (1993) Influence of irritants on lymph node cell proliferation and the detection of contact sensitivity to metal salts in the murine local lymph node assay. Contact Dermatitis 29:128
22. Jansén CT, Wennerstein G, Rystedt I, Thune P, Brodthagen H (1982)The Scandinavian standard photopatch test procedure. Contact Dermatitis 8:155-158
23. Jung EG (1974) Die photoallergische Testung. Ther Umsch 31:313-316
24. Jung EG (1979) In vitro-Untersuchungen zur Chlorpromazin (CPZ)-Photoallergie. Arch Klin Exp Dermatol 237:501-506
25. Jung EG (1980) Photoallergien. Zbl Hautkr 144:169-176
26. Jung EG (1981) Die belichtete Epikutantestung. Akt Dermatol:163-165
27. Kahn G, Fleischaker B (1971)Evaluation of phototoxicity of salicylanilides and similar compounds by photohemolysis. J Invest Dermatol 56:91-97
28. Kaidbey KH, Kligman AM (1980) Photomaximization test for identifying photoallergic contact sensitizers. Contact Dermatitis 6:161-169
29. Kimber I, Dearman RJ, Scholes EW, Basketter DA (1994)The local lymph node assay: developments and applications. Toxicology 93:13
30. Kimber I, Weisenberger C (1989) A murine local lymph node assay for the identification of contact allergenes. Assay development and results of initial validation study. Arch Toxicol 63:274
31. Knudson EA (1985) The Candida phototoxicity test. The sensitivity of different strains of Candida, standardization attempts and analysis of the dose-response curves for 5- and 8-methoxypsoralen. Photodermatol 2:80-85
32. Lehmann P (1990) Die deutschsprachige Arbeitsgemeinschaft Photopatch-Test (DAPT). Hautarzt 41: 295-297
33. Lehmann P (1992) Photodiagnostische Testverfahren in der Dermatologie. In: Macher E, Kolde G, Bröcker B (Hrsg) Jahrbuch der Dermatologie 1992/1993, Biermann Verlag, Zülpich, 81-100
34. Lehmann P (1993) Principles of photo testing and photopatch testing: A European perspective. Retinoids Today and Tomorrow 31: 36-42
35. Lehmann P (1997) Principles of photo testing and photopatch testing. In: P. Altmeyer, K. Hoffmann, M. Stücker (Eds.): Skin Cancer and UV Radiation, Springer-Verlag Berlin Heidelberg
36. Lehmann P, Hölzle E, Plewig G (1988) Photoallergie auf Neotri mit Kreuzreaktion auf Teneretic Nachweis durch systemische Photoprovokation. Hautarzt 39: 38-41
37. Lehmann P, Hölzle E, von Kries R, Plewig G (1986)Übersicht - Neue Konzepte. Lichtdiagnostische Verfahren bei Patienten mit Verdacht auf Photodermatosen. Zbl Hautkr 152:667-682
38. Lehmann P, Scharfetter K, Kind P, Goerz G (1991) Erythropoetische Protoporphyrie: Synopsis von 20 Patienten. Hautarzt 42:570-574
39. Magnusson B, Kligman AM (1969) The identification of contact allergens by animal assay. The guinea pig maximization test. J Invest Dermatol 52:268
40. Maguire HC (1973)The bioassay of contact allergens in the guinea pig. J Soc Cosmet Chem 24:51
41. Maguire HC, Chase Jr and MW (1972) Studies of the sensitization of animals with simple chemical compounds. 13. Sensitization of guinea pigs with picric acid. J Exp Med 135:357
41a. Maier K, Schmitt-Landgraf R, Siegmund B (1991) Development of an in vitro test system with human skin cells for evaluation of phototoxity. Toxicol in vitro: 5/6, 457-461
42. Maurer T (1986) Experimentelle Modelle des photoallergischen Ekzems. Allergologie 9:3-7
43. Maurer T (1987) Phototoxicity testing - in vivo and in vitro. Fd Chem Toxic 25:407-414
44. Maurer T, Thomann P, Weirich EG, Hess R (1975) The optimization test in the guinea pig. Agents and Actions 5:174
45. Maurer T, Weirich EG, Hess R (1980)The optimization test in the guinea pig in relation to other predictive sensitization methods. Toxicology 15(3):163-171

46. Maurer T, Weirich EG, Hess R (1980)Photokontaktallergie. Zur Epidemiologie und prädiktiven tierexperimentellen Erfassung. Derm Beruf Umwelt 28:70-81

47. McKenzie RC, Sauder DN (1990) The role of keratinocyte cytokines in inflammation and immunity. J Invest Dermatol 95:105

48. Moissen P Yu CL, Ziff M (1984) Lymphocyte chemotactic activity of human interleukin-1. J Immunol 133:2007

49. Neumann NJ, Fritsch C, Goerz G, Ruzicka T, Lehmann P (1997) d-Aminolevulinic Acid in the Photo Hen's Egg Test. Arch Dermatol Res 289 (suppl): A49

50. Neumann NJ, Hölzle E, Lehmann P, Benedikter S, Tapernoux B, Plewig G. (1994) Pattern analysis of photopatch test reactions. Photodermatol Photoimmunol Photomed 10(2):65-73

51. Neumann NJ, Hölzle E, Lehmann P, Rosenbruch M, Klaucic A, Plewig G (1997) Photo hen's egg test: A model for phototoxicity. Br J Dermatol 136:326-330

52. Neumann NJ, Klaucic A, Hölzle A, Lehmann P (1995)Evaluation of the phototoxic potential of ciprofloxacin in the phot hen's egg test. Arch Dermatol Res 287:384

53. OECD (Organisation for Economic Cooperation and Development) (1992) Guideline 406 for Testing Chemicals. Adopted 1992

54. Przybilla B, Schwab-Przybilla U, Ruzicka T, Ring J (1987)Phototoxicity of non-steroidal anti-inflammatory drugs demonstrated in vitro by a photo-basophil-histamine-release test. Photodermatol 4:73-78

55. Raab O (1900)Über die Wirkung flourescierender Stoffe auf Infusorien. Z Biol 39:524-546

56. Rosenbruch M (1990) Toxizitätsuntersuchungen am bebrüteten Hühnerei. Derm Beruf Umwelt 38:5-11

57. Rünger TM, Lehmann P, Neumann NJ, Matthies C, Schauder S, Ortel B, Münzberger C, Hölzle E (1995) Empfehlung einer Photopatch-Test Standardreihe durch die deutschsprachige Arbeitsgruppe "Photopatch-Test". Hautarzt 46:240-243

58. Schilling C, Homey B, Ruzicka T, Lehmann P, Schuppe HC, Vohr HW (1996) Characterization of the induction phase of contact hypersensitivity in murine epidermal and local draining lymph node cells. J Eur Acad Dermatol Venerol 7:A37

59. Schürer NY, Hölzle E, Plewig G, Lehmann P (1992)Photosensitivity induced by quinidine sulfate: experimental reproduction of skin lesions. Photodermatol Photoimmunol Photomed 9: 78-82

60. Schürer NY, Lehmann P, Plewig G (1991)Chinidininduzierte Photoallergie. Eine klinische und experimentelle Studie. Hautarzt 42: 158-161

61. Shivji GM, Gupta AK, Suder DR (1994)Role of cytokines in irritant contact dermatitis. In: Alternative Methods in Toxicology Series, Volume 10: In Vitro Skin Toxicology: Irritation Phototoxicity, Sensitization. A. Rougier, A.M. Goldberg, H.I. Maibach, eds. Mary Ann Liebert, Inc., Publishers, New York, NY, 13-21

62. Thune A, Jansén C, Wennersten G, Rystedt I, Brodthagen H, McFadden N (1988) The Scandinavian multicenter photopatch study 1980-1985: final report. Photodermatology 5:261-269

63. Vinson LJ, Borselli VF (1966) A guinea pig assay of photosensitizing potential of topical germicides. J Soc Cosmet Chem 17:123

64. Vinson LJ, Borselli VF, Singer EF (1968) Realistic methods for determining photosenzitization potential of topical agents. Amer Perfum Cosmet 83:37

65. Vohr HW., Homey B., Schuppe H.C., Kind P (1994) Detection of photoreactivity demonstrated in a modified local lymph node assay in mice. Photodermatol Photoimmunol Photomed: 10, 57-64

CHAPTER 23

Comedogenesis

C. Piérard–Franchimont, G.E. Piérard

Introduction

Comedogenesis refers to the abnormal differentiation with excessive cornification of the follicular infundibulum that results in the formation of a horny plug called microcomedo [1]. Clinical comedones evolve from precomedones and microcomedones, the initial stage being visible only at the microscopic level. Among the distinct types of pilosebaceous units, both the sebaceous follicle and the vellus follicle are prone to comedogenesis. Such abnormality may affect a limited number of follicles, but it may also involve the vast majority of them in certain areas of the body.

The abnormal cornification affects the acroinfundibulum corresponding to the upper one-fifth of the duct and/or the infrainfundibulum corresponding to the lower four-fifths. Both parts of the duct are lined with keratinizing epithelium continuous with the overlying epidermis. It is striking that the typical follicular hypercornification of comedones is almost never associated with interadnexal hyperkeratinization of the epidermis.

Acnegenesis and comedogenesis are two distinct types of skin reactions that are frequently confused with each other. Acnegenesis is a term suggesting that lesions are inflammatory and look similar to those of acne. In fact, two distinct and unrelated situations have been called acnegenesis. On the one hand, this term is applied to a micropustular folliculitis which appears in a matter of days following applications of the offending agent. In such a situation, comedones are absent and lesions are unrelated with acne but rather reflect some follicular toxicity and irritation. By contrast, true acnegenesis should refer to a real induction or flare up of acne. The time course for such a reaction is much longer than for the induction of pustular folliculitis. It takes weeks to occur.

Clinical Presentation

Chloracne of industrial and agricultural origins is a typical disease caused by chemical comedogenesis and acnegenesis. It is of outstanding medical importance because many of the offending agents are also hepatotoxic. The disease is caused by chlorinated aromatic hydrocarbons, in particular chlorinated dioxines (tetrachlorodibenzodioxine), which are the most potent acnegenic agents [2–4]. The epidemiological pattern of chloracne has changed much since the first cases occurred in the early years of the twentieth century. The most typical chloracnegens are listed in Table 1. Lesions almost similar to chloracne were reported following contacts with fluoride toothpastes [5].

Table 1. Chloracnegens

Chloronaphthalenes (CNs)
Polychlorinated dibenzofurans (PCDFs)
Contaminants of chlorophenols
  2,3,7,8-Tetrachlorodibenzo-*p*-dioxin (TCDD)
  Hexachlorodibenzo-*p*-dioxin
  Tetrachlorodibenzofuran
Chlorobenzenes
  Crude trichlorobenzene
  Crude benzene hexachloride
  3,4,3',4' Tetrachlorozoxybenzene

Oil acne is now very uncommon. It resulted from the skin contact with insoluble cutting oils which were impure paraffin-oil mixtures used in the engineering industry. Nowadays, crude petroleum is still acnegenic in oilfield and refinery workers. Contacts with a variety of other chemicals have also been reported uncommonly as a cause of industrial acne. They include DDT, heavy coal-tar, especially pitch and creosote, asbestos and heavy water distillate.

The description of acne cosmetica induced by cosmetics goes back to the end of the Second World War in France [6–8]. Comedones predominated on the face of subjects using poorly purified brilliantine. Twenty-five years later, pomade acne was reported in American Blacks applying capillary creams and vegetable oils on their skin [9]. A similar problem arose in other communities as a consequence of applications of white petrolatum [10]. Such induced acne is still prevalent in India and in many countries of Black Africa. The salts of fatty acids in conventional soaps also proved to be acnegenic when used extensively [11]. It is noteworthy that cosmetic products available to the public of Western countries are for the most part noncomedogenic [12, 13]. However, comedogenicity related to personal care products remains of great concern for the cosmetic industry [14, 15]. Nowadays, cosmetics are not identified as a major reason for the persistence of acne in adults. Nevertheless, the assumption that these agents are the cause of adult acne [12] may be valid in some regions of the world where local production of skin care products may contain ingredients which prove to be strongly comedogenic or acnegenic. Switching to reputed noncomedogenic cosmetics helps but does not however bring about rapid clinical changes.

Patterns of Follicular Cornification

The mechanism of comedo formation is still disputed and is not necessarily identical in all cases. The transformation of a normal infundibulum into a precomedo, a microcomedo and a comedo is a continuous process with no sharp definition. It is important to appreciate that these steps in comedogenesis do not inevitably evolve in full blown clinical lesions. In fact, they do not since precomedones are common in subjects with seborrhea and rosacea without, however, exhibiting comedones.

During maturation of the sebaceous duct and infundibulum, cornified material is progressively shed in the lumen. Cells from the deepest part of the sebaceous follicule are inevitably pushed toward the central axis of the duct during their ascent toward the skin surface. Cornified cells from upper portion of the duct progressively encase the material originating from below.

The basic defect in comedogenesis is thought to be a decreased dehiscence of corneocytes inside the follicular infundibulum. Precomedones are made of an outer envelope of compacted corneocytes originating from the infundibulum, encasing a softish amalgam of sloughed empty sebocytes and flimsy corneocytes from the sebaceous duct. Such material glides with little resistance in the duct towards the follicular opening. With progressive accumulation of cells near the acroinfundibulum, the precomedo has a cone shape with a deep tapering end.

Microcomedones represent a stage through which the sebaceous follicles pass on their way to comedo formation. The key change is the marked increase in cohesion between corneocytes of the infrainfundibulum and/or acro-infundibulum. The infrainfundibulum alone or in conjonction with the acroinfundibulum is the major target of endogenous comedogenesis as seen in acne. The acroinfundibulum represents the main target of exogenous (chemical) acne. The spontaneous outward glide of microcomedones is apparently slow allowing the accumulation of corneocytes through the cell production in the infundibulum. At the stage of comedones, the cornified material sticks firmly to the infundibular wall and forms a solid compact mass which steadily expands. It exhibits an exceedingly slow outward move before being eroded away.

Both microcomedones and comedones may exhibit three distinct shapes. They have a cone shape with a narrow base when the acroinfundibulum is primarily involved in retention hyperkatosis. They have a bulky base and a narrow tip when the infrainfundibulum is the kernel of the matter. They become more cylindrical as the orifice dilates during the slow protrusion of the deep comedo.

At the base of comedones, the sebaceous lobules shrink but usually continue to secrete sebum which streams through tortuous channels inside the horny mass [16]. The retention of the cornified material enriched with lipids allows the entraping of microorganisms within the core of microcomedones and comedones.

It should be emphasized that comedogenesis affects usually a minority of follicles on a given area of skin. Startling comedogenesis is often due to exogenous and chemical exposures.

Biological Aspects of Endogenous Comedogenesis

During comedognesis, corneocytes of the infundibulum remain tied together. Keratinosomes are numerous in the normal infrainfundibulum and have been reported to decrease when comedones form. As a result, the tight cohesion of corneocytes through corneosomes fails to loose and prevent the cells to slough normally [17, 18]. The upper follicular epithelium may be also the site of increased cell proliferation in comedones [19, 20]. In addition, apparently normal follicles of acne-prone patients exhibit increased cell proliferation compared with those of areas of skin unaffected by acne. Hence, both processes characterized by increased production and retention of epithelial cells may contribute to the comedo formation. Desmosomal proteins and keratin expression are unlikely altered in the hypercornification [21, 22].

It is the better part of wisdom not to offer any other biologic explanation for comedogenesis. However, several hypotheses have been lauched to further explain the origin of the disturbed process of corneocyte dehiscence. It seems likely that several distinct pathomechanisms may be involved in endogenous and exogenous comedogenesis.

One of the mechanisms responsible for endogenous comedogenesis may be androgen-mediated. The type I isozyme of 5α-reductase has been reported to be more active in infrainfundibular keratinocytes than in the epidermis [23]. The data suggest that the infundibulum has the capacity to metabolize and respond to androgens locally. Whether such production affects follicular keratinization remains to be determined.

Other hypotheses linking comedogenesis with the sebum content has been put forward for many years. Free fatty acids, which are derived almost exclusively from the hydrolysis of sebum triglycerides by microbial lipases, were felt to be themselves comedogenic [24, 25]. As other candidates, squalene and its peroxides have also been implicated as a possible cause of comedogenicity [26, 27]. Experimental data yielded a good correation between lipid peroxide levels and the size of comedones [28]. Ultraviolet irradiation was shown to enhance the capacity of human sebum and squalene to produce comedones [29]. Thus, if excess of some sebum components are in any way involved in comedogenesis, free fatty acids and squalene appeared to be less comedogenic than their peroxides. These hypotheses are, however, weakened by the fact that the amount of such sebum components needed to elicit a response in the rabbit ear model exceeds what exists normally in sebum [30]. No firm support of these hypotheses has developed recently. Hence, there have been no accepted mechanisms that relate excess of comedogenic lipids to human comedogenesis.

Still another hypothesis linking sebum production and comedogenesis was put forward implicating an essential fatty acid deficiency in the comedo-forming epithelial cells. Evidence was brought two decades ago that patients with acne had lower levels of linoleic acid in sebum than normal [31]. An inverse relationship between the sebum output and the linoleate content at the skin surface was also shown [32–35]. Although a systemic deficiency of linoleic acid was not proposed as a comedogenic factor in acne, it seemed possible that the effects of the local deficiency might be operative. In fact, the linoleate content of sebum depends on the amount of linoleic acid present in each sebocyte and on the extent to which this initial charge is diluted by the subsequent synthesis of sebum in each sebocyte and by the elevated sebum flow. The linoleate deficient sebum thus produced could impose a relative essential fatty acid deficiency on the cells of the follicular epithelium [32–35]. The keratinization of the infundibulum should then be disturbed resulting in formation of comedones.

Proinflammatory Cytokines in Ex Vivo Comedogenesis

It has been shown in experimental comedogenesis that infundibula isolated by microdissection respond in vitro to IL-1 by entering premature and terminal differentiation [36]. As a result, hypercornification appeared similar to that seen in comedones. IL-1α had not any effect on the expression of ICAM-1 while IFN-γ, IL-6 and TNF-α stimulated the expression of ICAM-1. TGF-α caused a disorganisation of the keratinocytes of the infundibulum that resulted in rupturing similar to that seen in inflammatory acne.

Experimental Comedogenesis in the Animal : the Rabbit Ear Model

The rabbit ear has long served as a model for assaying comedogenic materials [1, 8, 37–51]. Despite some obvious benefits accrued through the test, various barriers to its acceptance were raised regarding the value of hazard prediction and risk assessment. In fact, validation was not obtained because both the reliability and relevance of the model were not firmly established.

The rabbit ear model yields comparative data between products. However, no correlation with the human skin reactivity could be proven. On review of the available data, it is evident that the results have been subject to protocol variability. Different investigators have reported different results with the use of the same material [1, 49]. Discrepancies appeared to arise when visual inspection alone, even through a stereomicroscope, was used to rate the reaction. In fact, it was difficult to distinguish true comedogenesis from post-inflammatory follicular hyperkeratosis in the rabbit ear model. Hence, the comedogenic and irritating potentials of products were not always clearly interpreted. With increasing consumer concern about testing on animals, this model is no more available to most companies for developing cosmetics and other personal care products.

Assessment of Spontaneous and Induced Comedogenesis in Humans

The clinical assessment of acnegenicity may prove to be difficult [52]. Apart from the ethical objections towards the use of animals there is also a scientific viewpoint in criticizing the heavy reliance on animal data in comedogenesis. Important sources of incertainty can be found in qualitative and quantitative differences between physiological processes in the rabbit ear and human face.

Several human comedogenic assays have been proposed in the literature [53–55]. These new methods are still in a non-regulatory phase of development, only driven by information of scientific researchers. They await for validation and acceptance into regulatory practice. There are basically two main designs according to the body site choosen for the assay. Open or occlusive applications of products are made once daily or on alternate days for 4 to 6 weeks on the upper back. In our experience, thighs might be more prone to comedogenesis than the back. The other modality consists of an in-use test whereby panelists apply twice daily a cosmetic product to the face for at least two months.

Human comedogenic assays are often combined with objective quantitative assessments. The most popular relies on harvesting cyanoacrylate skin strippings [30, 56, 57] followed by digital image analysis of the follicular casts [54]. The system is non-biased and allows for the mathematical treatment of results. The same material illuminated under the microscope with ultraviolet light (400 nm) reveals the fluorescence of porphyrins produced by bacteria colonizing microcomedones. In our hands, such procedure brings no advantage to the casual observation of cyanoacrylate skin surface strippings. In fact, there may be a bias due to the unpredictable density of bacteria inside the follicular casts.

Assessment of Comedolysis in Humans

The same protocols as those designed for human comedogenesis can be applied to show comedolysis induced by topical products or oral drugs [58, 59]. Image analysis of cyanoacrylate skin surface strippings offers the ability to accurately rank order the comedolytic activity of formulations with unknown clinical activity relative to well accepted standards. This method provides a timely and cost effective feedback on clinical efficacy potential of drugs and cosmetics.

References

1. American Academy of Dermatology (1989) Invitational symposium on comedogenicity. J Am Acad Dermatol 20:272–277
2. Tindall JP(1985) Chloracne and chloracnegens. J Am Acad Dermatol 13:539–558
3. Moccarelli P, Marocchi A, Brambilla P (1986) Clinical laboratory manifestations of exposure to dioxin in children. A six-year study of the effects of an environmental disaster near Seveso, Italy. J Am Med Assoc 256:2687–2695
4. Vazquez ER, Macias PC, Tirado JGO, Solana CG, Casanova A, Moncada JFP (1996) Chloracne in the 1990s. Int J Dermatol 35:643–645
5. Saunders MA (1985) Fluoride toothpastes : a cause of acne like eruptions. Arch Dermatol 121:327–329
6. Garnier G (1944) Boutons d'huile du visage par brillantine. Bull Soc Fr Dermatol Syph 51:28–29
7. Gougerot H, Carteaud A, Grupper E (1945) Epidémie de comédons par les brillantines. Bull Soc Fr Dermatol Syph 52:124–125
8. Tzanck A, Sidi E (1945) Nombreux cas d'éruptions acnéiformes provoquées par une brillantine de fabrication récente. Bull Soc Fr Dermatol Syph 52:131–133
9. Plewig G, Fulton JE, Kligman AM (1970) Pomade acne. Arch Dermatol 101:580–584
10. Frankel EB (1985) Acne secondary to white petrolatum use. Arch Dermatol 121:589–590
11. Mills OH, Kligman AM (1975) Acne detergicans. Arch Dermatol 111:65–68
12. Kligman AM, Mills OH (1972) Acne cosmetica. Arch Dermatol 110:843–850
13. Bedane C, Souyri N (1990) Les acnés induites. Ann Dermatol Venereol 117:53–58
14. Mills OH, Berger RS (1989) Assessing acnegenic and acne-aggravating potential. J Toxicol Cut Ocul Toxicol 9:353–360
15. Mills OH, Berger RS (1991) Defining the susceptibility of acne prone and sensitive skin populations to extrinsic factors. Dermatol Clin 9:93–98
16. Piérard GE (1987) Rate and topography of follicular sebum excretion. Dermatology 175:280–283
17. Woo-Sam PC (1977) Cohesion of horny cells during comedo formation. Br J Dermatol 97:609–615
18. Maeda T (1991) An electron microscopic study of experimentally induced comedo and effects of vitamin A on comedo formation. J Dermatol 18:397–407
19. Plewig G, Fulton JE, Kligman AM (1971) Cellular dynamics of comedo formation in acne vulgaris. Arch Dermatol Forsch 242:12–29
20. Knaggs HE, Holland DB, Morris C, Wood EJ, Cunliffe WJ (1994) Quantification of cellular proliferation in acne using the monoclonal antibody Ki-67. J Invest Dermatol 102:89–92
21. Knaggs HE, Hughes BR, Morris C, Wood EJ, Holland DB, Cunliffe WJ (1994) Immunohistochemical study of desmosomes in acne vulgaris. Br J Dermatol 130:731–737
22. Hughes B, Morris C, Cunliffe W (1996) Keratin expression in pilosebaceous epithelia in truncal skin of acne patients. Br J Dermatol 134:247–256
23. Thiboutot D, Knaggs H, Gilliland K, Hagari S (1997) Activity of the type I 5α-reductase is greater in the follicular infrainfundibulum compared with the epidermis. Br J Dermatol 136:166–171
24. Kanaar R (1971) Follicular-keratogenic properties of fatty acids in the external ear canal of the rabbit. Dermatologica 142:14–22
25. Lavker RM, Leyden JJ, McGinley KJ (1981) The relationship between bacteria and the abnormal follicular keratinization in acne vulgaris. J Invest Dermatol 77:325–330
26. Tronnier H, Brunn G (1972) Vergleichsuntersuchungen des Hautober-flächenfettes Hautgesunder und Aknekranker. Berufsdermatosen 20:79–88
27. Saint-Léger D, Bague A, Lefebvre E, Cohen E, Chivot M (1986) A possible role for squalene in the pathogenesis of acne. In vitro study of squalene oxidation. Br J Dermatol 114:535–542

28. Mitoyoshi K (1983) Enhanced comedo formation in rabbit ear skin by squalene and oleic acid peroxides. Br J Dermatol 109:191–198
29. Mills OH, Porte M, Kligman AM (1978) Enhancement of comedogenic substances in ultraviolet radiation. Br J Dermatol 98:145–150
30. Mills OH, Kligman AM (1983) The follicular biopsy. Dermatologica 167:57–63
31. Morello AM, Downing DT, Strauss JS (1976) Octadecadienoic acids in the skin surface lipids of acne patients and normal subjects. J Invest Dermatol 66:319–323
32. Wertz PW, Miethke MC, Long SA, Strauss JS, Downing DT (1985) The composition of the ceramides from human stratuum corneum and from comedones. J Invest Dermatol 84:410–412
33. Stewart ME, Grahak MO, Cambier LS (1986) Dilutional effect of increased sebaceous gland activity on the proportion of linoleic acid in sebaceous wax esters and in epidermal acylceramides. J Invest Dermatol 87:733–736
34. Perisho K, Wertz PW, Madison KC, Stewart ME, Downing DT (1988) Fatty acids of acylceramides from comedones and from the skin surface of acne patients and control subjects. J Invest Dermatol 90:350-353
35. Downing DT, Stewart ME, Wertz PW, Strauss JS (1986) Essential fatty acids and acne. J Am Acad Dermatol 14:221–225
36. Guy R, Green MR, Kealy T (1996) Modeling acne in vitro. J Invest Dermatol 106:176–182
37. Hambrick GW Jr, Blank H (1956) A microanatomical study of the response of the pilosebaceous apparatus of the rabbits ear canal. J Invest Dermatol 26:185–200
38. Kaidbey KH, Kligman AM (1974) A human model of coal tar acne. Arch Dermatol 109:212–215
39. Kligman AM, Kwong T (1979) An improved rabbit ear model for assessing comedogenic substances. Br J Dermatol 100:699–702
40. Frank SB (1982) Is the rabbit ear model, in its present state, prophetic of acnegenicity. J Am Acad Dermatol 6:373–377
41. Marker PC (1983) Comedogenic testing. Relevancy of animal models. Cosmet Toilet 98:27–34
42. Morris WE, Kwan SC (1983) Use of the rabbit ear model in evaluating the comedogenic potential of cosmetic ingredients. J Soc Cosmet Chem 34:215–225
43. Fulton JE Jr, Pay SR, Fulton JE III (1984) Comedogenicity of current therapeutic products, cosmetics, and ingredients in the rabbit ear. J Am Acad Dermatol 10:96–105
44. Durupt G, Leger E, Montastier C (1985) Etude du pouvoir comédogène des produits cosmétiques. Nouv Dermatol 4:216-219
45. Lanzet M (1986) Comedogenic effects of cosmetics raw materials. Cosmet Toilet 161:63–70
46. Tucker SB, Flannigan SA, Dunbar M Jr, Drotman RB (1986) Development of an objective comedogenicity assay. Arch Dermatol 122:660–665
47. Fulton JE Jr (1989) Comedogenicity and irritancy of commonly used ingredients in skin care products. J Soc Cosmet Chem 40:321–333
48. Kligman AM (1989) Improved procedure for assessing acnegenicity (comedogenicity) in rabbit ear model. J Toxicol Cutan Ocul Toxicol 9: 395–410
49. Kligman AM (1989) Updating the rabbit ear comedogenic assay. In: Marks R, Plewig G (eds) Acne and related disorders. Dunitz, London, pp 97–106
50. Choi EH, Ahn SK, Lee SH (1997) The changes of stratum corneum interstices and calcium distribution of follicular epithelium of experimentally induced comedones by oleic acid. Exp Dermatol 6:29–35
51. Mezick JA, Thorne EG, Bhatia MC, Shea LM, Capetola RJ, Raritan NJ (1987) The rabbit ear microcomedo prevention assay. A new model to evaluate anti-acne agents. In: Maibach HI, Lowe NJ (eds) Models in dermatology, vol 3. Karger, Basel, pp 68–73
52. Jackson EM (1989) Clinical assessment of acnegenicity. J Toxicol Cutan Ocul Toxicol 9:387–393
53. Mills OH, Kligman AM (1982) A human model for assessing comedogenic substances. Arch Dermatol 118:903–905
54. Piérard GE, Piérard-Franchimont C, Goffin V (1995) Digital image analysis of microcomedones. Dermatology 190:99–103
55. Katoulis AC, Kakepis EM, Kintziou H, Kakepis ME, Stavriancas NG (1996) Comedogenicity of cosmetics: a review. J Eur Acad Dermatol Venereol 7:115–119
56. Marks R, Dawber RPR (1971) Skin surface biopsy. An improved technique for the examination of the horny layer. Br J Dermatol 84:117–123
57. Holmes RL, Williams M, Cunliffe WJ (1972) Pilosebaceous duct obstruction and acne. Br J Dermatol 87:327–332
58. Mills OH, Kligman AM (1982) A human model for assaying comedolytic substances. Br J Dermatol 107:543–548
59. Letawe C, Boone M, Piérard GE (1998) Digital image analysis of the effect of topically applied linoleic acid on acne microcomedones. Clin Exp Dermatol 23:56–58

CHAPTER 24

Antimicrobial and Preservative Efficacy

M. Heinzel

Antimicrobial and Preservative Efficacy

Consumer safety of cosmetics is determined by many different factors. The exclusion of chemical risk factors contribute to the safety of these products probably in the most important way. However, their microbiological properties may also impair the product quality considerably and everyone who is familiar with product development or manufacture of cosmetics has experienced microbiological problems with them. On the other hand consumer complaints due to microbiological spoilage of cosmetics are really rare events compared to food, for instance. This may give evidence that the microbiological risk management of cosmetics in general works sufficiently well.

The microbiological properties of cosmetics are determined by:
- Their quality, i.e. their content of microorganisms/viruses/biotoxins
- Their preservation, i.e. their stability in use conditions
  and in cases of special product claims
- Their antimicrobial efficacy.

Microbiological quality is ensured by good manufacturing practice (GMP) and good hygiene processing (GHP). In a more general quality management a fault minimization effect analysis (FMEA) will consider not only safety aspects of production but also of product development and vending. As these aspects will not be covered by this chapter the reader is conferred to the literature, e.g. [20, 22], or technical guidance documents, e.g. by the CTFA [6], the Council of Europe [4], or COLIPA [3]. Especially the books of Orth [16] or Brannan [1] thoroughly describe all aspects of cosmetic microbiology and are strongly recommended for detailed studies.

Stability and Preservation of Cosmetics

Cosmetics are preserved mainly in order to stabilize them during their use by the consumer, i.e. to prevent spoilage or microbial adulterations under normal conditions of use (secondary product safety). For this purpose the intrinsic properties of the product should at least inhibit the growth of microorganisms, which will contaminate the product through the normal way of usage. Often, however, a certain microbicidal effect will be necessary. Preservation cannot yet compensate heavy duty contaminations through product abuse.

The improvement of microbiological product quality in manufacture (primary product safety) may not be the main target of preservation although it is of course an important contribution to the production safety in manufacturing processes, which are not normally run under sterile conditions.

It should be mentioned, however, that there are no legal requirements to preserve cosmetics! The supplier has "only" to ensure the safety and stability of his products and he can freely decide in which way he meets these requirements. Technology is principally available for manufacturing cosmetics unpreserved under sterile conditions like pharmaceuticals. Thus, the consumer would receive a primarily safe product, i.e. a sterile product. However, this sterility could not be maintained under usual conditions of application and the product would be recontaminated and spoiled by microorganisms during use. Therefore, the secondary product safety would have to be ensured in other ways, e.g. by product presentation in a form of packaging, which is safe against recontaminations. Otherwise their limited stability would have to be declared to the consumer.

Microbial Adulteration and Spoilage of Cosmetics

Microbial spoilage of cosmetics may affect the health of the consumer and/or the functional properties and the appearence of the product. As already mentioned case reports on health complaints due to microbiologically spoiled cosmetics are extremely rare. Table 1 presents a list of possible microbial agents, which may be harmful to consumers. Preliminary investigations [17] have revealed that contaminations by viruses are probably of no importance. Even the risk of product contamination by the BSE-agent or the probability of infections arising from such a hypothetical contamination in cosmetics is minimal. On the other hand mycotoxin contamination of some raw materials, especially of cereal origine, may sometimes be observed [15]. Due to the lack of references it is, however, difficult to assess this risk for human health. However, some of these mycotoxins, e.g. zearalenones or trichothecenes, are known to cause severe

Table 1. Potential microbial risk factors for human health by cosmetics

Causative agent	Possible complaints
Bacteria	
Staphylococcus aureus	Pus, sepsis, toxic shock syndrome
Strepotoccus pyogenes	dto
Enterococcus spec.	Infections
Clostridium tetani	Tetanus
Clostridium perfringens	Gas gangrene
Pseudomonas aeruginosa	Conjunctivitis, pyodermia, pus, infections
Klebsiella spec.	Conjunctivitis, infections
Enterobacteriaceae	Enteritis
Fungi	
Candida albicans	Stomatomycosis, conjunctivitis
Candida parapsilosis	Conjunctivitis
Microsporum spec. }	Dermatomycoses
Pityrosporum ovale	
Trichophyton spec. }	Pyodermia, inflammations
Fusarium and *Trichoderma* toxins	
Aspergillus spec	Conjunctivitis, allergic effects
Viruses and other infective agents	
Enteroviruses	Enteritis
e.g. Hepatitisviruses	Hepatitis
Adeno virus	Conjunctivitis
Papilloma virus	Verrucosis
Herpes virus	Herpes simplex
BSE-agent	Creutzfeld-Jacob syndrome

dermal complaints. Contamination of raw materials with clostridial spores may also be possible. In the 1930s such contamination was reported as common in pharmaceutical alcohol in Germany, while American investigations could not confirm this finding at the same time. In the 1980s another investigation in hospitals of Berlin/Germany also revealed no apparent risk of spore contamination of pharmaceutical alcohols but the author knows from his personell experience reports on contaminations of alcohols by clostridial spores. Principally even highly concentrated alcohols bear the risk of contamination by bacterial spores due to their complete inefficiency against these dehydrated resting forms of microorganisms.

However, microbial adulterations are more frequent in cosmetics and impair product properties. Table 2 gives a list of examples. It should be mentioned that some of these phenomena may hardly be observed by the consumer because they interfere with other product properties. For instance, malodour due to metabolic products may often be covered by the perfume of the cosmetic. Liquification due to enzymatically caused

Table 2. Microbial adulterations of cosmetics

Spoilage by:	Causative agent
Formation of gas	
CO_2, H_2	Clostridia
CO_2	Lactic acid bacteria
CO_2, H_2, N_2	Enterobacteriaceae
N_2, N_2O	Denitrifiers
Deformations of plastic bottles	
Consumption of residual O_2	All aerobic microorganism
Acidification	
Butyric acid	Clostridia
Lactic acid, acetic acid	Lactic acid bacteria
Acetic acid, formic acid	Enterobacteriaceae
Lactic acid, acetic acid	Yeasts
Alcalisation	
Proteolytic NH_3 formation	Clostridia
dto.	Pseudomonads
	Bacilli
Respiratory NH_3 formation from NO_3 {	Enterobacteriacea
	Pseudomonads
Changes in colour	
Black discoloration due to FeS-formation	Sulfate reducers
Discoloration	Pseudomonads, Flavobacteria and other pigmented forms
Changes in odour	
H_2S	Sulfate reducers
Rancidity	Lipolytes
H_2S, amines	Proteolytes
Alcohols, acids	Fermentative microorganims
Changes in viscosity	
Increase in viscosity	Slime formation/secretion
Decrease in viscosity	Polysaccharide degradation
Decrease in viscosity	Lipid degradation
Separation of oil/water-phases in emulsions	
Degradation of emulsifiers	Different microorganisms
Formation of alcohol	Fermentative microorganisms
Visible growth of microorganisms	
Stocks and spots	Molds
Slime flocculation	Slime formers

decrease of viscosity can also hardly be realized by the consumer. On the other hand this process may continue even after inactivation of those microorganisms which have been responsible for the secretion of these extracellular enzymes.

Preservation of Cosmetics

Product preservation is necessary, and may principally be achieved in two ways: (1) Addition of chemical preservatives – which is the most frequent way, or (2) development of formulae which are self-preserving due to their specific composition.

Preservatives are chemical substances which are added to a formulation with the purpose of preservation. But when there are no preservatives used in a formula and even when there is no import by the preservation from raw materials, nevertheless such a product may be preserved! There may be yet some ingredients in a formulation which are not added with the intention of preservation, but which have antimicrobial properties or which contribute to an antimicrobial efficiency of the complete formulation. That means the formula would comprise antimicrobial ingredients for any "other use". Table 3 gives some examples. For instance, alcohols may be necessary as solvents or as adstringent, H_2O_2 is used as bleaching agent, salicylic acid as keratolytic agent and Triclosan for deodoration. Many essential oils used as perfumes have antimicrobial properties, too. All these substances may contribute to the preservation, but they are not used as preservatives. Therefore, the intended main purpose of an ingredient should be always decisive in these considerations.

Table 3. "Other use" factors in cosmetic formulations contributing to their microbial stability (i.e. their preservation)

Extreme pH-values
Ingredients minimizing the a_w-value, e.g. salts, alcohols (glycerol, sorbitol, PEG), or high-concentrated detergents
Anionic or cationic detergents
Active ingredients for other purposes, e.g. H_2O_2, ethanol or salicylic acid
Phenolic antioxidants, e.g. BHA, BHT, TBHQ
Sequestering agents, e.g. EDTA, citrate, phosphonic acids
Essential oils and perfumes

The strongest effect on the microbial stability of a product, however, results from its pH- and a_w-values. By extremes in these parameters an additional preservative may become unnecessary. Table 4 summarizes the risk conditions with respect to a_w- and pH-value.

Thus, as a conclusion, there are three ways to ensure the microbiological safety of cosmetics:

- Sterile manufacture of unpreserved products and prevention of in-use-risks
- Product preservation by self-preserving formulae
- Product preservation by chemical preservatives.

There is a fourth way feasible, which may become important in the future: By the use of preservatives, which decompose to harmless reaction products, and a product

Table 4. Risk assessment of microbial spoilage by physicochemical parameters. (Modi acc to [8])

1. Gram-negative bacteria

Minimal risk	a_w<0.92 or pH <2.5/>10.5
	a_w 0.92–0.95 and pH <5.5
Low risk	a_w 0.92–0.95 or pH 2.5–3/9–10
	a_w 0.92–0.95 and pH >5.5
	a_w 0.95–0.98 and pH <5.5
	a_w0.95–0.98 and pH 5.5–8
High risk	a_w>0.98 and/or pH 3.5–8

2. Fungi

Minimal risk	a_w<0.70 or pH <2/>10.0
Low risk	a_w 0.70-.080 or pH 2–3/9–10
Moderate risk	a_w 0.80–0.90 or pH 3.0–3.5/8–9
High risk	a_w >0.90 and/or pH 3.5–8

presentation in a way which minimizes in-use-recontaminations, the product would be microbiologically protected during production and use, but the consumer would receive a preservative-free product. H_2O_2 or dimethyldicarbonate have proven the feasibility of this "temporary preservation" in preliminary test models.

Preservatives for Cosmetics

Preservatives are active ingredients which must be safe and may not impose any risk on the consumer. In some countries, e.g. the European Community (EC), they have to be approved for the use in cosmetics. In the EC, approved preservatives and their conditions of use and declaration are listed in annex 6 of the EC Cosmetic Directive 76/768 (positive list). In the United States (US) there is only a positive list for active ingredients in OTC (over-the-counter)-drugs but not for antimicrobials which are used exclusively for preservation.

Preservatives have to be not only safe but also effective and compatible with other ingredients of a formula. These informations can not be derived from the positive list or the literature, but must be obtained experimentally. It is strongly recommended to verify efficacy and compatibility not only for each new formula, but also for each relaunch and each modification of a basic formula, e.g. by colour or perfume.

The efficacy of some preservatives depends on the pH of a formula. Organic acids, for example, are active only in their undissociated forms. That means, they work best at pH-values below their pKs-value. At higher pH's, which are preferred in many cosmetics, their efficacy decreases rapidly. The dissociation dymanics of benzoic, sorbic and dehydroacetic acid run in the pH-range between 5 and 6 as shown in Table 5.

Table 5. Percentages of undissociated form at diffent pH-values of benzoic acid, sorbic acid and dehydroacetic acid

pH value	Benzoic acid	Sorbic acid	Dehydroacetic acid
pH 5.0	13	37	65
pH 5.5	5	15	37
pH 6.0	2	6	16

On the other hand the precision in production may normally be assumed at Δ pH of ±0.5 units and a dosage accuracy of ±5%–10% with small volume ingredients, like preservatives. The amount of active and available preservatives may also be influenced by its partition coefficient between oils and water and by adsorption phenomena. Mineral pigments, sealants or packaging materials may adsorb preservatives, thus withdrawing them from the pool of active molecules.

Finally, the antimicrobial efficiency, i.e. the spectrum of activity, determines the efficacy of a preservative in a product. *The efficiency is the antimicrobial property of a preservative, while the efficacy is the performance of a preservation in a formulation. Literature data can help to estimate the efficiency of a substance but efficacy tests are absolutely necessary in the final product formulation for assessment of the performance.* A very simple and common measure for the antimicrobial efficiency is the minimum inhibitory concentration (m.i.c.). Table 6 summarizes the efficiency data as m.i.c.'s. of some preservatives commonly used in cosmetics. Such data depend strongly on the test methodology. Therefore, literature data may differ considerably, are difficult to compare and should be used only to estimate the potency of a preservative against different types of microorganisms. Bacteria, especially Gram-negatives, should preferably be covered by the efficiency, because contaminations of raw materials or final produtcs are mostly caused by Gram-negative bacteria. Yeasts and molds are comparatively rarely responsible for spoilage of cosmetics.

Table 6. Efficiency of cosmetic preservatives (INCI) and some preservative preparations

Preservative	m.i.c. Gram-positives	m.i.c. Gram-negatives	m.i.c. Yeasts	m.i.c. Molds
Benzoic acid (pH 6.0)	20–>2000[a] ppm	100–500 ppm	100–7000 ppm	50–5000 ppm
Salicylic acid (pH 3.2)	>1000 ppm	1000–2500 ppm	~2500 ppm	~2500 ppm
Sorbic acid (pH 6.0)	50–7000[a] ppm	50–10,000[b] ppm	50–3000 ppm	200–3000 ppm
Dehydroacetic acid (pH 6.0)	~1%	>2%	~200 ppm	~1500 ppm
Undecylenic acid (pH 6.0)	500–1000 ppm	1%–>2%	~200 ppm	50–200 ppm
Methylparaben	750–4000 ppm	750–4000[c] ppm	500–2000 ppm	500–1000 ppm
Propylparaben	250–1000 ppm	250–>2000[c] ppm	100–600 ppm	50–1000 ppm
Ethanol	8%–10%	5%–10%	12%–18%	5%–8%
Benzylalcohol	2000–5000 ppm	2000–6000 ppm	~3000 ppm	~5000 ppm
Phenoxyethanol	~2000 ppm	~4000 ppm	~5000 ppm	~5000 ppm
Formaldehyde	75–150 ppm	100–500 ppm	100–500 ppm	100–500 ppm
Imidazolidinyl urea	~1000 ppm	1000–>4000 ppm	>8000 ppm	>8000 ppm
Quaternium 15	50–200 ppm	50–>1000[c] ppm	>3000 ppm	>3000 ppm
DMDM Hydantoin	300–800 ppm	250–1000 ppm	250–1000 ppm	50–~1500 ppm
Triclocarban	~2 ppm	~10–~1000[c] ppm	~500 ppm	50–~500 ppm
Triclosan	0.01–30 ppm	0.1–>1000[c] ppm	1–10 ppm	1–30 ppm
Chlorhexidine-digluconate	1–65 ppma	20–>1000[c] ppm	5–50 ppm	10–500 ppm
Benzalkonium chloride	1–5 ppm	10–~600[c] ppm	5–50 ppm	10–200 ppm
Bronidox	20–80 ppm	20–200 ppm	20–80 ppm	50–250 ppm
Bronopol	20–80 ppm	20–100 ppm	20–200 ppm	20–200 ppm
Kathon CG	150–600[a] ppm	150–600 ppm	150–300 ppm	150–600 ppm
JMActiCare	100–200 ppm	100–200 ppm	100–800 ppm	100–200 ppm

[a] Lactic acid bacteria.
[b] *Salmonella* sp.
[c] *Pseudomonas* sp.

Adaption and Resistance Phenomena

Microorganisms differ in their intrinsic susceptibility to antimicrobial agents, such as antibiotics, preservatives (see Table 6) or disinfectants. This is called natural *toleran-ce*. However, they have or develop mechanisms to protect themselves from the anti-microbial action which may result in an increased tolerance. This is called *adaption* if it is acquired only transiently and lost more or less rapidly by changing the physiolo-gical conditions. It is called *resistance* if it is a permanent property (although depen-ding on the selective pressure in some way), especially when it is genetically determi-ned on the chromosome or by plasmids. Resistance is frequently transferable from one bacterium to another, even between different species. This is called *acquired resistance* while an *increased resistance* may be generated either artificially or in situ by the sel-ective pressure.

Transferability implies the epidemiological dissemination of a resistance once it has occurred. In antibiotics this is a well known phenomenon, which could be experienced already with the first antibiotics shortly after their introduction. In recent years evi-dence has increased that biocide resistances are also evolving [12, 18], for instance against preservatives. As paradigms, the mechanisms of resistance against formalde-hyde in enterobacteriaceae and quaternary ammonium compounds (QAC) in staphy-lococci have been elucidated, which are both plasmid mediated.

Formaldehyde resistant enterobacteriaceae have a strong glutathione (GSH)-de-pendent formaldehyde dehydrogenase (Enzyme Commission 1.2.1.1.), which is secre-ted from the cells to metabolise formaldehyde outside [14]. The plasmid coding for this enzyme is transferable to and has been isolated from different genera of the enterob-acteriaceae, thus giving evidence for a dissemination of the resistance plasmid. The en-zyme is unspecific for low-molecular aldehydes and this explains the cross resistance to other aldehydes and formaldehyde releasers. Formaldehyde resistance is also well known from pseudomonads but other mechanisms are responsible here.

Heir et al. [13] showed that QAC-resistance in staphylococci is caused by an exchan-ge of a single amino acid in a protein of the cytoplasmic membrane, thus making the cells impermeable for the toxine. The authors were able to detect the responsible plas-mid in staphylococci-isolates from various branches of the food industry which also demonstrates that the plasmid has already disseminated.

There are further reports concerning genetically determined resistance to other ac-tive ingredients or preservatives, for instance chlorhexidine or metal compounds like silver, but mostly the mechanisms are not very clear. Although the fact that most of the-se resistance phenomena are plasmid mediated and even strong evidence is given for a transferable exchange, up to now there are no case reports that this really happens in practice, as in the clinical situation with antibiotics. Most reports on increased tole-rances to preservatives which come from the practice confer only to a transient in-crease. That means they are results of adaptive processes which may be caused by in-sufficient disinfection of manufacturing equipment or by use of sublethal concentra-tions of preservatives. However, this should give rise to the development of alternative preservation systems for each product which could be introduced in such cases.

Efficacy Testing of Preservations

In most countries so far, there are no legal requirements for the assessment of the preservation in cosmetics although the EC was about to develop such demands [11] which have been withdrawn in the meanwhile. However, there are some recommendations, e.g. from norms (ASTM) or pharmacopoeiae (BP [2], EP [5], USP [21]), which can serve as technical guidance also for cosmetics, but it should be emphasized that the supplier is principally free in which way he validates the safety of his products. The CTFA technical guidelines [6], therefore, give detailed recommendations for the test methodology of preservation tests, but leave the interpretation and evaluation of the test results to the producer. The CTPA recommendations [7], however, joined the BP evaluation criteria.

The efficacy of a product preservation may be assessed either by artificial challenge tests or in-use tests with a test panel. The challenge test shall simulate the practical conditions of manufacture and usage, but it can never model them exactly. Therefore, a certain safety margin has to be calculated. Challenge tests are carried out in a microbiological laboratory. As they are less expensive, they are usually used to select the best preservation from a few alternatives which is then finally tested in an in-use test. Many parameters of a formula and the production conditions of a specific plant influence the efficacy of a preservation. Even the hardness of water or technical details of the production equipment may have an impact. Therefore, it may be necessary to re-evaluate the preservation in a challenge test when the formula is modified even in marginal details or the production is shifted from one plant to another, e.g. to a contractor. The challenge test should also be used to validate the stability of a preservation system under different storage conditions. According to the European Cosmetic Directive 76/768, for example, it is necessary to declare a stability when it is lower than 30 months and it is required to document the stability assessment in the product dossier.

The test strategy for preservative efficacy validation consists of: (1) The test methodology and (2) the evaluation of the experimental results following acceptance criteria.

It is recommended to define criteria of acceptance before experimental results are generated in order to have a common understanding of the requirements independently from certain test results. However, the acceptance criteria for pharmaceutical preservations as required in the different pharmacopoeiae (Table 7) are generally not

Table 7. Acceptance criteria of different challenge tests

Methodology	Bacteria	Fungi
ASTM E640	$10^7 \rightarrow 10^4/7d +$ bacteriostasis/28d	Yeasts $10^6 \rightarrow 10^3/7d +$ fungistasis/28d Molds $10^6 \rightarrow 10^5/28d$
Brit. Pharm. (topica)	$10^6 \rightarrow 10^3/2d$ and $10^3 \rightarrow <10^0/7d$	$10^6 \rightarrow 10^4/7d$ and $10^4 \rightarrow <10^0/28d$
Eur. Pharm. (topica, "A" criteria)	$10^5 \rightarrow 10^3/2d$ and $10^5 \rightarrow 10^2/7d$ + bacteriostasis/28d	$10^5 \rightarrow 10^3/14d +$ fungistasis/28d
EC-draft XXIV/1878/96:		
For general cosmetics	$10^5 \rightarrow 10^3/14d +$ bacteriostasis/28d	$10^5 \rightarrow 10^5/28d$
For baby and eye cosmetics	$10^5 \rightarrow 10^2/14d +$ bacteriostasis/28d	$10^5 \rightarrow 10^4/14d +$ fungistasis/28d
US Pharm.	$10^5 \rightarrow 10^2/14d +$ bacteriostasis/28d	$10^5 \rightarrow 10^5/28d$

sufficient for cosmetics. They require only a slight microbicidal effect followed by a lon-glasting inhibition. This may be suitable for pharmaceuticals, even for topical drugs, which are used only by a single applier for a limited time, but the common conditions of use and presentation of cosmetics require a stronger effect of preservation.

Challenge Tests

In challenge tests product samples are inoculated artifically with microorganisms and their further behaviour is monitored as to whether: (a) They continue to propagate, (b) they are inhibited or (c) they are killed.

The following parameters determine the performance of the test and the results generated. It is recommended to describe the details of the test methodology used in operation procedures in order to meet the requirements of good documentation practice.

Inoculum

Only pure cultures should be used, which can be classified as a definite taxon. They can be derived from culture collections, e.g. ATCC[1], or by isolation from contaminated products or manufacturing facilities. "House bugs", although initially often appearing by a striking tolerance, tend to change their sensitivity to preservatives during or soon after isolation. Their tolerance may, however, be maintained a long time, when they are kept in the product where they have appeared originally. If it is a pure culture, this product may be used as direct inoculum in order to test the preservation with resistant bacteria. In contrast, the tolerance of strains from culture collections is principally stable, but may be influenced by growth conditions. Therefore, the comparability of test results over a long time is better when strains from culture collections are used. Another advantage is that they are replaceable at any time by a new strain of the same identity. Common species used for challenge tests are:
- Gram-positive bacteria:
  - *Staphylococcus aureus*
- Gram-negative bacteria:
  - *Escherichia coli, Pseudomonas aeruginosa*
- Fungi (yeast and molds):
  - *Candida albicans, Aspergillus niger.*

This selection is derived from pharmacopoeiae and mainly represents pathogens which are relevant for topical drugs. For cosmetic purposes, however, it is recommended to supplement this set by a selection from the following species which rather represent the causative agents of microbial adulterations in cosmetics: Lactic acid bacteria, e.g. *Enterococcus faecium* or *Leuconostoc mesenteroides,* enterobacteriaceae, e.g. *Enterobacter gergoviae, Proteus* spec. or *Klebsiella* spec., non-fermenters, esp. *Burkholderia cepacia, Pseudomonas putida* or Ps. *fluorescens,* yeasts, e.g. *Candida parapsilosis* molds, e.g. *Penicillium* spec., *Fusarium* spec. or *Trichoderma* spec.

It is recommended not to use spore forming bacteria (Bacillus spec., Clostridium spec.) in challenge tests although these species may frequently be found as contami-

---

[1] ATCC, American Type Culture Collection, 12301 Parklawn Drive, Rockville, USA

nants in cosmetics. In their sporulated form they are resistant to any preservative (except H_2O_2!), but their vegetative form show the same sensitivity as other Gram-positives. That means in effect, their spores will not be affected by the preservation but when they should grow out in the product their vegetative cells would be killed. The formation and germination of the spores hardly are to control and therefore they produce ambiguous results in challenge tests.

Inoculation

The amount of microorganisms inoculated in the test sample represents the main challenge for preservation because they consist of organic matter and react in any way with the preservative. High amounts will stress the preservation more than low amounts. Commonly initial inocula of 10^6 colony forming units (cfu)/g are used. This is far more than a product contamination can be expected to amount under normal conditions of use but this is the safety margin for the validation. In repetitive challenge tests or capacity tests the product sample is stressed up to ten times with inocula of 10^5 cfu/g, thus representing in total the same amount as by a single inoculation of 10^6. Because each re-inoculation is normally carried out after one week of incubation these repetitive challenge tests are expensive and time consuming but they give no further information about the capacity of a preservation-system than a single inoculation test.

Also for the simulation of the storage stability of preservations they are not necessary as this question can be assessed by single challenges of samples which have been stored for different times at different temperatures.

The precultural conditions (e.g. temperature, time, nutrients, liquid/solid media) may influence the physiological status and thus the sensitivity of the test strains. Therefore, it is necessary to maintain definite growth conditions. Using liquid grown inocula the organic challenge for the preservation will be higher if the cells are not washed and resuspended in buffered NaCl-solution.

The inoculum volume should not exceed more than 1% of the sample volume in order to maintain the physicochemical conditions of the product. In w/o-emulsions even 1% may be too much. In cases of product-to-product inoculations 10% should not be exceeded. The homogenization of the inoculum in the sample is very important to avoid "nests" and inhomogenity in the test results. Normally the inoculum is homogenized by the inoculation loop in the sample, but some test institutes spend much effort by using drum-mills or potters for an optimized homogenization.

The test organisms can either be inoculated as single strains in each sample or as mixtures of bacteria and fungi in different samples. Of course, the informative value of the test is higher using single strain inoculations but on the other hand this will increase the costs. Using mixtures of bacteria or fungi, it must be ensured that they are compatible vice versa and require the same conditions of growth. Therefore, it would not be acceptable to mix bacteria with fungi. Using selective media for subcultivation the informative disadvantage of mixed inocula may partially be compensated.

Incubation

The inoculated samples may be incubated either at room temperature or increased temperatures in order to simulate the climate in a warm toilet room. Temperatures between 20–40°C favour microbial growth but also the reaction between preservatives and the organic matter. After certain test periods aliquots are withdrawn from the sample

Fig. 1. Calculation of D-value from the 24-h death curve. Cross, theoretical inoculum density calculated from the viable count of the inoculum; triangles, recovery data from an insufficient medium; dots, data from an optimized recovery medium

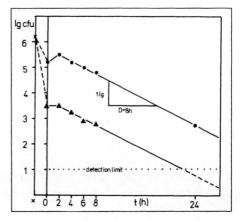

in order to assay them for viability of the test organisms. Common test periods are 1–2, 7–14, 21–28 days.

Subculture
The growth conditions used for the subcultures must sufficiently allow to recover the test strains. These are stressed by the preservative and may be damaged sublethally. Therefore, it is normal that the recovery rate is lower than it would be expected theoretically from the concentration in the inoculum. However, t-0-readings more than 1 log below the theoretical value indicate inadequate conditions of recovery. Figure 1 shows two examples of good and critical recovery conditions, respectively.

The viability can be determined qualitatively or quantitatively in recovery subcultures. A quantitative recording permits to follow the kinetics of killing and to calculate D-values[2] from the death curve, where single strain inoculation has been used. In both ways, however, it is essential to ensure the inactivation of preservatives which are carried over in small amounts by the inoculation procedure into the subcultural media where they can cause inhibitory effects. This may lead to false-negative results, i.e. lack of growth, which is not caused by the death of the test organisms but by the inhibition of their growth in the subculture. Especially, chlorhexidine or high concentrations of QACs can cause problems in inactivation. Gram-positive bacteria are normally more sensitive to inactivation problems than Gram-negatives. Commonly the subculture media are supplemented with the following inactivation cocktail:
- 3.0% Tween 80
- 0.3% lecithine
- 0.1% histidine
- 0.5% thiosulfate or cysteine.

The successful inactivation should be verified by a re-inoculation step of the test strains (at least a Gram-positive) into subcultures with primarily negative results. If the re-inoculated strain will grow in the subculture, this is proof for a successfull inacti-

---

[2] D-value is the time (in hours) necessary to reduce the cfu for 1 log

vation. However, if the re-inoculum will not grow, the inactivation is inadequate and the result recorded from this subculture must be considered as false-negative.

Determination of D-values

Under certain conditions the evaluation of a challenge test can be accelerated by the calculation of D-values from the viable counts in the first hours ($\leq$ 24 h) of the test (see Fig. 1). In this way it is possible to estimate at which time the acceptance criteria would be met without performing the test up to that date. However, this saving of time has to be bought expensively as at least ten parallels of the first readings are necessary in order to generate enough data for a sufficient statistical basis. The limiting conditions are:

1. Single strain inoculation has been used
2. The subcultures are evaluated quantitatively
3. The preservation is strong enough to generate D-values of <24 h
4. The death curve follows a linear regression
5. There are sufficient data of the first readings allowing to develop a linear regression graph.

Especially this last condition is critical as minor subpopulations of the test strain developing a delayed dominance even after two or three weeks cannot be detected within the first hours.

In-Use Tests

In a final safety assessment a pre-evaluated formula may be submitted to an in-use-test in order to validate its preservation under practical conditions. As this is a very time consuming test this fact has to be sufficiently respected in the time schedule of product development.

The test panel must be representative for that user group, which the product has in view, and should comprise a random sample of at least 50 items. Normally in-use-tests for cosmetics are performed as home-use-tests. That means the number of probands using the items will differ depending on the size of each household participating. The frequency of application, however, determines the consumption as well as the microbial challenge of the product. This has to be considered when selecting the test panels for different product types. The test design must also take into account specific forms of usage, for instance with seasonal articles, e.g. sun protective products.

The users have to be instructed on the product application but it is commendable not to inform them about the hygienic backgrounds of the test in order to preserve their normal behaviour of usage. They have to be instructed to send back the product samples when approximately 3/4 of the initial volume have been consumed and to note the date of the last usage.

To the users product samples have been supplied which were controlled for their microbiological quality before release. On return the samples must immediately be controlled:

– Visibly for appearent adulterations (see Table 2)
– Microbiologically for:
  – Aerobic total counts
  – Spore forming bacteria
  – Yeasts and molds.

The time between last use and the test is documented. Frequently, samples will be found to be contaminated at that time. This is quite normal as the preservation needs some time to reduce these contaminations. Therefore, it will be necessary to repeat the microbiological controls after that time interval which can be expected from the results of the challenge tests to reduce the contamination to the acceptance level.

As in the challenge test the supplier is free again in setting his evaluation criteria of the test results. Return samples with heavy contaminations (i.e. »10^3 cfu/g), however, indicate that the preservative system only controls insufficiently contaminations. Microbial charges of 10^2–10^3 may be acceptable when they are reduced in a reasonable time to ≤ 100 cfu/g.

Claim Support of Antimicrobial Cosmetics and Toiletries

In some types of cosmetics antimicrobial effects may contribute to the product performance considerably. This is the case for instance in anti-perspirants (see Chap. 8) or anti-dandruff products (see Chap. 11).

These product types are not yet discussed here. There is, however, an increasing group of products which claim especially antimicrobial properties. This may range from antimicrobial soaps, hygienic mouthwashs or tooth pastes to special products, which are claimed for bacteriologically caused skin impurities, for instance.

Considerations of the Legal Status

Such products move along the borderline between pharmaceuticals, antiseptics disinfectants and cosmetics. In some countries they are regarded as pharmaceutical drugs or disinfectants not only when they are intended to treat but also by prevent infectious diseases, i.e. when they claim an efficacy against pathogens.

In the EC the major intended use of a product is only decisive for its juridicial definition and primarily not its active ingredients. If, in this regard, a product has to be defined as a pharmaceutical drug it comes under the regulations of the EC Directive 65/65 on pharmaceuticals requiring product approval. This is is case for antiseptics. Disinfectants are covered either by the EC Directive 93/42 on Medical Devices (requiring certification) or by the EC Directive 98/8 on Biocidal Products (requiring product approval or registration). Only when the exclusive or major purpose of a product is *to clean, to perfume, to correct body odors, to change the appearance or to protect or maintain of the body in good condition* it meets the definition of a cosmetic product according to EC Cosmetic Directive 76/768 which demands neither a product approval nor a registration or certification. Nevertheless, the EC Cosmetic Directive quite permits antimicrobial product claims, even preventive claims against pathogens, as long as they not refer to the prevention or treatment of a disease. Taking all these directives together it must be stated that the actual European regulations of antimicrobial skincare products are not very clear.

In the US the Food, Drug and Cosmetic Act regards these products as OTC drugs. Among others, these may be cosmetics which are also intended to prevent or to treat diseases. They are differed from pharmaceutical drugs as they must not contain substances as active ingredients which are recognized in the US Pharmacopoeia [21], the National Formulatory or the Homeopathic Pharmacopoeia. Monographs are prepared for the different sorts of OTC drugs describing conditions which are generally regarded as safe and effective (GRAS/E) for these products. These conditions comprise a positive list of active ingredients and specific labelling claims which shall be used. Following these GRAS/E conditions the supplier needs no further authorization. The use of other active substances or labelling, however, would require the supplier to apply for a new drug application (NDA). "OTC topical antimicrobial drugs" comprise the following categories: antimicrobial soaps, health care personnel hand washs, surgical hand scrubs, preoperative skin preparations, skin antiseptics, skin wound cleansers, and skin wound protectants. In other words, products which are mostly regarded by the European legislation as medical devices or pharmaceutical drugs but not as antimicrobial skin care products.

Antimicrobial Claims and Antimicrobial Effects

The spectrum of *effectiveness* may be limited to bacteria or fungi or it may comprise both. Accordingly it is called: *antibacterial, antifungal* or *antimicrobial* effectiveness. That only means that the product works in some way against bacteria, fungi or miroorganisms, respectively.

The *efficiency* of a product may be growth inhibiting or killing. Accordingly it is called:
- *Bacteriostatic, fungistatic* or *microbistatic* for inhibitory efficiencies or
- *Bactericidal, fungicidal* or *microbicidal* for killing efficiencies.

Effectiveness and efficiency are immanent product properties which may be tested by in vitro methods describing the product performance. *Efficacy* is what results from the (correct) application of an efficient product, i.e. the hygienic or antimicrobial effect on the skin of an user, for example. These effects do not always have to be positive as antimicrobial skin treatment may impair the autochtonic flora, too. Therefore, the efficacy can only be tested in vivo by application of the product to probands in clinical test studies.

In antimicrobial labelling of cosmetics and toiletries, however, these scientific terms aren't always used. Marketing prefers to express the product performance in claims like "hygienic", "degerming", "prevents/reduces significantly...", "against impurities of young skin", "anti-plaque" etc. The problem is to translate this marketing language into scientific terms in order to develop an appropriate test strategy to support these claims. Therefore, it is necessary at least to define effectiveness and efficiency in any way which determine the test requirements.

The minimum requirement supporting any "anti"-claim is an inhibition of specific target organisms (bacteria or fungi), but "cidal"-products meet this requirement, too. An antimicrobial mouthwash, for example, claiming an anti-plaque efficiency should at least inhibit specific plaque bacteria, like *Streptococcus mutans* or *Streptococcus sobrinus*. An anti-acne lotion should be bacteriostatic against *Propionibacterium acnes* and a product against athletes' feet should be fungistatic against *Trichophyton* and *Epidermophyton*. A hygienic handwash claimed especially to prevent cross-contaminations in kitchen or food processing should kill the most important agents of food infections/intoxications, like Enterobacteriaceae or *Staphylococcus aureus*.

The products' performance must meet these requirements in test conditions which correspond to the recommended application conditions: The mouthwash is normally a ready-to-use product but in the oral cavity it is diluted by the saliva by approximately 50% while an antibacterial skin lotion will not be diluted during application. The hygienic handwash will not only be diluted by application but it should also kill the target organisms within a reasonable time.

Efficiency Tests

There are many standardized methods and norms for validating the efficiency of disinfectants or antiseptics. Most of them are in vitro methods testing the performance of "cidal"-products in suspension tests with different types of microorganisms [e.g. AFNOR, AOAC(Association of Official Analytical Chemists, USA), BSI, DGHM (Deutsche Gesellschaft für Hygiene und Mikrobiologie, Germany) methods]. Only the ASTM E1115 and the new EN methods (EN 1499, EN 1500) have also provided for a validation of the in vivo performance, i.e. the efficacy, of antimicrobial hand washing products or hand disinfectants, respectively. Test assays for disinfectants or antiseptics may fit also for antimicrobial toiletries. However, the requirements to the performance of disinfectants/antiseptics are not an appropriate scale of evaluation in cosmetics.

The inhibitory efficiency is tested in dilution assays, e.g. following the DGHM methodology[9]. Doubly concentrated culture media are diluted 1:1 with doubly concentrated aqueous solution of the test substance/test product and growth inhibition is monitored with different test strains. Thus, m.i.c.'s can be determined. Methodological problems arise with products which are not sufficiently soluble in water or which are presented ready to use, i.e. application in undiluted form. Under such conditions the ratio of medium : test-solution can be increased from 1:1 up to 1:9 which would permit testing a 90% concentrated product, but a further increase is not possible due to the solubility of ingredients in tenfold concentrated media. This assay also serves for the determination of the best inactivation cocktail which is necessary to know for all "cidal"-tests. For this purpose the medium is supplemented with doubly concentrated inactivation mixtures and no growth inhibition should result in those tubes where the inactivation of antimicrobial agents was successful. For many purposes the mixture given on page 285 is suitable.

The "cidal" efficiency is tested in vitro by different suspension tests. In the past the AFNOR normes 72–150/72–151 or 72–170/72–171 for bactericidal or fungicidal claims, respectivly, have frequently been used besides the German DGHM-tests [9],. Recently these tests have been harmonized by EN 1040 and EN 1275, respectively, which describe for the first time European requirements to support the claims "bactericidal" or "fungicidal". Both norms represent basic assays which comprise only *Staphylococcus aureus* and *Pseudomonas aeruginosa* as bacteria (EN 1040) and *Candida albicans* and *Aspergillus niger* (EN 1275) as fungal representatives. In both cases the maximum contact time is 60 min. A log-reduction of a factor of 5 or 4 is required for bacteria and fungi, respectively. These are no very high requirements but the norms demand them to be met in at least two further dilutions of geometrical progression. The highest concentration possible is 90% of product.

In additional norms, which are currently in preparation, the spectrum of effectiveness is broadened and assessed with special bacterial or fungal species for disinfectants applied for public health (prEN 12054), food industry (EN 1276, EN 1650) or veterinary use (prEN 1656, prEN 1657). Cosmetic applications are not provided for but it should not be a problem for a microbiologist to adapt the test spectrum of EN 1040 and EN 1275 to species relevant for special claims of cosmetics and toiletries (see Tables 1 and 2).

Claim supports by in vivo efficacy tests in cosmetics make the development of product specific test designs and assays necessary. As not only the antimicrobial, but also dermatological effects have to be evaluated, cooperation with a dermatologist is essential. Furthermore, the legal situation in some countries requires supervision by a physician in clinical tests.

References

1. Brannan DK (ed) (1997) Cosmetic microbiology. CRC, New York
2. British Pharmacopoeia (1980) vol. II, appendix XVIc, A193–194, London
3. COLIPA (The European Cosmetic Toiletry and Perfumery Association, Bruxelles) (1997) Guidelines on microbial quality management
4. Council of Europe (1995) Guidelines for good manufacturing practice of cosmetic products (GMPC). Strasbourg
5. Council of Europe (1997) European pharmacopoeia, 3rd edn. Strasbourg, pp 286–287
6. CTFA (Cosmetic, Toiletry and Fragrance Association) (1985) Technical guidelines. Washington
7. CTPA (The Cosmetic Toiletry and Perfumery Association) (1990) Microbial quality management
8. Curry J (1991) Microbiological aspects of cosmetics and toiletry manufacturing. Cosmet Toiletries, special issue on manufacture 202, 205, 206, 208
9. DGHM (1997) List of disinfection procedures tested according to the "Guidelines for Testing Chemical Disinfectants" and found effective by the German Society for Hygiene and Microbiology. mhp, Wiesbaden
10. EC Decision of the Commision (8th May 1996) 96/335 establishing an inventory and a common nomenclature of ingredients employed in cosmetic products. OJ 39: Nr. L132/1
11. EC (1996) Microbiological quality of the finished cosmetic product. Draft for an annex 7 of the EC-cosmetic directive 76/768. EC-Commission, DG XXIV/ Doc. 1878/96
12. Heinzel M (1998) Phenomena of biocide resistance in microorganisms. Int Biodete. Biodegrad; 41:225–234
13. Heir E, Sundheim G, Holck AC (1995) Resistance to quaternary ammonium compounds in Staphylococcus aureus spp. isolated from the food industry and nucleotide sequence of the resistance plasmid pST827. J Appl Bacteriol 79:149–156
14. Kümmerle N, Feucht HH, Kaulfers PM (1996) Plasmid-mediated formaldehyde resistance in Escherichia coli. Characterization of resistance gene. Antimicrob Agents Chemother 40:2276–2279
15. Meyer B, Gedek B, Heinzel M (1992) Mycotoxins. Relevance to cosmetics. Cosmet Toilet 107:75–79
16. Orth DS (1993) Handbook of cosmetic microbiology. Cosmetic science and technology, vol.12. Marcel Dekker, New York
17. Rheinbaben Fv, Heinzel M (1992) Studies on the stability of selected viruses in cosmetics. Int J Cosmet Sci 14:235–244
18. Russel AD (1997) Plasmids and bacterial resistance to biocides. J Appl Microb 82:155–165
19. Russell AD, Hugo WB, Ayliffe GAJ (1982) Principles and practice of disinfection, preservation and sterilisation. Blackwell Sci, London, pp 134–157
20. Umbach W (1991) Cosmetics and toiletries. Development, production, use. Ellis Horwood, New York (Ellis Horwood series in applied science and industrial technology)
21. United States pharmacopoeia (1995) 23rd edn. Rockville
22. Williams DF, Schmitt WH (1996) Chemistry and technology of the cosmetics and toiletries industry. Blackie Academic, London

CHAPTER 25

Mutagenicity

R. D. Combes

Introduction

Scope of Chapter

The background to mutagenicity (genotoxicity) studies in toxicology is summarised, followed by an explanation of tier-testing strategies in the context of current European regulatory requirements, including data on photomutagenicity. Other topics covered include: the principles of the main *in vitro* tests, as well as adjunct assays; ways of improving the basic testing package; refinement of *in vivo* (short-term) animal assays, including the use of transgenic rodent strains; the detection of non-genotoxic carcinogens; the use of human data, and the application of structure/activity approaches to screening. Some examples of recent studies on mutagenicity testing of cosmetics and ingredients are also given, and the relatively new requirement for photomutagenicity is discussed. Also, a scheme is proposed for the mutagenicity testing of cosmetics involving minimal animal usage, without compromising the regulatory process. Finally, some likely future developments are considered, particularly in relation to efforts to develop non-animal strategies for cosmetics testing, to support current and future EC legislative initiatives to ban the use of animals.

Definition of Genotoxicity

Genotoxicity is defined here as: *the induction of DNA damage caused by either covalent interaction with DNA (the formation of specific DNA base adducts), or by physical alteration in DNA, for example nucleotide strand breakage.* Such damage can lead to replicable changes in nucleotide base sequence and therefore mutation. The mechanistic relationship between DNA damage and mutation has resulted in the widespread adoption of mutagenicity assays to predict other endpoints in toxicity, particularly carcinogenicity, due to the fact that the latter is known to involve somatic mutation. A recent text on mutagenesis and genotoxicity was edited by Phillips and Venitt [74]; general reviews have been published by [10] and Fielder et al. [36], and one on cosmetics testing by Combes [18]. The following journals specialise in the subject, containing review-type and original papers on fundamental aspects of mutagenesis and also cover regulatory genotoxicity testing: *Mutation Research; Environmental and Molecular Mutagenesis, Mutagenesis, Teratogenesis, Mutagenesis and Carcinogenesis.*

Regulatory Testing Requirements

Introduction

Information on the mutagenicity of cosmetics products (final formulations) and on their separate ingredients is generally required by regulatory authorities throughout the world, including the Scientific Committee for Cosmetology (SCC) in Europe. Such testing is an essential pre-requisite for further studies culminating in volunteer testing. The reader is referred to respective regulatory documents for details of specific guidelines and requirements[40].

Tier-testing Strategies

Mutagenicity testing generally involves the application of initial screens consisting of gene mutation in bacteria and a test for chromosomal damage [69]. These two endpoints are used as some chemicals exert one effect specifically. Confirmation of any genotoxicity observed *in vitro*, particularly negative data, is obtained with a short-term rodent in vivo test. The need for *in vivo* assays is, however, usually considered greater when the intended usage of the chemical concerned is expected to result in high and continuous human exposure [32]. In the case of cosmetics, it should be remembered that contact with the body is intended, mainly via the skin, but also that occupational exposure occurs via a variety of potential routes, often to high concentrations over prolonged periods.

In screening tests, emphasis is placed on a high degree of sensitivity, there being little, if any, concern to reproduce *in vivo* conditions accurately. The aim is to detect and define any inherent genotoxic potential of a test chemical, and then to consider whether this potential can be realised in vivo.

Principles of Regulatory Genotoxicity Tests

Exogenous Metabolism

To compensate for the usual lack of metabolising capacity of the indicator cells used in these *in vitro* screens, mammalian enzyme preparations, usually the post-mitochondrial supernatant from rat liver (S9 fraction), are added exogenously, most often in the presence of the test material. Such enzyme preparations contain a preponderance of induced, phase-I enzymes [17]. Since these enzymes often activate chemicals to mutagenicity *in vitro* screens tend to be oversensitive, especially for identifying *in vivo* rodent mutagens and carcinogens.

Core In Vitro Tests

Bacterial gene mutation assays [14, 90] comprise treating tester/indicator strains which are hypermutable, due to their possession of defective cell envelopes, to enhance uptake of test chemicals, and to their deficiency in one or more aspects of DNA repair [41]. Both reverse and forward mutation systems are available, the most widely used being the Ames test. This involves selecting *his* revertants on minimally supplemented agar using a battery of tester strains carrying different *his* mutations in *Salmonella typhimurium.* Some care needs to be exercised in choice of tester strains due to specific effects of certain chemicals [31]. A less widely used bacterial mutation system is based on *trp* reversion in *Escherichia coli* strain WP2, and some repair-defective derivatives of this strain.

In cytogenetic assays, the most widely used approach is to screen for structural chromosomal abnormalities in metaphase-spread preparations of exposed mammalian cells using light microscopy, and a variety of staining techniques and other visual aids. Regulatory *in vitro* assays are divisible into tests using permanent cell lines, usually derived from Chinese hamsters (eg ovary (CHO) or lung (CHL)) cell lines, and those using primary cells usually of human origin (e.g. lymphocytes). There is no overall consensus as to which indicator cells are best to use, since both have advantages and disadvantages, depending on the study in question [69]. Exposure can be either in culture suspension using tubes or flasks or on slides of coverslips in dishes. Cells have to undergo DNA replication for chemically-induced DNA lesions to be detected as chromosomal damage resulting in structural aberrations, micronuclei or sister chromatid exchanges (SCEs).

In summary, dividing cells are exposed to test material (in the presence and absence of S9), then cultured for ca 1.5 cell cycles before treating with a spindle inhibitor, such as colcemid or colchicine, to collect cells in metaphase for harvesting by trypsinization and subsequent fixation and chromosomal staining. The total aberrations/cell, and the frequency of cells with aberrations, are scored. A statistically significant increase in the latter, compared with the frequency in concurrent control cultures, is usually considered indicative of genotoxicity.

Although structural aberrations are the main focus, numerical aberrations (polyploidy and hypodiploidy/hyperdiploidy), indicative of aneuploidy should also be noted [71]. Protocols for cytogenetics testing can be found elsewhere [64, 69, 81].

Short-term In Vivo Animal Genotoxicity Assays

The most widely used short-term animal test is the mouse bone marrow micronucleus assay, although chromosomal damage using metaphase preparations is an alternative method [43, 77]. These *in vivo* tests last usually only a few weeks at most, and involve acute dosing of small numbers of animals [19]. It is now considered that it is only necessary to conduct one or other of these assays. However, the micronucleus test has the advantage of allowing detection of a wide spectrum of changes in chromosomal integrity, as micronuclei arise from both acentric fragments (genotoxicity), and from dislocation of chromosomes from the mitotic spindle (non-disjunction resulting in aneuploidy). This is useful as aneuploidy is a non-genotoxic process, possibly leading to carcinogenesis [4, 72].

Additional Tests

Many different *in vitro*, and non-rodent tests, as well as different rodent *in vivo* assays, have been developed, the latter in response to a need to increase the range of tissues that can be analysed for the induction of genotoxicity (discussed later). Adjunct assays include gene mutation in a variety of cells, including cultured mammalian cells [15], differential DNA repair, unscheduled DNA synthesis (UDS), used both *in vitro* and *in vivo* [26], mitotic recombination, gene conversion/mutation in yeast (Saccharomyces cerevisiae) and Drosophila, as well as mammalian cell transformation [50, 69].

There have been calls for inclusion of mammalian cell gene mutation assays, particularly the mouse lymphoma gene mutation assay, in the core battery of tests. This suggestion has received further endorsement by the International Conference on Harmonisation of Technical Requirements for Registration of Pharmaceuticals for Human Use (ICH), which at its last international meeting [49] agreed to include the mouse lymphoma assay in its recommended basic screening battery of genotoxicity tests. This followed the results of a recent collaborative trial in Japan which demonstrated the equivalence of both cytogenetics and mouse lymphoma gene mutation assays for detecting the activity of a range of chemicals.

The mouse lymphoma assay involves measuring forward mutation at the thymidine kinase locus in L5178Y cells which are heterozygous for this locus. Such cells are sensitive to the nucleoside base analogue, trifluorothymidine (TFT), which is converted by thymidine kinase to a toxic form. Homozygous mutant cells for the tk locus, arising from forward mutation at the wild type allele, are resistant to TFT, and therefore grow in the presence of the base analogue. It has been shown that such mutations can arise as a result of a variety of genotoxic molecular events, including both point mutations (base pair changes) and chromosomal damage [69].

There is currently much interest in developing an *in vitro* micronucleus assay for regulatory purposes, especially since this endpoint is potentially useful for detecting aneugenicity *in vitro*, and scoring micronuclei is less labour-intensive and lengthy than conventional metaphase analysis [2, 75]. An acceptable protocol has yet to emerge, however, although the results of recent collaborative trials indicate that the *in vitro* micronucleus test is a reliable substitute for the chromosomal aberration test, with the advantage of being able to detect aneugens [22, 39, 67, 83]. In the case of cosmetics testing, it is noteworthy that micronuclei are induced in cultured human keratinocytes, which can be used to study metabolic activation [88].

Chromosome Painting Techniques in Cytogenetics

Methods for detecting numerical and structural chromosomal aberrations have been improved by introducing 'chromosome painting' techniques into cytogenetic analysis [71]. The method involves fluorescence *in situ* molecular hybridisation (FISH) to differentially highlight structural and numerical chromosomal aberrations as fluorescing signals, sharply contrasting with a counterstained total DNA background [33].

Some Recent Studies Involving Genotoxicity Testing of Cosmetics

Some examples of recent studies involving genotoxicity testing of cosmetics and cosmetics ingredients are given in Table 1.

Photomutagenicity

Many new products are being produced to incorporate sun protection factors, some of which possess properties allowing them to be applied for long periods of time as sunscreens. These products contain novel ingredients, designed to reflect, or specifically

Table 1. Some recent genotoxicity studies on cosmetics and cosmetic ingredients (Pos positive (genotoxic), neg negative non-genotoxic; Sal Salmonella mutagenicity assay, gm gene mutation, Dros SLRL Drosophila sex-linked recessive lethal assay, SOS SOS-inducible DNA repair, bm mn mouse bone marrow micronucleus test, uds unscheduled DNA synthesis, ca *in vitro* cytogenetics, gm moly gene mutation in mouse lymphoma cells, gm V7 gene mutation in V79 chinese hamster fibroblasts, dd DNA damage, sce sister chromatid exchange, ct cell transformation)

Test material	Endpoint	Call	Notes	Reference
Kathon CG	sal	pos	Activity attributed to methylchloroisothizoline	[23]
Kathon 886	sal	pos	Activity attributed to methylchloroisothizoline	[23]
Kathon CG	sal	pos		[62]
Kathon CG	gm	pos	Hereditary bleaching test in *Euglena gracilis* for extranuclear mutation	[62]
Triethanolamine	gm	neg	Hereditary bleaching test in *Euglena gracilis* for extranuclear mutation	[62]
Diamine silver tetraborate	gm	neg	Hereditary bleaching test in *Euglena gracilis* for extranuclear mutation	[62]
Musk ambrette	sal Dros SLRL	pos	TA100, required metabolic activation pos in Drosophila in mature sperm	[34]
Musk ambrette	SOS rep bm mn		(all 5 musks contained nitro groups) neg for mn after i.p. or oral dosing of male/ female mice	[34, 48]
Musk xylene	sal/ca/ uds *in vitro*/ vivo SOS rep gm moly/	neg		[34, 48]
Musk moskene	sal/ca/ uds *in vitro*/ vivo SOS rep gm moly/	neg		[34]
Musk tibeten	sal/ca/ uds *in vitro*/ vivo SOS rep gm moly/	neg		[34]
FDC Red No. 3 (Erythrosine)	sal/ca/ dd/ct/ gm moly	neg		[57]
FDC Red No. 3 (Erythrosine)	gm V79/ mn/sce	pos	For mn only	[79]
Bromophenol Blue	sal/moly/ dd/ bm mn	neg	dd=DNA damage assayed by mitotic recombination in *Saccharomyces cerevisiae* D5; also neg in mouse micronucleus test	[57]
Tetra-Bromophenol Blue	sal/moly/ dd/ bm mn	neg	dd=DNA damage assayed by mitotic recombination in *Saccharomyces cerevisiae* D5; also neg in mouse micronucleus test	[57]
Carminic acid (Natural Red 4)	sal/ca/ sce/ bm mn	neg	Cytogenetics assayed in CHO cells	[59]

absorb, UV light of particular wavelengths. Such ingredients might possess intrinsic toxicity, or be converted to toxic, or more toxic, forms in the presence of light (phototoxicity). As a consequence, various methods for measuring phototoxicity in vitro have been developed, by investigating the effects of UVA (320–400 nm) and UVB (280–320 nm), separately and variously in combination with each other, and with candidate sunscreens. Several of these methods have been subjected to an EU/COLIPA validation study, the results of which have been published [82], and it is anticipated that a guideline protocol will be adopted by the OECD in 1998.

Photomutagenicity is another toxic endpoint which has now been introduced as a regulatory requirement for the safety assessment of cosmetics by the SCC in its revision of the notes of guidance for testing of cosmetic ingredients for their safety evaluation (revision CSC/803–5/90) [60, 61]. This requirement applies only to chemicals which are not completely stable to solar-simulated radiation (UVA and UVB) for at least ten hours. In the absence of such evidence of photostability, a potential sunscreen must be tested for gene mutation in bacteria and chromosomal aberrations in cultured mammalian cells, with and without metabolic activation. The need for any confirmatory *in vivo* photomutagenicity testing has yet to be clarified, although it is unclear how this would be achieved, except by using transgenic mutation animal models.

A suggested approach to photomutagenicity testing was developed by Dean et al. [27], involving the use of a bacterial mutation assay in E. coli WP2 (trp reversion in soft agar), and a cytogenetics assay in CHO cells, with and without UV from a sunlamp source using three well-established photomutagens, 8-methoxypsoralen (8-MOP), para-aminobenzoic acid (PABA) and chlorpromazine (CP) as positive control chemicals (see Table 2). These authors subsequently demonstrated that three sunscreen ingredients (Table 2) were not photomutagenic, using the above complementary assays [28]. Henderson et al. [44] obtained similar data, using either agar plate incorporation or liquid suspension protocols with Salmonella and E. coli, although PABA proved nonmutagenic.

Other strategies for photomutagenicity testing have been developed. Thus, 8-MOP, CP and PARSOLR, a sunscreen ingredient, were tested in bacterial and yeast assays [11, 12], with a good dose-related mutagenic response being observed for 8-MOP. Also, the Comet assay, and a test using the green alga Chlamydamonas, have been utilized to detect photomutagenicity (Table 2).

Factors affecting the development of protocols for photomutagenicity testing include the exact nature of the UV source, the doses of UV and the chemical, exposure conditions, and the indicator strains. A COLIPA Taskforce on Photomutagenicity was established in April, 1991, with the objective of establishing validated, standard protocols for detecting photomutagenicity. Apart from the problems of standardising UV sources and type of indicator strains, choice and application of controls were two other issues discussed. Thus, it is necessary to assess the effects of UV, the sunscreen, the combination of the two, and any modulation of activity due to filtering effects of the sunscreen. Also, there is a need to agree on which bacterial tester strains to use, and to determine the optimum exposure conditions to both chemical and UV for each strain. Seven laboratories in the taskforce participated in a ring trial involving the use of both liquid pre-incubation and plate incorporation bacterial mutation protocols with three different *Salmonella* tester strains, and two strains of E. coli [45]. The following recommendations were made by the taskforce: (a) the light source must simulate sunlight; (b) it is necessary to use a combination of tester strains; (c) exposure can be either in suspension culture or on agar; (d) non-phototoxic chemicals can be assayed at different concentrations with a single UV dose; (e) phototoxic chemicals should be tested over a range of concentrations and with different UV doses, the maximum dose being limited by toxicity or mutagenicity, and (f) it is only necessary to use a single test, where there is a clear positive or negative response. The report also suggests that the

Table 2. Some photomutagenicity studies on cosmetic ingredients (var variable; wk pos weak positive; bgm bacterial gene mutation; see also legend to Table 1)

Test material	Endpoint	Call	Notes	Reference
Khellin	SAL	pos	In TA102 (neg in TA1537); used 8-MOP and 4,5',8-trimethoxypsoralen (TMP) as pos controls; TMP pos in TA1537; Khellin required UVA to be mutagenic; classified as a weak photomutagen	[76]
Benzene sulphonic acid	bgm/ca	neg	E. coli trp and CHO cells used; UVA and UVB from OSRAM Ultra-Vitalux sunlamp;	[28]
4-[(4,7,7-trimethyl-3-oxo-bicyclo[2.2.1]Heptane-2-ylidine)methyl] = MEXORYL SL	bgm/ca	neg	3 Candidate sunscreens tested to max solubility/toxicity; all 3 were neg with/without UV; 8-MOP used as pos control in both assays	[28]
4-(2-oxo-3-bornylidinemethyl) Phenyl trimethyl ammonium methyl sulphate=MEXORYL SO	bgm/ca	neg	3 Candidate sunscreens tested to max solubility/toxicity; all 3 were neg with/without UV; 8-MOP used as pos control in both assays	[28]
3,3'-(1,4-phenylenedimethyl-ylidine)Bis[7,7-dimethyl-2-oxo-bicyclo[2.2.1]heptane-1-methane sulphonic acid]= MEXORYL SX	bgm/ca	neg	3 Candidate sunscreens tested to max solubility/toxicity; all 3 were neg with/without UV; 8-MOP used as pos control in both assays	[28]
Chlorpromazine	SAL/bgm	pos	SAL (TA98,TA102,TA1537); also E.coli WP2 and WP2(pkM101); exsposures in either suspension or on agar; were differences in sensitivity between the different strains, but all conditions able to detect photomutagenicity	[44]
8-MOP	SAL/bgm	pos	SAL (TA98,TA102,TA1537); also E.coli WP2 and WP2(pkM101); exsposures in either suspension or on agar; were differences in sensitivity between the different strains, but all conditions able to detect photomutagenicity	[44]
Para-aminobenzoic acid (PABA)	SAL/bgm	neg	SAL (TA98,TA102,TA1537); also E.coli WP2 and WP2(pkM101); exsposures in either suspension or on agar; were differences in sensitivity between the different strains, but all conditions able to detect photomutagenicity; neg under all conditions	[44]

Table 2. (Continued)

Test material	Endpoint	Call	Notes	Reference
3 Fluoroquinolines (fleroxacin (Fl), ciproflaxacin (Cp), lomefloxacin)	SAL/gm/ca/dd	var	weak pos (SAL TA104,TA100); neg (gm in Saccharomcyes cerevisiae); pos (ca in V79 cells and in mouse lymphoma cells using COMET assay); although chemicals were equipotent in SAL and COMET ssays, for ca was a gradation in potency: L >Fl >Cp; used solar-simulated UV (with reduced UVB component); free radicals implicated in mechanism of phototoxicity and photogenotoxicity	[13]
8-MOP	SAL/gm/dd	pos	pos for SAL in TA102; pos for gm and for dd (gene conversion in Saccharomyces cerevisiae; 8-MOP photomutagenicity correlated with O₂ partial pressure; β-carotene and α-to'opherol were protective	[9]
PABA	bgm	neg	neg in SAL and E. coli; weak pos in TA1537, clearly pos in TA102 and E.coli WP2	[87]
Octyldimethyl-PABA = EUSOLEX 6007	bgm	neg		[87]
4-Methylbenzylidine camphor =EUSOLEX 6300	bgm	neg		[87]
Dihydroxyacetone (DHA)	bgm	wk pos	DHA is active ingredient of some self-tanning lotions; pos in TA100,TA102 only at very toxic concs, and activity not potentiated by UV	[87]
12-Dimethylbenz[a]anthracene	bgm	pos	Tested with/without S9; pos in SAL (TA98,TA1537); spectrum of activity in different tester strains dependent on if S9 and UV used	[87]
8-MOP	SAL/gm	pos	gm (Saccharomyces cerevisiae); 8-MOP gave good dose-response	[11]
Chlorpromazine	SAL/gm	neg		
PARSOLR	SAL/gm	neg		
Khellin	gm	neg	arg reversion in Chlamydamonas reinhardtii with UVA (see [76])	[80]
Visnagin	gm	wk pos	arg reversion in Chlamydamonas reinhardtii with UVA (see [76])	[80]

SCC requirement for photomutagenicity testing should be reviewed periodically, particularly as few chemicals, if any, have thus far been shown to be mutagenic only in the presence of UV, and also because photomutagenicity testing of sunscreens is not requested by other regulatory authorities.

None of the protocols used in the studies discussed above involved using an exogenous source of mammalian activating enzymes, despite the need to take this into account, as stated in the SCC guidelines. Utesh and Splittgerber [87] have shown, however, that different results can be obtained with and without S9 mix for photomutagenicity of 12-dimethylbenzanthracene (DMBA), depending on the *Salmonella* tester strain used. This chemical might, therefore, be an appropriate positive control in photomutagenicity protocols in which S9 mix is added.

Other Approaches

Genetically Engineered Cells

Many attempts have been made to increase the sensitivity of mammalian cell lines by producing a variety of indicator cell strains, which express cloned cytochrome P-450 isozymes [17, 24, 51, 89]. Also, *Salmonella* tester strains possessing mammalian metabolising capacity have been produced [52]. The usefulness of such strains, and of the genetically engineered mammalian cell lines, for routine testing remains to be established, however, especially due to constraints on the versatility of the resulting systems to metabolise different substrates, and to differences in the inducibility of enzymes. Nevertheless, indicator strains with endogenous metabolising capacity allow active metabolites to be generated closer to DNA, the target site for genotoxicity.

Refining Animal Genotoxicity Assays

Bone Marrow Tests

Few potential target organs, other than the bone-marrow, are investigated routinely for genotoxicity using animal assays. Methods for detecting micronuclei in the skin, and in peripheral blood cells [42] have been developed, however. The *ex vivo/in vivo* rodent liver unscheduled DNA synthesis assay [68] is also now used as an adjunct to the bone-marrow cytogenetics test [54]. There are also methods for detecting UDS in extrahepatic tissues including the skin [86].

Another way of measuring DNA damage in any tissue is provided by the 'Comet' assay [3, 65, 85], which involves lysing cells and subjecting them to microgel electrophoresis, to visualise and quantitate tails of stained DNA migrated from the nucleus.

Although it is generally considered that routes of administration should be those that are applicable for the intended normal usage of a test chemical, bone marrow studies are often conducted using the i.p. route, so as to maximise the amount of chemical absorbed. Use of this route, however, can generate spurious data, particularly when testing cosmetics, where the principal target organ is the skin.

Transgenic Rodents

Methods for detecting gene mutation *in vivo* in different target organs have been feasible on a routine basis only comparatively recently, with the development of specific transgenic rodent strains for mutagenesis (see [37, 66] for reviews). Such transgenic organisms contain foreign DNA, usually at least one intact gene, from another organism, which has become stably integrated into the genome of all somatic and germ line host cells. The rationale for using transgenic strains is to develop methods for detecting mutagens in a range of different tissues, including germ cells, suitable for use with a variety of exposure conditions and regimens.

Mutamouse™ and Big Blue™ are currently the principle commercially available transgenic mouse models, although transgenic rat strains have been generated. Mutamouse™ and Big Blue™ strains contain the *E.coli lacZ* and lacI transgenes respectively, which are cloned in bacteriophage lambda vectors integrated in the genome. Following exposure of the transgenic mice to a test chemical, the integrated bacteriophage vectors are rescued from the total genomic DNA by *in vitro* packaging. Mutant phage, with disrupted *lac* genes, are recognised by their ability to grow on susceptible *E. coli* host strains, and by the colour of the resulting plaques growing on the agar plates. Thus, the foreign phage DNA has a defined base sequence and acts as the target for *in vivo* mutagenesis.

Such transgenic systems would seem to be particularly suitable for testing cosmetics, providing opportunities for direct dosing of skin and scoring of mutation in the same target organ. In this respect, it is intereresting to note that acetic acid induced acute toxicity (ulceration) together with mutation after a single topical application to transgenic mice (S Dean and B Myhr 1994, personal communication).

Acceptable protocols for detecting mutation using these transgenic rodent strains are currently being developed as a result of several validation studies [66]. It would appear that strong mutagens are detected with a high degree of accuracy (high sensitivity), but the ability of these assays to correctly detect non-carcinogens requires further investigation (due to the questionable specificity so far obtained). There have also been concerns that chemicals causing mainly large deletions of DNA sequences are not readily detected in the standard strains. This has been attributed to limitations on the size of DNA fragment that can be packaged.

It is important that validation studies of these transgenic strains include an assessment of their suitability for the simultaneous detection of micronuclei, acute lethal potency, and metabolic fate, where aspects of protocol design, such as dosing and sampling time, permit. Using the same animals to detect more than one endpoint simultaneously not only increases sensitivity of testing strategies, but also will contribute to an overall reduction in the numbers of animals required for mutagenicity testing. Moreover, although some species-specific genotoxins have been identified [1], the extent of this phenomenon is insufficient to justify the automatic use of both rat and mouse transgenic strains. Further developments in the application of transgenic rodents for *in vivo* mutagenicity testing will also be influenced by the outcome of efforts to develop and validate transgenic strains for carcinogenicity testing, and should also take account of the ethical issues and animal welfare implications associated with their usage [66].

Use and Interpretation of Human Data

Prospective cosmetics products are subjected to volunteer studies, as well as efficacy assessment, during patch testing, for example. Such studies are designed usually to confirm safety in use, following on from earlier investigations used to obtain evidence of non-toxicity. Increasingly, the need for animal testing before using volunteers is being phased out, especially in the development of new finished products containing reformulations of existing ingredients for which animal test data are available. This has been possible for two principal reasons: the development and use of alternative methods for predicting the overall toxicity of new combinations of ingredients, and also increased knowledge concerning the mechanisms whereby different components of mixtures can interact to modulate toxicity.

There are surprisingly few published *in vitro* toxicity studies showing possible synergistic and antagonistic interactions between chemicals, although interestingly, the majority of those studies which are available are concerned with genotoxicity (see eg [25]). In view of this fact, it is suggested that investigations into possible interactions between ingredients in new formulations should commence with *Salmonella* mutagenicity studies, and this should be combined with an assay for basal cytotoxicity in cultured mammalian cells. It is, of course, feasible that synergistic effects can be manifested *in vivo* uniquely because the presence of one ingredient can enhance the skin penetration, and possibly also the enzymatic transformation, of another. This phenomenon should be detectable in an *in vitro* percutaneous absorption assay, especially one incorporating metabolising skin cells [46].

With regard to volunteer testing, the genotoxic effects of topical exposures to cosmetics could be undertaken via non-invasive analysis of blood and urine [16], for chromosomal damage in peripheral lymphocytes, and for the presence of mutagenic metabolites. Such information can be interpreted in conjunction with levels of compound and metabolites in body fluids, as well as other data on sampling time and other possible exposures to minimise the possible effects of confounding factors and levels of inter-individual variation. In three studies conducted on volunteers using hair colourants, there was no definitive evidence for an increased incidence of chromosomal aberrations in peripheral lymphocytes taken from exposed individuals, compared with matched controls [47].

Human data can also contribute to risk assessment of occupational exposure to cosmetics and cosmetic ingredients via biomonitoring and the detection of biomarkers of internal exposure. Babish et al. [7] found that a cohort of cosmetologists had a significantly higher frequency of urinary mutagens compared with that found using a complementary group of dental hygienists. The cause of this difference between the two cohorts was unclear, however. Thus, the possible genetic effects from occupational exposure of hairdressers, beauticians and barbers to cosmetics, especially hair dyes, has received some attention, although the evidence to date for an association between exposure and increased endogenous levels of genotoxins is equivocal [47].

Structure–Activity Relationships

The prediction of activity from molecular structure, on the basis of chemical similarity with known toxicants, is known as structure-activity relationships (SAR). Several different computer methods, known as expert systems, have been developed for predicting toxicity from physico-chemical properties, based on a number of different criteria, information and rules [21, 27, 53]. Perhaps the most widely used of these for mutagenicity prediction are CASE-TOX, DEREK and TopKat, although there is increasing usage of such systems in conjunction with others designed to predict metabolic pathways and major metabolites.

For example, DEREK (Deductive Estimation of Risk from Existing Knowledge) has an extensive rulebase for the identification of toxicophores for mutagenicity in chemical structures [58, 78]. Although these rules are based to a large extent on the earlier identification of structural alerts for mutagenicity in chemicals from the NTP database [5], they take account of many physicochemical factors. DEREK also has been used for predicting skin sensitisation [8, 73], with an extensive rule base for identifying toxicophores for this toxicity endpoint which, in common with mutagenicity, often involves chemical reactivity, in this case protein binding. This mechanistic relationship is emphasised by observation of a correlation between induction of lymphocyte proliferation, using the local lymph node assay in mice, and *Salmonella* mutagenicity, for a group of twenty structurally diverse chemicals [6]. The mechanisms of skin sensitisation are not fully understood, however, and thus it is very unlikely, that a simple mutagenicity test would be suitable for routine screening of potential sensitisers, although the link between sensitisation and mutagenicity has also been investigated by Thune et al. [84].

The use of such expert systems for mutagenicity prediction must be approached with caution, since rule bases are still being written, and predictivity depends upon the availability of high quality and unequivocal experimental mutation data, where the possible effects of any contaminating chemicals can be discounted, to provide the expert information required for the database. Nevertheless, it is clear that such computer prediction systems, coupled with increasingly sophisticated molecular graphical techniques, will play an ever increasing central role in mutagenicity testing, especially with the advent of enhanced combinatorial methods for chemical synthesis.

Discussion

A Possible Future Strategy

A possible strategy for genotoxicity testing of cosmetics is suggested in Figure 1 (see also [56]). This scheme assumes that *in vivo* animal studies are unnecessary, or only rarely required, under the following conditions: (a) in the absence of percutaneous absorption, and (b) if the chemical is genotoxic *in vitro*, since such a result automatically leads to rejection of the test compound. These assumptions are based on the fact that detoxification occurring before DNA is exposed in the target organ skin would be expected to be considerably less following topical treatment during human usage, compared with the detoxification occurring in standard *in vivo* protocols involving other routes of exposure. In comparison, the results of *in vitro* assays should, therefore, provide more relevant and reliable data for predicting human hazard, since phase-II (detoxification) reactions are generally absent, or of very low activity.

If a chemical is non-genotoxic *in vitro*, and whether or not percutaneous absorption occurs, there is a possibility of non-genotoxic carcinogenesis, which cannot be predic-

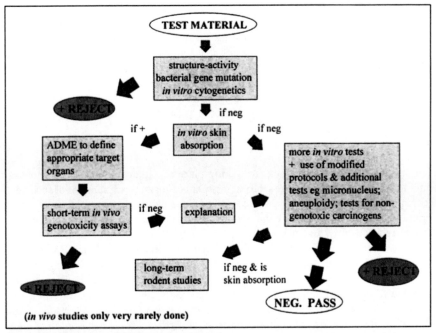

Fig. 1. Scheme for mutagenicity testing of cosmetics

ted by the standard mutagenicity assays. There is an urgent need, therefore, to develop a mechanistic understanding of how non-genotoxic carcinogens act, and for a battery of mechanistically-based *in vitro* tests and approaches covering all the relevant endpoints, rather than relying on further animal tests. Some progess is being made in this direction, including new understanding of structural features of molecules required for their binding to various cellular receptors, and also techniques for detecting aneuploidy mentioned earlier [20]. Thus, for chemicals that are non-genotoxic *in vitro*, and which do not penetrate skin, there may still be a need for further study, in view of the possibility for dermal effects, particularly when there is evidence of other toxicity, such as irritation, corrosivity or sensitisation, which could result in cell proliferation, a process considered to be involved in non-genotoxic carcinogenesis [55].

Recently, there have been suggestions that the basic genotoxicity testing package should include an *in vivo* assay for routine screening (see [19]). This is to take account of a small, but increasing, number of chemicals which apparently exhibit genotoxicity uniquely *in vivo*. It is, however, very likely that most, if not all, of these genotoxins could be detected *in vitro* using modified protocols, together with a few extra assays, especially for aneuploidy. In many cases, the modification involves the use of improved metabolic activation conditions. For example, Dillon et al. [30] showed that the azo dye, D&C Red No. 9, was activated to a mutagen in the *Salmonella* assay, only if the chemical was subjected to reductive metabolism afforded by incubating the dye with a rat caecal bacterial preparation. Thus, a more flexible approach to the use of *in vitro* tests and protocols needs to be adopted, especially for cosmetics testing. This is advisable for both scientific and animal welfare reasons, rather than using the existence of some so-called specific *in vivo* positives to justify the premature application of animal tests for genotoxicity, which are themselves insufficiently sensitive and versatile as screens.

In those rare cases where animal testing is considered unavoidable, it should not be undertaken without information from absorption, distribution and metabolism (ADME) studies, to enable usage of the most appropriate protocols and assays [63]. Such pharmacokinetic information should be obtained as an integral part of the testing strategy in view of its importance in influencing the nature of any subsequent animal testing [38], rather than being neglected as is often the case at present [35].

Conclusions

Many exciting new developments are taking place in mutagenicity testing, most of which are directly relevant to the safety assessment of cosmetics. Examples of such new techniques include genetically engineered cell lines expressing high levels of cytochrome P-450 isozymes, use of computer modelling and expert systems for structure-activity relationships, and utilization of new, highly sensitive and semi-automated cytogenetic techniques for the rapid detection and characterisation of chromosomal damage. Also it is likely that future advances will include the development of acceptable protocols for new *in vitro* assays, including those for the detection of micronuclei, aneuploidy, cell proliferation and cell transformation, based on human cell lines. The adoption of more flexibility in the use of protocols and complementary tests for genotoxicity *in vitro*, deployed in conjunction with *in vitro* tests for other endpoints, such as percutaneous absorption, will help to provide a reliable regulatory framework for cosmetics testing which makes minimal, or no, usage of animals, and which will help to satisfy emerging and future likely legislation.

On the rare occasions when animal tests are considered unavoidable, they should be used judiciously at the correct time in the overall safety assessment process, to facilitate data interpretation using related information on ADME, for example. This restriction should apply also to assays involving transgenic rodent strains, even though these allow the rapid detection of potential genotoxicity of topical exposures on skin cells, since in any case *in vivo* assays are unnecessary for cosmetics ingredient testing, unless there is evidence of skin penetration. It is also suggested that more reliable information on possible *in vivo* genotoxic hazard might be obtained from the analysis of blood and urine of volunteers for cytogenetic damage in lymphocytes and mutagenic metabolites, respectively.

References

1. Albanese R, Mirkova E, Gatehouse D, Ashby J (1988) Species-specific response to the rodent carcinogens 1,2-dimethylhydrazine and 1,2-dibromo-chloropropane in rodent bone marrow micronucleus assays. Mutagenesis 3:35–38
2. Albertini S, Miller B, Kirsch-Volders M (1996) The *in vitro* micronucleus assay as an alternative/replacement for the *in vitro* chromosome aberration assay: status and implications for testing strategies. EEMS Newsletter 27:13–14.
3. Anderson D, Plewa MJ (1998) The international Comet assay workshop. Mutagenesis 13:67–73
4. Anon (1997) Aneuploidy. (Monograph no 27) European Centre for Ecotoxicology and Toxicology of Chemicals (ECETOC), Brussels, p 172
5. Ashby J, Paton D (1993) The influence of chemical structure on the extent and sites of carcinogenesis for 522 rodent carcinogens and 55 different human carcinogen exposures. Mutat Res 286:3–74

6. Ashby J, Hilton J, Dearman RJ, Callander RD, Kimber I (1993) Mechanistic relationship among mutagenicity, skin sensitisation, and skin carcinogenicity. Environ Health Perspect101:62–67
7. Babish JG, Scarlett JM, Voekler SE, Gutenmann WH, Lisk DJ (1991) Urinary mutagens in cosmetologists and dental personnel. J Toxicol Environ Health 34:197–206
8. Barratt MD, Basketter DA (1994) Structure–activity relationships for skin sensitization: an expert system. In: Rougier A, Goldberg AM, Mailbach HI (eds) *In Vitro* Toxicology. Mary Ann Liebert, New York, pp 293-301
9. Bianchi L, Melli R, Pizzala R, Stivala LA, Rehak L, Quarta S, Vannini V (1996) Effects of beta-carotene and alpha-tocopherol on photogenotoxicity induced by 8-methoxypsoralen: role of oxygen. Mutat Res 369:183–194
10. Brusick D (1994) Genetic toxicology. In: Hayes AW (ed) Principles and methods of toxicology, 3rd edn. Raven Press, New York, pp 545–577
11. Chetelat A, Albertini S, Dresp JH, Strobel R Gocke E (1993) Photomutagenesis test development: I. 8-methoxypsoralen, chlorpromazine and sunscreen compounds in bacterial and yeast assays. Mutat Res 292: 241–250.
12. Chetelat A, Dresp JH, Gocke E (1993) Photomutagenesis test development: II. 8-methoxypsoralen, chlorpromazine and sunscreen compounds in chromosomal aberration assays using CHO cells. Mutat Res 292:254–258
13. Chetelat AA, Abertini S, Gocke E (1996) The photomutagenicity of fluoroquinolones in tests for gene mutation, chromosomal aberration, gene conversion and DNA breakage (Comet assay). Mutagenesis 11:497–504
14. Clare C (1995) Mutation assays in bacteria. In: O'Hare S, Atterwill CK (eds) In Vitro Toxicity Testing Protocols. Human Press, Totowa, pp 297–306
15. Clements J (1995) Gene mutation assays in mammalian cells. In: O'Hare S, Atterwill CK (eds) In Vitro Toxicity Testing Protocols. Human Press, Totowa, pp 277–286
16. Combes RD (1991) Use of clinical samples for biomonitoring of genotoxic exposure to pharmaceuticals. In: Nimmo W (ed) Clinical Measurement in Drug Evaluation. Wolfe Medical, London, pp 173–191
17. Combes RD (1992) The *in vivo* relevance of *in vitro* genotoxity assays incorporating enzyme activation systems. In: Gibson GG (ed) Progress in Drug Metabolism, vol 13. Taylor and Francis, London, pp 295–321
18. Combes RD (1995) Mutagenicity testing of cosmetics: current trends and prospects for the replacement, refinement, and reduction of animal testing. Comments Toxicol 5:247–270
19. Combes RD (1995) Regulatory genotoxicity testing: a critical appraisal. ATLA 23:352–379
20. Combes RD (1997) Detection of nongenotoxic carcinogens: major barriers to replacement of the rodent bioassay. In: van Zutphen LFM, Balls M (eds) Animal Alternatives, Welfare and Ethics. (Proceedings of the Second World Congress on Alternatives and Animal Use in the Life Sciences) Elsevier, Amsterdam, pp 627–634
21. Combes RD, Judson P (1995) The use of artificial intelligence systems for predicting toxicity. Pesticide Sci 45:179–194
22. Combes RD, Stopper H, Casary WJ (1995) The use of L5178Y mouse lymphoma cells to assess mutagenic, clastogenic and aneugenic acitivity of chemicals. Mutagenesis 10:403–408
23. Connor TH, Tee PG, Afshar M, Connor KM (1996) Mutagenicity of cosmetic products containing Kathon. Environ Mol Mutagen 28:127–132
24. Crespi C (1995) Use of genetically engineered cells for genotoxicity testing. In: Phillips DH, Venitt S (eds) Environmental Mutagenesis. Bios Scientific, Oxford, pp 233–260
25. Dashwood RH, Combes RD, Ashby J (1986) Mutagenicity to *Salmonella* of derivatives of the potent azo mutagen 5I: some implications for structure-activity data bases and the evaluation of combinations of mutagens. Mutagenesis 1:261–265
26. Dean S (1995) Measurement of unscheduled DNA synthesis *in vitro* using primary rat hepatocyte cultures. In: O'Hare S, Atterwill CK (eds) *In Vitro* Toxicity Testing Protocols. Human Press, Totowa, pp 267–276
27. Dean SW, Lane M, Dunmore RH, Ruddock SP, Martin CN, Kirkland DJ, Loprieno N (1991) Development of assays for the detection of photomutagenicity of chemicals during exposure to UV light. I. Assay development. Mutagenesis 6:335–341
28. Dean SW, Dunmore RH, Ruddock SP, Dean JC, Martin CN, Kirkland DJ (1992) Development of assays for the detection of photomutagenicity of chemicals during exposure to UV light. II. Results of testing three sunscreen ingredients. Mutagenesis 7:179–182
29. Dearden JC, Barratt MD, Benigni R, Bristol DW, Combes RD, Cronin MTD, Judson PM, Payne MP, Richard AM, Tichy M, Worth AP, Yourick JJ (1997) The development and validation of expert systems for predicting toxicity. The report and recommendations of an ECVAM/ECB workshop. (ECVAM workshop 24) ATLA 25:223–252

30. Dillon D, Combes R, Zeiger E (1994) Activation by caecal reduction of the azo dye D & C Red No 9 to a bacterial mutagen. Mutagenesis 9:295–299

31. Dillon D, Combes R, Zeiger E (1998) The effectiveness of *Salmonella* strains TA100, TA102 and TA104 for detecting mutagenicity of some aldehydes and peroxides. Mutagenesis 13:19–26

32. DOH (Department of Health) (1989) Guidelines for the Testing of Chemicals for Mutagenicity. HMSO, London

33. Eastmond DA, Rupa DS (1995) Fluorescence *in situ* hybridization: application to environmental mutagenesis. In: Phillips DH, Venitt S (eds) Environmental Mutagenesis. Bios Scientific, Oxford, pp 261-290

34. Emig M, Reinhardt A, Mersch-Sunderman V (1996) A comparative study of five nitro musk compounds for genotoxicity in the SOS chromotest and *Salmonella* mutagenicity. Toxicol Lett 85: 151–156

35. Fahrig R, Lang R, Madle S (1991) General strategy for assessment of genotoxicity. Mutat Res 252:161–163

36. Fielder RJ, Atterwill CK, Anderson D, Boobis AR, Botham P, Chamberlain M, Combes R, Duffy P, Lewis RW, Lumley CE, Kimber I, Newall DR (1997) BTS working party report on *in vitro* toxicology. Hum Exp Toxicol 16:S1–S40

37. Foster R (1995) Measuring genetic events in transgenic animals. in: Phillips DH, Venitt S (eds) Environmental Mutagenesis. Bios Scientific, Oxford, pp 291-314

38. Frantz SW, Beatty PW, English JC, Hundley SG, Wilson AGE (1994) The use of pharmacokinetics as an interpretive and predictive tool in chemical toxicology testing and risk assessment: a position paper on the appropriate use of pharmacokinetics in chemical toxicology. Regul Toxicol Pharmacol 19:317–337

39. Fritzenschaf H, Kohlpoth M, Rusche B, Schiffman D (1993) Testing of known carcinogens and non-carcinogens in the Syrian hamster embryo (SHE) micronucleus test *in vitro*; correlations with *in vivo* micronucleus formation and cell transformation. Mutat Res 319:47–53

40. Gatehouse D (1994) Mutagenicity. In: Cartwright AC, Mathews BR (eds) International Pharmaceutical Product Registration – Aspects of Quality, Safety and Efficacy. Ellis Horwood, New York, pp 474–552

41. Gatehouse D, Rowland IR, Wilcox P, Callender RD, Forster R (1990) Bacterial mutation assays. In: Kirkland DJ (ed) Basic Mutagenicity Tests: UKEMS Recommended Procedures. (UKEMS Sub-committee on Guidelines for Mutagenicity Testing Report, part I revised: Basic tests) Cambridge University Press, Cambridge, pp13–61

42. Hayashi M, Morita T, Kodama Y, Sofuni T, Ishidate M Jr (1990) The micronucleus assay with mouse peripheral blood reticulocytes, using acridine orange-coated slides. Mutat Res 245:245–249

43. Heddle JA (1995) *In vivo* assays for mutagenicity. In: Phillips DH, Venitt S (eds) Environmental Mutagenesis. Bios Scientific, Oxford, pp 141–154

44. Henderson L, Fedyk J, Bourner C, Windebank S, Fletcher S, Lovell W (1994) Photomutagenicity assays in bacteria: factors affecting assay design and assessment of photomutagenic potential of para-aminobenzoic acid. Mutagenesis 9:459–465

45. Henderson L, Gocke E, Utesch D, Brendler S, Gahlmann R, Pungier J, Gorelick N, Dean S, Clare C, Jones E (1996) Development of test methods for assessing the photomutagenic potential of sunscreens. In: Lisansky SG, Macmillan R, Dupuis J (eds) Alternatives to Animal Testing. (Proceedings of an International Scientific Conference Organised by the European Cosmetic Industry) CPL Press, Newbury, pp 303–305

46. Howes D, Guy R, Hadgraft J, Heylings J, Hoeck U, Kemper F, Mailbach H., Marty J-P, Merk H, Parra J, Rekkas D, Rondelli, I, Schaefer H, Täuber U, Verbiese N (1996) Methods for assessing percutaneous absorption. (ECVAM Workshop Report 13) ATLA 24:81–106

47. IARC (1993) Occupational exposures to hairdressers and barbers and personal use of hair colourants; some hair dyes, cosmetic colourants, industrial dyestuffs and aromatic amines. (IARC Monographs on the Evaluation of Carcinogenic Risk to Humans, vol 57) IARC, Lyon

48. IARC (1996) Printing processes and printing inks, carbon black and some nitro compounds. (IARC Monographs on the Evaluation of Carcinogenic Risk to Humans, vol 65) IARC, Lyon, France

49. ICH (1997) Reprt of the Fourth International Conference on Harmonisation, Brussels, July, 1997: Genotoxicity: Standard Battery of Tests, Step 4 Report, ICH

50. Isfort RJ, LeBoeuf RA (1996) Application of *in vitro* cell transformation assays to predict the carcinogenic potential of chemicals. Mutat Res 365:161–173

51. Josephy PD, Gruz P, Nohmi T (1997) Recent advances in the construction of bacterial genotoxicity assays. Mutat Res 386:1–23

52. Josephy PD, Evans DH, Parikh A, Guengerich FP (1998) Metabolic activation of aromatic amine mutagens by simultaneous expression of human cytochrome P450 1A2, NADPH-cytochrome P450 reductase, and N-aectyltransferase in *Escherichia coli*. Chem Res Toxicol 11:70–74

53. Judson PN (1997) Expert systems for hazard evaluation. In: Tennant DR (ed) Food Chemical Risk Analysis. Blackie Academic & Professional, London, pp 109–132
54. Kennelly JC, Waters R, Ashby J, Lefevre PA, Burlinson B, Benford DJ, Dean SW, Mitchell I. deG (1993) *In vivo* rat UDS assay. In: Kirkland DJ, Fox M (eds) Supplementary Mutagenicity Tests: UKEMS Recommended Procedures. UKEMS Sub-committee on Guidelines for Mutagenicity Testing: Report, Part II, revised, pp 52–77
55. Lai DY, Baetcke KP, Vu VT, Cotruvo JA, Eustis SL (1994) Evaluation of reduced protocols for carcinogenicity testing of chemicals: report of a joint EPA/NIEHS workshop. Regul Toxicol Pharmacol 19:183–201
56. Langley G, Fisher C (1995) New perspectives in cosmetics toxicology. Non-animal testing strategies. Ideal Publications, London, p 28
57. Lin GH, Brusick DJ (1986) Mutagenicity studies on FD & C Red no. 3. Mutagenesis 1:253–259
58. Long A, Combes RD (1995) Using DEREK to predict the activity of some carcinogens/mutagens found in foods. Toxicol In Vitro 9: 563–569
59. Loprieno G, Boncristiani G, Loprieno N (1992) Genotoxicity studies *in vitro* and *in vivo* on carminic acid (natural red 4). Fed Chem Toxicol 30: 759–764
60. Loprieno N (1991) *In vitro* assay systems for testing photomutagenic chemicals. Mutagenesis 6:331–333
61. Loprieno N (1992) Guidelines for safety evaluation of cosmetics ingredients in the EC countries. Fed Chem Toxicol 30:809–815
62. Macor M, Beno J, Grones J, Siekel P, Novotny J (1996) *Euglena gracilis* as a supplementary test organism for detecting biologically active compounds. Folia Microbiol Praha 41:48–52
63. Madle S, Lang R (1992) Assessment and evaluation of genotoxicity findings. Mutat Res 291:87–91
64. Marshall R (1995) Measurement of chromosome aberrations *in vitro* using human peripheral blood lymphocytes. In: O'Hare S, Atterwill CK (eds) In Vitro Toxicity Testing Protocols. Human a Press, Totowa, pp 287–296
65. McKelvey-Martin VI, Green MHL, Schmezer P, Pool-Zobel BL, DeMeo MP, Collins A (1993) The single cell gel electrophoresis assay (comet assay): a European perspective. Mutat Res 288:47–63
66. Mepham TB, Combes RD, Balls M, Barbieri O, Blokhuis HJ, Costa P, Crilly RE, de Cock Buning T, Delpire VC, O'Hare MJ, Houdebine L-M, van Kreijl CF, van der Meer M, Reinhardt CA, Wolf E, van Zeller AM (1998) Use of transgenic animals in the European Union – the report and recommendations of ECVAM workshop 28. ATLA 26:21–43
67. Miller BM, Pujadas E, Gocke E (1995) Evaluation of the micronucleus test *in vitro* using Chinese Hamster cells: results with four chemicals weakly positive in the *in vivo* micronucleus test. Environ Mol Mutagen 26:240–247
68. Mirsalis JC (1995) Assays for unscheduled DNA synthesis *in vivo*. In: Phillips DH, Venitt S (eds) Environmental Mutagenesis. Bios Scientific, Oxford, pp 219–232
69. Mitchell I deG, Combes RD (1996) In vitro genotoxicity and cell transformation assessment. In: Castell JV, Gomez-Lechon MJ (eds) *In vitro* Methods in Pharmaceutical Research. Academic Press, London, pp 317–352
70. Müller K, Kasper K, Muller L (1993) An assessment of the *in vitro* hepatocyte micronucleus assay. Mutat Res 292:213–224
71. Parry, EM, Parry JM (1995) *In vitro* cytogenetics and aneueploidy. In: Phillips DH, Venitt S (eds) Environmental Mutagenesis. Bios Scientific, Oxford, pp 121–139
72. Parry EM, Henderson L, Mackay JM (1995) Procedures for the detection of chemically induced aneuploidy: recommendations of a UK Environmental Mutagen Society Working Group. Mutagenesis 10:1–14
73. Payne MP, Walsh PT (1994). Structure–activity relationships for skin sensitization potential: development of structural alerts for use in knowledge-based toxicity prediction systems. J Chem Inform Comput Sci 34:154–161
74. Phillips DH, Venitt S (eds) (1995). Environmental Mutagenesis. Bios Scientific, Oxford
75. Ramirez MJ, Surallés J, Puerto S, Creus A, Marcos R (1997) Aneugenic activity in human cultured lymphocytes. An overall study with colchicine using the micronucleus assay and fluorescence *in situ* hybridisation techniques. Mutagenesis 12:405–410
76. Riccio ML, Coratza G, Bovalini L, Martelli P (1992) Investigation of the mutagenic activity in *Salmonella typhimurium* of the furochrome khellin, proposed as a therapeutic agent for skin diseases. Mutat Res 279:103–108
77. Richold M, Ashby J, Bootman J, Chandley A, Gatehouse DJ, Henderson L (1990) *In vivo* cytogenetics assays. In: Kirkland DJ (ed) Basic Mutagenicity Tests: UKEMS Recommended Procedures. UKEMS Sub-committee on Guidelines for Mutagenicity Testing, Report, Part I, Revised: Basic tests. Cambridge University Press, Cambridge, pp 115–141

78. Ridings JE, Barratt MD, Cary R, Earnshaw CG, Eggington CE, Ellis MK, Judson PN, Langowski JJ, Marchant CA, Payne MP, Watson WP, Yih TD (1996) Computer prediction of possible toxic action from chemical structure: an update on the DEREK system. Toxicology 106:267–279

79. Rogers CG, Boyes BG, Matula TI, Heroux-Metcalf C, Clayson DB (1988) A multiple endpoint approach to evaluation of cytotoxicity and genotoxicity of erythrosine (FD and C Red no 3) in a V79 heptocyte-mediated mutation assay. Mutat Res 205:415–423

80. Schimmer O (1997) Studies on the photobiological activity of two naturally occurring furochromones, visnagin and khellin, in *Chlamydamonas reinhardtii*. Mutagenesis 12:141–145

81. Scott D, Dean BJ, Danford ND, Kirkland DJ (1990) Metaphase chromosome aberration assays *in vitro*. In: Kirkland DJ (ed) UKEMS Sub-committee on Guidelines for Mutagenicity Testing, Report, Part I, Revised: Basic tests. Cambridge University Press, Cambridge, pp 62–86

82. Spielmann H, Balls M, Dupuis J, Pape WJW, Pechovitch G, de Silva O, Holzhütter H-G, Clothier R, Desolle P, Gerberick F, Liebsch M, Lovell WW, Maurer T, Pfannenbecker U, Potthast JM, Csato M, Sladowski D, Steiling W, Brantom P (1998) The international EU/COLIPA *in vitro* phototoxicity validation study: results of phase II (blind trial). I. The 3T3 NRU phototoxicity test. Toxicol In Vitro 12:305–327

83. Stopper H, Müller SO (1997) Micronuclei as a biological endpoint for genotoxicity: a minireview. Toxicol In Vitro 11:661–667

84. Thune P, Sandberg M (1987) Allergy to lichen and compositae compounds in perfumes. Investigations on the sensitizing, toxic and mutagenic potential. Acta Derm Venereol Suppl (Stockh) 134:87–89

85. Tice RR (1995) The single cell gel/Comet assay: microgel electrophoretic technique for the detection of DNA damage and repair in individual cells. In: Phillips DH, Venitt S (eds) Environmental Mutagenesis. Bios Scientific, Oxford, pp 315–339

86. Tungal A, Bonin AM, He S, Baker RSU (1991) Micronuclei induction by dichlorvos in the mouse skin. Mutagenesis 6:405–408

87. Utesh D, Splittgerber J (1996) Bacterial photomutagenicity testing: distinction between direct, enzyme-mediated and light-induced effects. Mutat Res 361:41–48

88. Van Pelt FNAM, Haring RM, Weterings PJJM (1991) Micronucleus formation in cultured human keratinocytes: involvement of intercellular bioactivation. Toxicol In Vitro 5:515–518

89. Wiebel FJ, Andersson TB, Casciano DA, Dickins M, Fischer V, Glatt H., Horbach J, Langenbach RJ, Luyten W, Turchi G, Vandewalle A (1997) Genetically engineered cell lines: characterisation and applications in toxicity testing. ATLA 25: 625–639

90. Zeiger E (1995) Mutagenicity tests in bacteria as indicators of carcinogenic potential in mammals. In: Phillips DH, Venitt S (eds) Environmental Mutagenesis. Bios Scientific, Oxford, pp 107–119

Subject Index

Springer
and the
environment

At Springer we firmly believe that an
international science publisher has a
special obligation to the environment,
and our corporate policies consistently
reflect this conviction.
We also expect our business partners –
paper mills, printers, packaging
manufacturers, etc. – to commit
themselves to using materials and
production processes that do not harm
the environment. The paper in this
book is made from low- or no-chlorine
pulp and is acid free, in conformance
with international standards for paper
permanency.

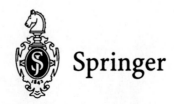 Springer

Druck: KN Digital Printforce GmbH · Schockenriedstraße 37 · 70565 Stuttgart